# Motor Skills Acquisition in the First Year

## *An Illustrated Guide to Normal Development*

Lois Bly, M.A., PT

Photographs by Lois Bly, M.A., PT

**PEARSON**

Pearson
19500 Bulverde Road
San Antonio, TX  78259
800-211-8378

Published by Pearson

# PEARSON

19500 Bulverde Road
San Antonio, TX  78259
800-211-8378

ISBN 0761642285

# Dedication

This book is dedicated to the memory of my parents, Ellen Lucy Bly and Harold Kenneth Bly. They helped me acquire my skills.

# Acknowledgments

My sincere thanks go to the children who are featured in this book and in my lecture slides—Christina, Christina, Michael, Matthew, Elisabeth, Jessica, Lorraine, Rebecca, Suzanne, and Heidi. Without them there would be no book. My deepest appreciation is also extended to the parents of these children who enthusiastically participated with me in all of the photography sessions.

I am also especially grateful to many friends and colleagues who encouraged me and prayed for me and this work all along the way:

Joan Mohr, PT, and Renee Leimgruber, PT, who encouraged me to undertake this project many years ago

Rona Alexander, Ph.D., CCC-SP, Regi Boehme, OTR, and Jane Sweeney, Ph.D., PT, who assisted me with editing early drafts of the manuscript

Mary Ann Loschi, who typed the original draft of this manuscript on a typewriter, not a word processor or a computer

Dorothy Voss, PT, who taught me many things, one of which was how to look at components of movement

Berta Bobath, PT, who taught me about unending possibilities in the treatment of children with cerebral palsy by challenging me to look at normal motor development

Mary Quinton, PT, who taught me to take another look at movement and motor development. She taught me to look with an inner eye and an outer eye. Her knowledge of infant development is remarkable.

Madonna Nash, OTR, Laura Vogtle, OTR, and Diane Fritts, OTR, who shared their knowledge of fine motor development with me

Marsha Dunn Klein, M.Ed., OTR, who volunteered to be my cheerleader during this process and encouraged me to resurrect the original manuscript and continue what I had started many years ago

Carole Sussi, PT, who kept me laughing

Most of all I want to thank our Creator for, through the process of writing this book, I continually concurred with the psalmist that we "are fearfully and wonderfully made; your works are wonderful, I know that full well" (Psalm 139:14).

# About the Author

**Lois Bly,** M.A., PT, received the B.A. degree in biology from Thiel College in Greenville, Pennsylvania, and a certificate of physical therapy from the D. T. Watson School of Physiatrics in Leetsdale, Pennsylvania. She did graduate work in pathokinesiology at New York University, New York, and received the M.A. degree in motor learning from Teachers College, Columbia University, New York.

Ms. Bly received her initial training in Neuro-Developmental Training (NDT) from Dr. and Mrs. Bobath in London, England. She has attended numerous NDT courses, including the NDT baby course with Ms. Mary Quinton and Dr. Elsbeth Koeng in Bern, Switzerland, after which she worked and studied at the Inselspital Bern, Zentrum fur Cerebrale Bewegungsstorungen in Bern.

Following a ten-week course with Ms. Quinton and Dr. Koeng in Seattle, Ms. Bly became an NDT coordinator instructor and was certified to teach eight-week NDTA, Inc., courses. She is the author of the monograph, *The Components of Normal Movement during the First Year of Life.*

Ms. Bly has worked for many years as a physical therapist, treating babies with developmental disabilities and children with cerebral palsy. Since 1980, she has taught numerous seminars, workshops, NDT certification courses, and advanced baby courses throughout the United States and Australia. Currently she continues to teach, consult, and maintain a small private practice in New Jersey.

# Contents

# Preface

"The interest in the development of the normal child is now widespread, and as a result, knowledge of his development is ever increasing: yet there is still a great deal to be learnt—and I expect there always will be" (Illingworth 1975, Preface).

This manuscript is a descriptive presentation of normal motor development and skill acquisition during the first year of life. The impetus to write this book was generated by my frustration and a desire for a greater understanding of normal motor development and normal movement in infants, in order to treat infants with delayed or aberrant movements. After searching the literature and seeing that little information existed, I began my own independent study. This study was greatly influenced by the many continuing education courses I took from skilled clinicians, especially Dorothy Voss, Berta Bobath, and Mary Quinton.

I have used most of the content of this book while teaching in conferences, workshops, and Neuro-Developmental Treatment courses. It was the professionals whom I met in these courses and close colleagues who encouraged me to write down this analysis and information and share it with others. The goal of this book, through its text and photographs, is to inform and enhance your knowledge, understanding, and observational skills in the assessment of normal motor development.

This book is not the product of a research project, but it is the result of many years of personal study, observations, analysis, and clinical experiences as a physical therapist working with a population of pediatric patients with various movement disorders. I followed, observed, and personally photographed many babies as they progressed from one milestone to another in the first year of life. This enabled me to analyze the development of the movement components associated with these milestones. I have also evaluated and worked with many infants and children who have developmental delays, cerebral palsy, and other neurological and orthopedic problems.

For this book, eight full-term babies who were developing normally were photographed every two weeks (usually in their homes) throughout their first year of life. As noted in the text, several of the photographs were taken by Joan Mohr, who was generous enough to share them with me. These babies were located through friends and acquaintances. They all come from middle-class Caucasian families. Unfortunately the photographs do not include a mix of infants from different ethnic groups. I apologize for this.

There are numerous books from reputed authors which identify and sequence the milestones of normal motor development. It is not my intent to try to rewrite or resequence these developmental scales. The milestones and their predictable normal timing provide a standard or reference point. However, there is no source or reference that describes how these milestones are performed and how they evolve into skills.

The goal of this book is to present an analysis of the motor components that babies use to achieve each milestone normally. Hopefully this book will provide a background for enlarging the scope of kinesiological analysis and will serve as a stimulus for others to further investigate and analyze the kinesiological aspects of motor development.

There are 13 chapters in this book. The first chapter is devoted to the neonate, and the following chapters each cover one month of motor development during the first 12 months of life.

Each chapter begins with a general overview, which presents an introduction and summary of the developmental characteristics of that particular month. The chapter is then divided into sections which relate to specific positions: supine, prone, side lying, sitting, and standing (which also includes the pull-to-sit test, rolling, and walking). The milestones and movements under each heading are analyzed, and the subheadings are organized to discuss the movements of the head, trunk, upper extremities, and lower extremities.

With this type of organization, the book can be studied or used on many different levels. Because of the format, specific information can be retrieved readily. For example, a comprehensive overview of each month can be obtained from the introductory section of each chapter. Specific activities and skills in each position can be traced through each month (such as Prone: Upper Extremity Weight Bearing, Rolling: Prone to Supine, or Supported Sitting).

In the developing baby, there is no distinct line between normal and abnormal movement unless the problem is severe and/or congenital or traumatic. Therefore, indications of possible disturbances in motor development and subtle deviations from the normal and their possible consequences are highlighted to help the clinician determine the difference between normal variations and pathology. The subject of abnormal motor development should be considered only as being highlighted. The specific process of abnormal motor development needs further investigation.

Throughout each chapter, photographs capture the essence of each movement and illustrate and document the text. The photographs can also heighten visual understanding and observational skills.

Many theories of motor development are proposed currently. It is not the purpose of this manuscript to endorse or support a specific theory but to take a more global perspective in which maturation, environment, behavior, biomechanics, kinesiology, perception, learning, and goal direction are considered to be important.

The neurological aspects of development have traditionally been considered to be the primary driving force. Until recently, motor development has been viewed as being due entirely to maturation of the nervous system. In the maturation model, it is theorized that progressive encephalization of the brain and spinal cord changes the primitive reflexes to voluntary actions (Gesell and Amatruda 1947; McGraw 1945).

More contemporary theories on motor development consider maturation as only one—although important—facet of the process. Concomitant to and parallel with maturation of the nervous system, the infant is detecting (perceiving) affordances (which are described as perceptual steps in which the viewer determines whether an object is useful to the viewer for some purpose [Gibson and Schmuckler 1989; Gibson 1986]), establishing goals, and learning and problem solving how to interact with the environment. These problem-solving sessions seem to give variability to the developmental process.

Traditionally, reflexes were considered as the foundation of infant movements. Reflexes were used to determine the maturational level of the nervous system (Fiorentino 1972a, 1972b, 1981). Although reflexes are discussed and described in this book, they are not presented as a primitive level of maturation of the nervous system.

A more contemporary view looks at reflexes as coordinative structures, which are muscle linkages or "a group of muscles often spanning several joints that is constrained to act as a single functional unit" (Tuller, Fitch, and Turvey 1982, 253). Coordinative structures are used by the nervous system to limit the degrees of freedom. *Degrees of freedom* refers to the number of planes of motion possible at a joint. In coordinative structures, specific muscle synergies are used by the nervous system to link the joints and reduce the number of variables in a movement. (Fixing also reduces the degrees of freedom [Bernstein 1967].)

Various sensory systems (labyrinthine/vestibular, visual, tactile, somatosensory, proprioceptive) are individually recognized according to their influence on the developmental sequence: labyrinthine righting, optical righting, body righting on the head, body righting on the body, and the asymmetrical tonic neck response (ATNR). The work of Nashner, Horak, Shumway-Cook, Woollacott, and others has provided further insight into the three primary redundant sensory systems (vestibular, visual, and somatosensory) that affect posture (Woollacott, Shumway-Cook, and Williams 1989).

Although the role of feedback from the sensory systems is discussed in depth, the role of feedforward postural adjustments is also emphasized. Feedforward control is used in anticipation of a postural disturbance. Thus it is critical that a baby learn this control early in the developmental process.

The behavioral aspects include the milestones which are presented as age-appropriate functional skills. These milestones, documented in many studies, are used as guidelines to assess a baby's developing skills. The milestones also express the infant's functional level.

Other behavioral aspects include the infant's increasing ability to detect affordances and to problem solve ways in which to interact with the environment. These behavioral changes (milestones) are actually a demonstration of skill development. Infants are performing "age-appropriate" skills that are functional and meaningful to them in their limited experience with the world. Many of these behavioral activities are probably not meaningful or functional to an older infant, child, or adult.

Infants develop skills as they spend much time experimenting with what their arms and legs can do, how they can swipe at objects, how they can reach to mommy's face. When they are in supine, they discover how they can move their bodies by rolling to the side. They also discover their limitations, such as reaching for a toy while sitting unsupported and falling because trunk control is insufficient. Eventually, infants discover that they can pull themselves up on furniture, cruise around it, or climb on it.

The kinesiological aspects of motor development are presented as a hypothesis. No EMG studies were conducted. (However, these would be very useful to document or refute the hypotheses of muscle use that are presented.) The kinesiological information was developed in reverse of the usual manner. I observed a baby's movements and positions, mimicked them, and analyzed which muscles seemed to be active. Numerous kinesiological books were consulted to understand and explain which muscles are active.

Throughout the text, theories are presented regarding the developmental activation of individual muscles as they respond to gravity and move specific body parts. Discussions also cover how muscle activation influences and conversely is dependent upon joint mobility, stability, and positioning.

The book offers explanations as to how the components of antigravity extension, flexion, lateral flexion, and rotation that develop in prone, supine, and side lying are integrated with each other, and how they are used in other positions such as sitting and standing. Synergistic muscle activity is emphasized. Movements are also analyzed as they occur on the sagittal, frontal, and transverse planes. The kinesiology is presented with the assumption that you have searched or will search out basic kinesiological information.

It is understood that specific muscle activation is quite variable depending on the baby's orientation to gravity. The concomitant synergistic muscle activity also varies depending on the baby's purpose or goal for the movement. These differences need to be investigated.

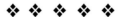

By introducing the kinesiological aspects of motor development, I hope to stimulate you to observe and evaluate beyond motor milestones. These kinesiological aspects are especially important in treating infants with motor problems.

Reading the text and looking at the photographs can provide only a limited understanding of movement. A person's perception and understanding of movement is usually enhanced by mimicking the movement. Therefore, to more fully appreciate the developmental process described in this book, I recommend that you get on the floor and mimic the movements. Put yourself in all of the positions. Feel where control is needed and where mobility is needed. Once you can reproduce a movement, you can understand it (Quinton 1976, 1977, 1978).

Treatment is not a focus of this book. However, I would like to make some comments regarding the use of this information in treatment. The information should be especially helpful in the treatment of infants during the first year of life. It is hoped that the therapists who read this book will be able to extrapolate treatment ideas which will enrich and refine their present treatment techniques. Treatment needs to be dealt with in another volume.

When using this information for patients beyond the first year of life, many additional variables must be considered: age, body size, joint and muscle mobility, muscle strength, habit patterns of movement, perception, current goal-oriented behaviors, and interest. Although a baby who is developing normally goes through a specific developmental process, there is little evidence to suggest that patients older than one year should go through this same developmental sequence (prone, supine, side lying) during rehabilitation. There is nothing "magical" in the developmental sequence. It just seems to fit the kinesiology-biomechanics (for example, joint mobility, muscle action) and perception-action facets (such as affordances) that are available to the baby. Beyond the first year of life, the infant's, child's, and adult's biomechanics change. The reactive forces are different. Perception-action has matured. Interests and goals are different. Treatment must be designed around these changes. On the other hand, it is hoped that the analysis of movements will be helpful in seeing and planning for these differences.

In conclusion, this book is a beginning. Even as I write the final sentences, I know that there is so much more to add, so much more to know. I agree with Illingworth (1975, Preface):

There is still a great deal to be learnt—and I expect there always will be.

# The Neonate: Birth to Ten Days

The full-term newborn comes into this world after 38 to 42 weeks of fetal development which has been influenced primarily by genetic coding and nervous system maturation. The infant has had minimal experience with extrauterine environmental factors (such as gravity, sound, and light). These will now begin to have a potent effect on development.

The full-term neonate is gravity-controlled, with many random extremity movements but little independent control of any part of the body. Posture is dominated by flexion of the extremities. The elbows, hips, knees, and ankles have strong flexor tone which causes recoil of the extremities into flexion when passively extended (Saint-Anne Dargassies 1977).

Although this physiologically normal flexor tone is the result of central nervous system maturation during fetal life (Saint-Anne Dargassies 1977), it is not sufficient to resist or overcome the pull of gravity. Consequently, flexor tone will be reduced by gravity and by the development of extensor muscle control during developmental maturation. Extensor muscle activation enables flexor muscles to be systematically elongated. This elongation occurs before efficient antigravity flexor control is developed.

The effect of gravity on the fetal posture is first seen proximally in the neck, shoulders, and hips, by the head being rotated further to the side, and by the extremities becoming more externally rotated and abducted. The effects of the gravitational forces are most obvious when the baby is at rest. Sudden backward movement of the infant's head elicits a proprioceptive reaction in the neck muscles, the **Moro reflex,** which results in wide abduction and extension of the upper extremities, followed by adduction and flexion (Saint-Anne Dargassies 1977).

Newborns are not passive. They are usually moving when awake. This is especially obvious in the extremities, which move with random, wide-ranged, exaggerated, and vigorous movements. These movements are seen primarily in supine where the extremities are optimally positioned for independent movement. Other movements may be highly organized and resemble, or be part of, more complex movements (such as crawling or walking) seen later in development.

1

The full-term neonate's lower extremities are usually more active and have firmer muscle tone than the upper extremities (Saint-Anne Dargassies 1977). Muscle tone in the fetus and premature baby develops in a caudal-cephalic progression, beginning in the ankles at 28 weeks of gestation and progressing to the upper extremities by 37 weeks of gestation (Saint-Anne Dargassies 1977). This direction of muscle development and antigravity activation reverses when the child is born and has to deal with gravity.

Head movements have a significant influence on subsequent motor development. Through the movements of the head, spinal mobility is initiated. If head turning is vigorous or sustained, it may cause the baby to roll onto the side. From birth, head rotation in supine is utilized by the baby to locate a food source. This is a reflex action (**rooting reflex**) caused by tactile stimulation to the area around the mouth, which is vital to the baby's survival (Prechtl 1977). Head rotation in prone is also a lifesaving reaction because it can prevent suffocation.

The neonate's spine is generally flexed. Cailliet (1977) attributes this curved posture to the absence of intervertebral disks. However, it may also be related to the in-utero position and to inactivity of the paraspinal muscles (neck and back extensors). Spinal mobility in the neonate is limited to the cervical and lumbar vertebrae. The chest shape and horizontal position of the ribs limit thoracic vertebrae mobility (Crelin 1973). Cervical mobility enables head lifting and turning in prone.

Spinal flexion enables lateral and rotational mobility between the lumbar vertebrae and at the lumbosacral joint, which are not possible when the spine is extended (Cailliet 1968). Because of this spinal flexion, the neonate is able to assume many different asymmetrical lower extremity postures in prone which are lost as lumbar extension increases. Lumbar mobility also enables lower trunk weight shifting in prone.

When pulled to sit, the neonate is not able to assist. The infant has a total head lag, unopposed elbow extension, and positional flexion of the lower extremities. Once in sitting, the head falls forward, although the neonate may make fleeting attempts to lift it. The back is rounded but the pelvis is perpendicular, enabling the weight to be borne on the ischial tuberosities.

When held in the fully erect, vertical position, the neonate is capable of extending the legs and taking weight on them (**primary standing**) (Fiorentino 1981). If subsequently tipped forward in standing, the neonate will respond with well-organized, reciprocal walking movements in the lower extremities (**automatic walking**) (Prechtl 1977; Fiorentino 1981). In the full-term baby, these two activities—primary standing and automatic walking—usually become inactive around the fourth week of life.

Neonates are not very interested in toys but will attend to black and white contrasting patterns (Fantz, Faga, and Miranda 1975). They enjoy tactile and vestibular stimulation. They are interested mainly in eating and being held, cuddled, and talked to. This is the time during which they develop trust in their caregivers.

# Supine

In supine, the neonate's posture is dominated by flexion, especially in the ankles, knees, hips, and elbows. The extremities are usually held close to the body, and the head is turned slightly to the side (figure 0.1).

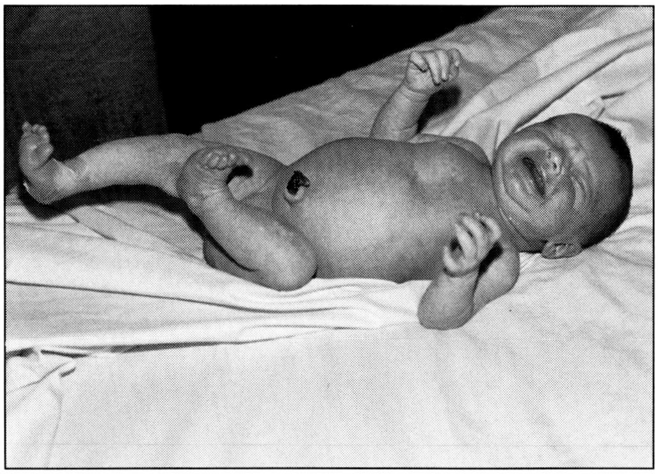

## *Head*

In most full-term neonates, the head rests in a slightly rotated position because of its round shape and lack of sufficient muscle control to keep it in midline (figure 0.1). Babies with low muscle tone have more mobility; therefore their heads often turn further to the side (Saint-Anne Dargassies 1977).

*Figure 0.1. When the neonate is in supine, the extremities are held in flexion. The neonate kicks vigorously with rhythmical and reciprocal patterns.*

During active head turning, a neonate may actually roll to the side due to the **neonatal neck righting reaction.** This reaction occurs as a result of the head and neck position in relation to the rest of the body and the lack of dissociation between the neck and trunk. Rotation of the head and neck causes the body to follow in a log-rolling pattern (Barnes, Crutchfield, and Heriza 1978). There is no segmentation in the body during the roll.

There may be a kinesiological reason for this total body response. At this age, the neck is not dissociated from the trunk, and spinal rotational mobility is limited. Therefore, head rotation causes immediate concurrent rotation of the cervical vertebrae and, subsequently, the whole trunk. The **neck righting reaction** does not occur as spontaneously or as dramatically in babies with low muscle tone or ligamentous laxity because there is little soft tissue or structural resistance to the movement. However, it can be elicited in a test situation.

Rooting is one of the first stimuli for head turning. This reflex reaction occurs as a result of tactile stimulation in the perioral area (Saint-Anne Dargassies 1977). Such stimulation causes the baby to orient the head, mouth, and tongue toward the stimulation, thus enabling the baby to take the mother's breast or bottle (Twitchell 1965; Prechtl 1977). The baby's head movements may include flexion, extension, and rotation, depending on which area is stimulated, demonstrating the newborn's ability to move the head in all directions. According to Mueller (1972), this response is integrated around three months of age. Babies who do not and cannot demonstrate this reflex response in all directions should be watched.

## *Vision*

It is easiest for the baby to orient visually when in supine with the head supported. A newborn can fixate and track an object briefly (Allen 1991). It is easiest for a neonate to fixate a moving object laterally and vertically (Saint-Anne Dargassies 1977). For tracking, therefore, it is best to capture a baby's vision at the side and track toward midline. According to Allen (1991), neonates see best when an object is 8″ to 9″ away.

The newborn fixates best on objects with strong contrasts (Fantz, Faga, and Miranda 1975; Brazelton 1973; Taylor 1992; Inatsuka 1979), preferring black and white patterns over colors.

## Upper Extremities

During quiet periods, the neonate's upper extremities usually rest in slight shoulder adduction and external rotation, elbow flexion, and forearm pronation. The arms will be quickly affected by the pull of gravity. The hands are loosely flexed (figure 0.1).

The neonate frequently brings a hand to the mouth. This is possible because of the flexed elbow and rotated head. The hand-to-mouth reaction is the result of a strong "oral state" which stimulates flexion of the upper extremity on the side to which the mouth is oriented, in both supine and prone (Saint-Anne Dargassies 1977).

Although the arms are kept close to the body during quiet times, the neonate is capable of wide, shoulder-originating movements of the upper extremities. Although these wide movements are traditionally described as "random movements," von Hofsten (1990) suggests that the arm movements of a neonate are often coordinated with visual fixation on a target and thus may be the beginning of eye-hand coordination. Elbow, wrist, and finger movements of flexion and semiextension occur, but rarely is full elbow extension or full shoulder external rotation seen.

The baby's hand positions vary between being flexed and being slightly open. The hand movements are usually related to the arm movements. When the arms are held close to the body, the fingers are flexed and adducted. Wrist extension and finger extension with abduction increase when elbow extension and shoulder abduction occur. According to von Hofsten (1990), movements of the newborn's arms and hands are synergistically coupled. As the arm extends, the hand opens; as the arm flexes, the hand closes.

Strong finger flexion occurs when tactile stimulation is applied to the palm of the hand, especially on the ulnar side (Erhardt 1984). This response develops early in fetal life and can be elicited in a premature infant of 28 weeks (Saint-Anne Dargassies 1977). This response is called a **palmar grasp reflex.**

A second part of this reflex occurs as a response to traction (Saint-Anne Dargassies 1977). When traction is applied to the infant's arm, the entire limb responds with contraction of the flexor muscles, and the infant may be able to be lifted from the table. According to Twitchell (1965), the finger flexion that occurs with traction of the neonate's arm is not a true grasp reflex but is the result of synergistic flexion of all of the joints of the arm and hand (von Hofsten 1990).

## Lower Extremities

The neonate has soft tissue tightness which holds the hips in flexion, abduction, and external rotation (Bleck 1987; Staheli 1980), the knees in flexion, and the ankles in dorsiflexion (Walker 1991; Drews, Vraciu, and Pellino 1984) (figure 0.1). The flexion may increase with activity and/or stress. During quiet times, however, the feet usually rest on the supporting surface with the knees and thighs remaining in the air (figure 0.1). In this unsupported position, the lower extremities are vulnerable to the pull of gravity.

Due to the physiological flexor tone in the lower extremities, there is resistance and recoil of the hips, knees, and ankles when they are passively extended (Saint-Anne Dargassies 1977). During active periods, the neonate's legs kick vigorously with rhythmical and reciprocal patterns (figure 0.1) (Thelen and Fisher 1983; Thelen 1985). Movements alternate between hip and knee flexion and semiextension while maintaining some degree of hip abduction and external rotation. Ankle dorsiflexion usually remains constant throughout the kicking.

Although the soft tissue tightness holds the hips in a position of flexion, abduction, and external rotation, skeletal characteristics of the hips include medial femoral torsion, femoral anteversion, femoral bowing, femoral coxa valga, and a shallow acetabulum. Other skeletal characteristics of the neonate's lower extremities include genu varum, tibia varum, tibial torsion, calcaneal varus, forefoot varus, and occasionally metatarsus adductus (Walker 1991; Bleck 1987; Tachdjian 1972; Tax 1985; Beats 1969; Staheli 1980).

# Prone

In prone, the neonate rests with the head rotated to the side but is capable of lifting and turning it. Because rotation mobility of the neck is limited (Saint-Anne Dargassies 1977), it is usually the cheek, not the ear, which rests on the surface. In prone, head lifting and rotation help to prevent suffocation and to stimulate sensory feedback during the weight shifting which occurs when the head is lifted or turned.

In keeping with the neonate's antigravity cephalo-caudal progression (in utero the direction was the reverse) (Saint-Anne Dargassies 1977), head and neck extensors are the first muscles to exhibit antigravity activation. Thus head and neck hyperextension are the first components of antigravity postural control.

Head lifting and turning (extension and rotation) appear to exercise the head (capital) and neck (cervical) extensor muscles (see Cailliet 1964, page 21), activate lower spinal extensors, provide vestibular stimulation, and initiate the process of spinal (axial) rotation. These are all critical to the baby's normal development in the future. In addition, head extension causes a slight posterior weight shift, and head turning causes a lateral weight shift in the trunk.

## *Upper Extremities*

In prone, the neonate's upper extremity positions change very little because of the weight that is shifted onto them. However, most neonates at some time assume a flexed, adducted posture, with the upper extremities close to, if not adducted under, the body. The elbows are markedly flexed so that the hands are close to the shoulders. When the baby is at rest, the forearms and hands may be in contact with the surface, or only the hands may be in contact, with the forearms and elbows slightly elevated (figure 0.2).

When the upper extremities are adducted and flexed close to the body and weight is shifted anteriorly by elevation of the pelvis, the scapulae tip forward, causing rounding of the shoulders. Forward tipping of the scapula is accompanied by elevation, adduction, and downward rotation. Downward rotation of the scapula causes the glenoid fossa to face posteriorly and downward (Brunnstrom 1979),

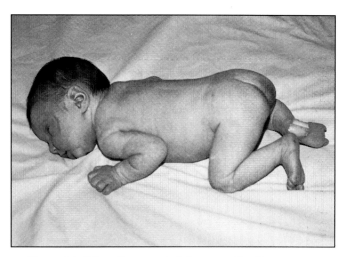

*Figure 0.2.* When the neonate is in prone, the elbows are flexed, the hands are close to the shoulders, and the elbows and forearms are elevated. The baby's knees are flexed and the ankles are dorsiflexed.

which subsequently influences the humerus to internally rotate and hyperextend. This causes elevation of the elbow and forearm (figure 0.2), which then shifts more weight onto the hands.

The shoulder girdle muscles seem to provide the synergistic stability for head lifting and turning. Because of the elevated position of the hips, the baby's weight is shifted forward onto the shoulders and face. Therefore, in order to lift the head, the baby must shift the weight posteriorly. The weight is shifted as far as the shoulder girdle, and the shoulders and chest are pressed into the supporting surface. The neonate demonstrates marked effort to provide muscular stability for this head lifting; therefore, vigorous and exaggerated random movements in the lower extremities often accompany head turning. This action during head lifting and turning creates subtle weight shifting and thus sensory feedback to the muscles and body parts involved.

Shoulder depression into the supporting surface causes scapular tipping, which subsequently causes lifting of the elbows from the support and extends the wrist as the hands press into the support. The hands, therefore, also may act as a fulcrum during head lifting and turning.

### Lower Extremities

In prone, the neonate's hips are usually flexed, slightly abducted, and externally rotated. The knees are flexed and the ankles are strongly dorsiflexed (figure 0.2). The flexed position of the lower extremities causes the pelvis to be elevated, shifting much weight forward onto the baby's face, shoulders, upper extremities, and hands. This anterior weight shift permits more random movements in the lower extremities than in the upper extremities.

Babies with lower muscle tone will be capable of more hip abduction and external rotation. They may even have sufficient mobility to permit the pelvis to rest on the supporting surface. Thus, the weight is not shifted forward in the trunk but is more evenly distributed.

Random kicking could cause the baby to crawl forward or pivot in a circle. Crawling may occur if the baby's toes contact a firm surface during kicking. The pivoting is usually a result of foot contact when the pelvis is laterally tilted. These movements diminish as lumbar and hip extension increase and the positions of the lower extremities change. As hip extension increases, the feet are no longer in a favorable position to push.

# Sitting

The pull-to-sit test is a useful way of analyzing progressive development of the antigravity flexor muscles as well as the baby's recognition and response to the changing sensory feedback that occurs as the head position changes.

When the full-term neonate is pulled to sit, the baby's facial expressions usually indicate an awareness that something is wrong. There may be visible contraction in the neck flexor-shoulder elevator muscles (sternocleidomastoid) (Brazelton 1973; Saint-Anne Dargassies 1977). However, the weight and size of the head prevent the baby from lifting it. Therefore there is a head lag.

There is no upper extremity, abdominal, or lower extremity activity during the pull-to-sit test. There may appear to be active lower extremity flexion at the hips and knees, but this is due to physiological flexor tone rather than active antigravity movement (figure 0.3).

Recognition of and response to the changing sensory feedback that occurs when the position of the head is changed is a very important component of the pull-to-sit test. The visual and vestibular systems must be activated for the baby to sense that the head should be lifted. Therefore, it is important to watch the baby's face and eyes during the pull-to-sit test to evaluate whether the baby is aware of the changing head position. This becomes increasingly important in older babies who have a head lag. A head lag may occur as a result of muscle weakness and/or insufficient awareness of the sensory feedback. Different reasons for the head lag will necessitate different treatment strategies.

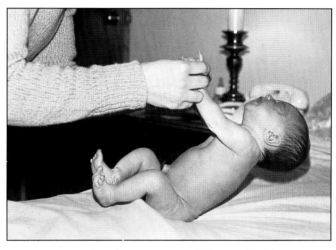

**Figure 0.3.** When the neonate is pulled to sit, head lag is pronounced. The upper extremities do not assist.

During the pull-to-sit exercise, the baby may hold on with a strong grip, the result of the grasp reflex. This reflex is stimulated when the examiner places a finger in the palm of the baby's hand and is reinforced by the traction applied to the entire upper extremity (Twitchell 1965). This reflex action should not be confused with voluntary hand control.

Sitting is not a functional position for the neonate. When supported, the baby may attempt to lift the head, but it quickly falls forward, with the chin resting on the chest because of weakness in the neck extensors. The back is round, giving a "C" shape to the spine, and there appears to be no control of the spinal extensor muscles. The lower extremities are flexed, abducted, and externally rotated at the hips, with the knees semiflexed and the ankles dorsiflexed. The upper extremities hang loosely when the trunk is supported (figure 0.4).

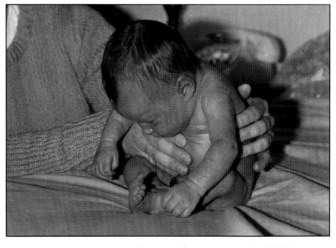

**Figure 0.4.** In supported sitting, the neonate's head falls forward and the back is rounded.

# Standing

When supported in the upright position, neonates respond with remarkable capability. They can take weight and extend their legs due to the **positive supporting reaction** (figure 0.5) (Touwen 1976; Saint-Anne Dargassies 1977; Capute et al. 1978). This response is also called primary standing (Fiorentino 1981). The increased extensor tone in standing helps the neonate to lift the head briefly.

In spite of the increase in extensor tone in standing, the range of lower extremity extension is limited by muscle and other soft tissue tightness (figures 0.5, 0.6). There may be semiextension at the knees, but the hips remain flexed and well behind the shoulders in the vertical position. The hips are also externally rotated. The feet are close together or crossed, but the knees are far apart, giving a bow-legged appearance. The ankles are dorsiflexed and everted. The feet are usually flat or pronated, but they may invert during walking movements so that the lateral aspect of the foot makes contact with the supporting surface.

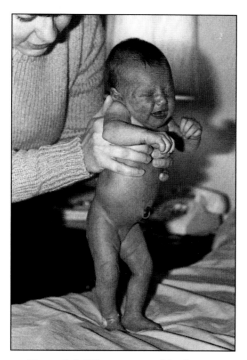

*Figure 0.5. When supported in the upright position, the neonate can take weight and extend the legs due to the positive supporting reaction (also termed primary standing).*

If the neonate is leaned forward while standing, the baby will respond with well-organized reciprocal walking movements (figure 0.6) (Andre-Thomas and Autgaerden 1966; Saint-Anne Dargassies 1977). There is synchronous flexion of all of the joints during swing, and synchronous extension of all of the joints (within available range of motion) after foot contact. Coactivation of the antagonistic leg muscles also occurs during this automatic walking (Forssberg 1992; Thelen and Fisher 1982; Thelen 1985).

Foot contact may be made with the heel first (Saint-Anne Dargassies 1977) or with the toes or forefoot first (Forssberg 1992; Forssberg, Hirschfeld, and Stokes 1992). The feet often cross. This response is called automatic walking (Andre-Thomas and Autgaerden 1966; Prechtl 1977; Barnes, Crutchfield, and Heriza 1978; Fiorentino 1981). In the full-term baby, automatic walking is strongest at around three weeks and then diminishes (McGraw 1945).

Although the movements are organized, they lack participation of two important muscle groups needed for dynamic support in standing: the hip extensors (gluteals and hamstrings) and the gastrocnemius-soleus group (Thelen and Cooke 1987). Not only are these muscle groups inactive, but they are maintained in a state of elongation by marked hip flexion and ankle dorsiflexion. The neonate also lacks postural and balance control during this early walking (Forssberg 1992).

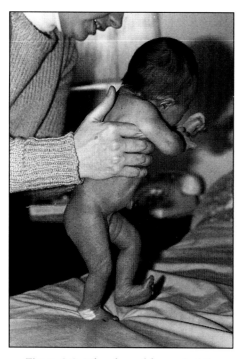

*Figure 0.6. When leaned forward while standing, the neonate will respond with well-organized reciprocal walking movements, called automatic walking.*

Traditionally, the automatic walking has been called the neonatal "stepping reflex" and has been attributed to a series of stretch reflexes (McGraw 1945; Andre-Thomas and Autgaerden 1966; Illingworth 1975). However, Thelen and Fisher (1982, 1983), Thelen (1984, 1985), Leonard, Hirschfeld, and Forssberg (1991), Forssberg,

Hirschfeld, and Stokes (1992), and Forssberg (1992) suggest that the automatic walking demonstrated by the neonate is due to spinal cord mechanisms such as a central pattern generator (CPG), or "coordinative structures." Thelen and Fisher (1982) suggest that movement patterns used in the automatic walking are the same as those used in neonatal supine kicking. They further suggest that the same neural networks are used in both actions.

# Indications of Possible Disturbances in Motor Development

Babies at this age who are suspect for developmental delays and who are referred for treatment usually have a profound medical history. Such a history could include significant prematurity, intraventricular hemorrhage (IVH) grades III or IV, bronchopulmonary dysplasia, very low birth weight (under 1500 grams), and perinatal asphyxia, among others (Moore 1984, 1986).

Feeding difficulties are usually the most serious problem. The baby who is unable to eat well is at risk for nutritional problems. Such problems are often accompanied by irritability. Therapy to address the oral motor difficulties is very important. However, oral motor problems are beyond the scope of this book.

Babies who have experienced significant neurological insult may be very stiff or very floppy. If the baby is very stiff, therapy should be directed to include movement through various positions and activities that will help to stretch out the muscles. If the baby is very floppy, therapy should be directed to increase muscle activity against gravity.

# The First Month

**M**any changes occur during the first month of life. The baby is more alert, has better visual awareness, and is beginning to respond and adapt to the vast environment. Increased alertness and visual awareness make head movements more purposeful in supine and prone.

The 1-month-old is more extended and more mobile than at birth. Head and cervical spine mobility have increased, enabling the baby to rotate the head further to the side. Proximal tone and tightness in the shoulders and hips have decreased sufficiently to permit the shoulders to externally rotate and the hips to extend. Therefore the extremities move away from the body and from each other. The elbows, hips, and knees have less flexor tone and less recoil when passively extended. Ankle dorsiflexion has changed very little.

Random extremity movements characterize the 1-month-old in supine. In prone, the baby's skills are still limited to head lifting and turning. This task continues to require the baby's maximum effort, even though it has been made slightly easier by the increased cervical spine mobility and the lowered pelvic position.

When pulled to sit, the 1-month-old's reactions are similar to those of the neonate. There is a total head lag, unresisted elbow extension, and lower extremities that are less responsive and less flexed than the neonate's.

When sitting, the baby's back is round but the pelvis continues to be perpendicular, enabling weight to be borne on the ischial tuberosities. The baby makes fleeting attempts to lift (right) the head in sitting but lacks the muscle control to sustain the lift.

Primary standing and automatic walking may still be present, but they have started to fade in their strength and predictability.

The 1-month-old enjoys the same play activities as the newborn (namely, eating and tracking a high-contrast, black and white object). The baby also enjoys being held, cuddled, talked to, sung to, and rocked.

# Supine

## *Head*

In supine, the 1-month-old's head turns farther to the side than it did at birth, suggesting that there is increased mobility in the cervical area. As a result of this increased mobility and lack of symmetrical neck muscle control, the baby's head is

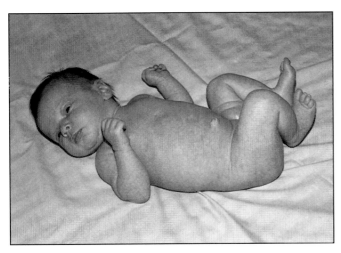

less frequently near midline (figure 1.1). Increased head and neck extension, seen as chin raising, is now common when the head is turned to the side. The **neck righting reaction** can still be elicited at one month and still may cause the baby to roll to the side spontaneously.

The **asymmetrical tonic neck reaction** (ATNR) may appear any time during the first three months (Egan, Illingworth, and MacKeith 1969; Touwen 1976), but it is most common during the second month (Touwen 1976). An ATNR is elicited through neck rotation, which subsequently causes the upper extremity fencing posture (Twitchell 1965). The arm on the face side is extended, while the arm on the skull side is flexed. Visual interest may cause the baby to turn the head far to the side and thus elicit the ATNR. This reflex is never obligatory.

*Figure 1.1. In supine, the 1-month-old's head turns farther to the side than does the neonate's.*

## *Vision*

In the 1-month-old, as in the neonate, the eyes are more accurate than the upper extremities and hands in reaching out to objects (von Hofsten 1990). Therefore the eyes start leading the way for the hands. Gibson (1986) and Gibson and Schmuckler

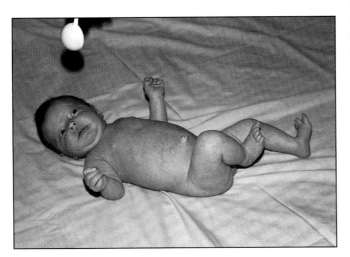

(1989) describe this process as one in which the eyes detect the "affordance" of an object. An affordance is described as a perceptual step in which the viewer determines whether an object is useful to the viewer for some purpose.

Like the newborn, the 1-month-old has better lateral vision than midline vision (Nash 1991). The baby can visually track an object or a face from the side to midline (Inatsuka 1979) (figures 1.2, 1.3). Although the tracking is not smooth, it is not as jerky as it was in the neonate (Nash 1991).

*Figure 1.2. The 1-month-old can visually track from the side to midline. Reciprocal kicking is noted.*

## Upper Extremities

The 1-month-old's arms no longer rest close to the body. Gravity has assisted in pulling the arms into increased external rotation, elongating the anterior chest and arm muscles (figures 1.2, 1.3). Active shoulder abduction is starting (figure 1.3).

Due to increased mobility, the 1-month-old is capable of wider ranges of shoulder movement and slightly more elbow extension than the neonate (figure 1.3). Although the fingers continue to be loosely flexed, they are capable of abduction and extension, which is noted particularly during strong elbow extension. Von Hofsten (1990) suggests that the movements of the arms and hands are synergistically coupled—all the joints of the arms and hands extend or flex together—until two months of age.

Although the 1-month-old demonstrates opening and closing of the hands and clenches objects as a result of tactile stimulation (**grasp reflex**), the baby has no hand control. The hand usually must be pried open to place a rattle in it. The baby may retain it briefly but soon drops it (figure 1.4). The **palmar grasp reflex** continues to be associated with traction of the arm, which subsequently stimulates synergistic flexion of all of the joints of the arm and hand (Twitchell 1965).

## Lower Extremities

During the first month, hip flexor tone appears to decrease, and the hips become more extended. Range in hip abduction and external rotation also increases, but active hip adduction and internal rotation do not occur. Active knee extension occurs more frequently, but the range of extension is still limited by soft tissue tightness (figure 1.3).

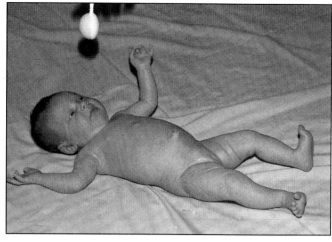

*Figure 1.3.* The 1-month-old displays visual tracking, increased range of shoulder movement, greater elbow extension, increased knee extension, and bilateral symmetrical kicking.

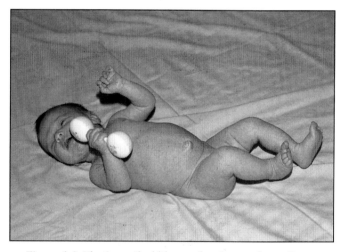

*Figure 1.4.* The 1-month-old has no hand control; an object placed in the baby's hand is soon dropped.

There is a slight decrease in the random activity of the lower extremities. Reciprocal kicking (figure 1.2) is interspersed with bilateral symmetrical kicking (figure 1.3). Although hip and knee extension have increased, kicking usually occurs with the legs in the air rather than on the surface. Hip rotation, hip abduction, and ankle dorsiflexion have changed very little during kicking.

Thelen (1985) suggests that the infant's kicking is not random and that the joint movements do not occur independently but occur as a result of linked muscle synergies (coordinative structures). In other words, these movements are not voluntary, but they are organized. The author suggests further that these same movements and linkages are seen in the automatic walking patterns (Thelen and Fisher 1983; Thelen 1985).

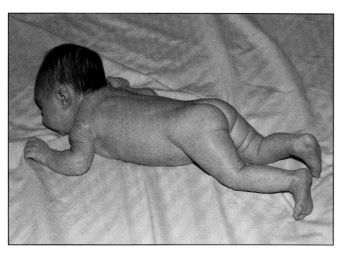

*Figure 1.5. In prone, there is decreased hip flexion and the pelvis is lowered. The extremities are moved away from the trunk, and there is less weight on the face, shoulders, and upper extremities.*

# Prone

In prone, physiological flexion is still present but less pronounced than it was in the neonate. Increased upper extremity external rotation, abduction, and increased hip and knee extension cause the extremities to move away from the trunk. With the extremities farther away from the trunk, the spine is less rounded and more extended (figure 1.5).

## *Head*

The head continues to be rotated to the side in prone. During quiet times the baby demonstrates decreased hip flexion and a lowered pelvis. Subsequently, there is less weight on the face, shoulders, and upper extremities (figure 1.5).

Head lifting and turning continue to be accomplished with hyperextension, suggesting continued use of head and neck extensor muscles. The 1-month-old can lift the head slightly higher and clear the nose better than during the neonatal period.

The head movements provide excitation to the vestibular system, which continues to provide stimulus for head righting (that is, head lifting in prone). This is described as the **labyrinthine righting reaction.** Stimulation of the labyrinths or vestibular system results in contraction of the neck muscles in an attempt to bring the head into the proper orientation in relation to gravity (Twitchell 1965; O'Connell and Gardner 1972; Barnes, Crutchfield, and Heriza 1978).

Head lifting or righting is also stimulated through **optical righting reactions.** Visual feedback is used to adjust and orient the head and eyes with the horizon (Twitchell 1965; O'Connell and Gardner 1972; Barnes, Crutchfield, and Heriza 1978). Adelson and Fraiberg (1974) suggest that vision may play a more important role in head righting than does labyrinthine stimulation.

## *Upper Extremities*

During quiet states in prone, the 1-month-old's upper extremities are more abducted and externally rotated than they were at birth (figure 1.5). As the arms move away from the body and the pelvis lowers, reducing the amount of anterior weight shift, the shoulders become less protracted. The active humeral abduction assists in abducting and rotating the scapula upward, causing the glenoid fossa to face laterally instead of posteriorly and inferiorly. Upward rotation of the scapula and increased humeral external rotation will enable further development of humeral flexion (Kapandji 1970a; Norkin and Levangie 1983; Soderberg 1986). Active elbow extension is increasing. The wrists extend and the fingers remain loosely flexed. The 1-month-old baby does not have functional use of the arms in prone.

Although hip flexion and pelvic elevation in prone have decreased when the baby is quiet, the baby's active movements result in increased hip flexion and pelvic elevation (figure 1.6). Subsequently, elevation of the pelvis shifts weight onto the upper extremities and inhibits their movements.

When the pelvis is elevated and weight is shifted forward, the upper extremities assume a primitive position in which the scapula is adducted, rotated downward, elevated, and tipped forward. The humeri subsequently assume a position of extension and internal rotation (figure 1.6). Pelvic elevation due to hip flexion subsequently results in regression of upper extremity positioning. Although this is a normal occurrence in the young baby, it is not normal in the older baby (five to six months). The gradual development of active hip extension in prone will contribute to further development of the shoulder girdle and upper extremities by providing an anchor or point of synergistic stability.

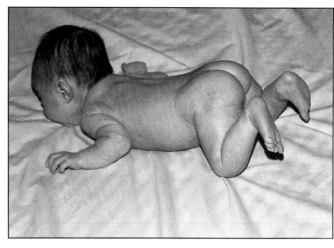

*Figure 1.6.* During activity in prone, hip flexion and pelvic elevation increase; weight is shifted onto the upper extremities, inhibiting their movement.

This primitive shoulder girdle/upper extremity position is also often assumed by the baby during active head lifting and turning (figure 1.6). This may suggest that the shoulder girdle muscles provide synergistic stability for early head lifting.

Synergistic stability for active head lifting in prone appears to be transferred caudally from the shoulders to the hips as humeral abduction, flexion, and horizontal adduction increase concurrently with increased range and control in spinal and hip extension.

## Lower Extremities

Random lower extremity kicking and crawling are still present but are much less vigorous than in the neonate. Extension in the lumbar spine appears to be increasing.

Hip flexion in prone has decreased, suggesting elongation of the hip flexor muscles (iliopsoas, rectus femoris) (figure 1.5). This elongation enables the pelvis to rest closer to the surface. Slight hip abduction and external rotation are still present due to the continued tightness of the soft tissue around the hip joints.

Increased knee extension is also evident in the prone position (figure 1.5). This suggests elongation of the hip flexors (iliopsoas, rectus femoris) and knee flexors (hamstrings), and some increased activity of the knee extensors (quadriceps femoris). Ankle dorsiflexion remains constant and seems to be affected very little by the proximal changes.

Although the lower extremities rest in extension during the baby's quiet times, hip flexion increases quickly when the baby becomes active. Lower extremity kicking is not as vigorous as during the neonatal period. However, it still results in hip flexion and pelvic elevation. When hip flexion and pelvic elevation occur during head lifting and turning, anterior shifting of the baby's weight is exaggerated, and the shoulders and upper extremities assume a primitive position.

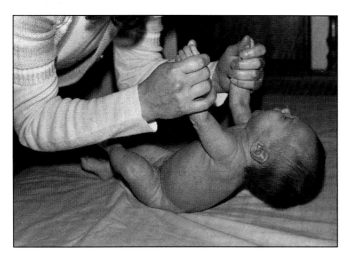

**Figure 1.7.** *During pull-to-sit, the head still lags, but the baby often seems to try to assist. There is less lower extremity flexion than at birth.*

# Sitting

When pulled to sit, the 1-month-old does not have any more observable muscle control than the neonate but is more alert and often seems to try to assist. The fleeting attempts to right the head are unsuccessful because the baby lacks the needed neck flexor control. However, the baby's desire indicates recognition of feedback from the vestibular and optical righting systems.

There is a total head lag and passive, unresisted extension of the upper extremities (figure 1.7). The abdominals and lower extremities do not actively participate. There is less lower extremity flexion and activity than there was at birth. This may be due to the increased elongation of the lower extremity musculature.

In supported sitting, the head falls forward, although the baby does make fleeting attempts to lift it. The desire to lift the head indicates activity in the vestibular and visual righting systems. Head lifting is accomplished with head and neck hyperextension (capital and cervical extensors). As with the neonate, the 1-month-old's back is flexed, and the pelvis continues to be perpendicular so that weight is borne on the ischial tuberosities (figure 1.8).

The upper extremities no longer hang loosely at the baby's sides. During active states (such as head lifting), there is retraction of the whole shoulder girdle, increased elbow flexion, forearm pronation, wrist extension, and loose flexion of the fingers (figure 1.9). The activity in the shoulder girdle may provide synergistic stability for head lifting.

The lower extremities are flexed, abducted, and externally rotated (figure 1.9). The external rotation is limited; therefore the lateral sides of the legs usually do not rest on the supporting surface. The knees are more flexed than in the neonatal phase. The ankles continue to be strongly dorsiflexed and slightly everted.

If the baby is carefully left unsupported, the head and trunk will fall forward until the head rests on the surface between the baby's lower extremities. The pelvic position is not affected by this exaggerated trunk flexion (figure 1.10).

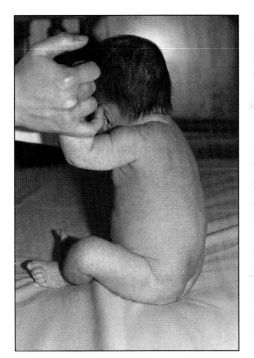

**Figure 1.8.** *In supported sitting, the head falls forward despite the baby's attempts to lift it. The back is flexed, as earlier, and weight is borne on the ischial tuberosities.*

# Standing

In standing, the general appearance of the 1-month-old does not differ significantly from that of the neonate. Although primary standing may still be present, automatic walking has usually diminished.

The upright posture is characterized by increased extensor tone which seems to reinforce attempts at head lifting (righting). Increased head and neck extensor muscle activity enables head lifting to be more frequent and more sustained than in the neonate (figure 1.11, page 18).

Upper extremity posture in standing is similar to the neonate's. Elbow flexion is present during standing, but increased activity and increased effort cause elbow extension, wrist extension, and partial finger extension (figure 1.12, page 18).

The hips are still flexed and well behind the shoulders in the vertical position. Hip external rotation and abduction have changed very little. The knees are still extended within their limited range of motion. Genu varum is still noted. The feet are still dorsiflexed and everted (pronated), resting flatly on the supporting surface. However, they are not as close to each other as in the neonate, and crossing of the feet is infrequent.

Automatic walking may still occur with reciprocal alternating movements of the lower extremities (figure 1.12). The baby still lacks postural and balance control and purpose in this activity. The 1-month-old continues to use the same walking pattern as described for the neonate (Forssberg, Hirschfeld, and Stokes 1992). During the hip flexion phase of walking, the foot dorsiflexes and inverts.

The 1-month-old moves the legs with synchronous joint movements. The hip, knee, and ankle flex together and the foot inverts. These three joints extend together just prior to initial contact. Co-activation of the antagonistic leg muscles also occurs during this automatic walking (Forssberg, Hirschfeld, and Stokes 1992).

As mentioned earlier, automatic walking usually diminishes between the fourth and sixth weeks of life in the full-term baby. Thelen, Fisher, and Ridley-Johnson (1984) attribute this loss of automatic walking to the baby's increase in body size and weight and the lack of concomitant increase in muscle strength to lift the legs. Forssberg, Hirschfeld, and Stokes (1992) suggest that the inactivity is due to increased supraspinal inhibition.

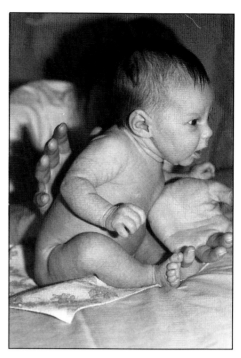

*Figure 1.9.* During activity in supported sitting, there is retraction in the shoulder girdle with increased elbow flexion, forearm pronation, wrist extension, and loose flexion of the fingers. Knees are more flexed than in the neonate.

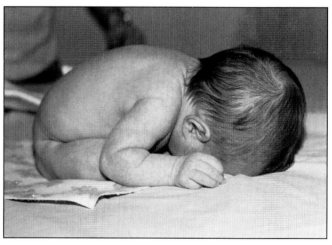

*Figure 1.10.* The 1-month-old's head and trunk fall forward during unsupported sitting.

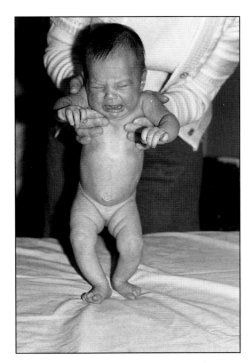

**Figure 1.11.** During standing, head lifting is more frequent and sustained than in the neonate.

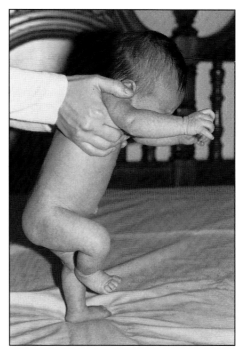

**Figure 1.12.** Increased upper extremity activity and effort cause elbow extension, wrist extension, and partial finger extension. Automatic walking may still occur.

# The Second Month

The 2-month-old is more alert and aware of people in the environment than the 1-month-old. The quality of movements has been modified, but the baby is not much more functional than at one month. The physiological flexor tone has been reduced by gravity and by increased asymmetrical extensor activity, but active antigravity flexor activity has not yet emerged. Therefore, the 2-month-old seems to have less muscle tone and appears to be more disorganized than at one month of age. The infant thus experiences a period of semihypotonia (Saint-Anne Dargassies 1977).

The 2-month-old's spine is slightly more extended than it was at one month. This increased extension is seen primarily in the cervical and upper thoracic spine. Increased spinal mobility, increased muscle control, and increased alertness make head movements easier and more goal-directed. Head and cervical spine movements have a ripple affect on the thoracic spine.

The baby's extended appearance in prone and supine is enhanced by the increased range of shoulder abduction and hip extension. As the upper and lower extremities continue to move farther apart, spinal extension increases. With extension developing more distally, the elbows and knees become more extended and have less primitive flexor tone, thus less recoil, when they are passively extended. Ankle dorsiflexion, however, has changed very little.

In prone, the 2-month-old has increased head control and a lower pelvis, which enables the baby to lift the head and turn it more easily. There is also increased stimulus for head righting from the labyrinthine and optical systems. Adelson and Fraiberg (1974) reported that blind babies do not lift their heads in prone until much later than sighted babies. This would suggest that visual (optical) righting may be the more important of the two systems for initial head lifting.

With increased visual awareness, the baby's head movements in supine are frequently directed by visual attention. Control of the neck muscles in supine is still undeveloped; therefore, the baby finds the greatest visual stability when the head is turned and resting to the side (gravity assisted). The side-rotated posture may stimulate neck receptors which produce an asymmetrical tonic neck reaction. The ATNR, with upper extremity extension on the face side, may be utilized to swipe at toys or to initiate eye-hand regard. However, this posture is never obligatory.

Random lower extremity movements and active reciprocal kicking have decreased. The movements the baby engages in are accomplished with less vigor and less exaggeration.

When pulled to sit, the 2-month-old attempts to assist with head lifting but continues to lack the capital (head) and cervical (neck) flexor muscle control. Therefore the baby still has a head lag. The upper extremities, however, respond with some elbow flexion, which may be due to the **grasp reflex traction response** (Twitchell 1965).

When supported in sitting, the 2-month-old's back continues to be flexed, but the baby does attempt to use the extensors to lift the head. Control of the head and neck extensors is still precarious; consequently, there is more head bobbing than sustained lifting.

In the vertical position, the 2-month-old demonstrates astasia abasia or motor incoordination for standing and walking (Touwen 1976; Capute et al. 1978; Barnes, Crutchfield, and Heriza 1978). Primary standing and automatic walking are not usually seen in the full-term baby at two months.

At two months of age, the baby is making obvious attempts to interact with and explore the world, swiping at toys while supine. Although babies will grasp a rattle that is placed in the hand, they do not attend to it. Mobiles, especially those with high visual contrasts and auditory feedback, usually capture the baby's visual interest (Aston 1974). The baby may even try to swipe at the mobile. Human faces with changing expressions, especially smiles, also interest the 2-month-old.

# Supine

Functional activity in supine is still quite limited, consisting of active head turning and random, semicontrolled extremity movements. Although limited, visual attentiveness and visual reaching are two of the baby's most functional activities.

## *Head*

The 2-month-old's head is rarely in midline, which may be due to the increased cervical spine/muscle mobility. The chin now comes to lie closer to the acromion process or the shoulder. This rotation is accompanied by increased head extension and chin lifting.

Head rotation may cause a subtle lateral weight shift of the body to the face side, or head rotation may elicit the **neck righting reaction.** In the latter case, head rotation is followed by rotation or rolling of the body, as a whole unit, to the side (log rolling) (Capute et al. 1978; Barnes, Crutchfield, and Heriza 1978). This early log rolling, as well as later log rolling, is usually associated with limited spinal rotational mobility and limited dissociation between the vertebrae. Segmental rolling occurs later as spinal mobility increases.

Head rotation may also stimulate the neck proprioceptors which elicit the ATNR, causing an increase in extensor tone in the face-side upper extremity and flexor tone in the skull-side upper extremity (figure 2.1) (Twitchell 1965; O'Connell and Gardner 1972; Barnes, Crutchfield, and Heriza 1978; Capute et al. 1978). The ATNR may also increase extensor tone in the neck and trunk.

The ATNR is never obligatory in the normal baby, and head rotation may frequently occur with no influence on the extremities (figures 2.3, 2.4). The ATNR is most evident during the second month of life. It is then that neck extensor activity is the least balanced by neck flexor activity or tone, and asymmetrical muscle activity is more prominent than symmetrical muscle activity.

Vision and eye muscle control are related to the head position and head control (Nash 1991). In these early months, the eyes move faster than the head (Vogtle and Albert 1985). Because the baby's head is frequently to the side, the eyes are also to the side. This enables the baby to notice the hand as the arm is abducted. This head, eye, and hand linkage enables the baby to notice and swipe at toys to the side of the body.

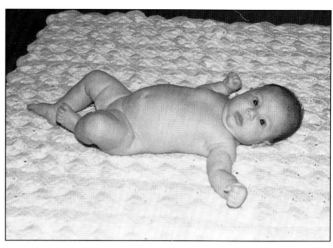

**Figure 2.1.** *In supine, the chin now comes to lie closer to the shoulder. This increased rotation may elicit the ATNR. Positional abduction and external rotation during quiet periods have changed little.*

The 2-month-old can briefly fixate in midline (figure 2.2). The baby can track from the side to midline, and from midline to the side, and is also beginning to track across midline. The baby may be able to track horizontally 180° with a favorite toy (Nash 1991). Binocular vision is also starting (Nash 1991).

In supine, the baby can visually follow a dangling ring past midline by simultaneously moving the head and eyes (Inatsuka 1979). Midline regard cannot yet be maintained, because the baby does not yet have the needed head or neck muscle control to stabilize the head in midline. Eye convergence in midline will be observed concurrently as midline control of the head and neck flexor muscles develops (Nash 1991). Eye convergence will be used more consistently in the next few months.

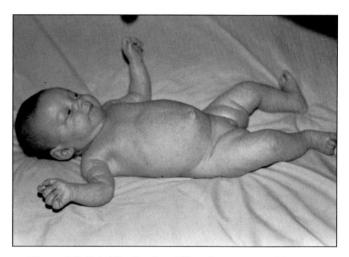

**Figure 2.2.** *Brief fixation in midline. Lower extremities show increased hip extension and knee extension. Ankle dorsiflexion has changed very little.*

The relationship between head control, head movements, and vision is especially important. The baby learns much about the world through vision. Visual awareness, detection of affordances, and interest motivate the baby to try to reach out into the environment (Gibson and Schmuckler 1989). Visual awareness is a significant step toward developing skills that will enable the baby to interact with the environment.

If the baby does not have good head control, ocular motor control will be affected. Subsequently, vision will be affected, and this may affect how the baby problem solves motor control in reaching out into the world. Head control thus has a significant effect on normal and abnormal motor development.

## *Upper Extremities*

By the second month, the upper extremities are quieter but move in wide and varied ranges (figures 2.1 to 2.4). They have increased mobility, especially for abduction and external rotation. Except for the asymmetrical fencing posture assumed as a result of the ATNR, the upper extremities demonstrate little significant difference from those of the 1-month-old.

Reaching is usually performed as an asymmetrical unilateral response (Fagard 1990; Corbetta and Mounoud 1990). Von Hofsten (1990) reports that the synergistic arm-hand action (arm extension with finger extension) that was seen in the newborn is no longer used by the 2-month-old. Instead, he reports that 2-month-olds fist their hands when they extend their arms.

Elbow mobility has increased as the elbow flexors (biceps brachii, brachio-radialis, and brachialis) are elongated by the increasing activity on the elbow extensors (triceps brachii). However, elbow flexion is still the most dominant upper extremity posture of the 2-month-old. Wrist extension is present, and the fingers are still loosely flexed. Wrist extension continues to elicit a tenodesis effect which causes finger flexion.

When it is elicited, the ATNR increases activity (or tone) in specific muscles or causes synergistic activity in specific muscles or coordinative structures (Easton 1972). There is increased extensor tone, causing elbow extension, in the upper extremity on the face side. Simultaneously, there is increased activation of the elbow flexors in the skull-side arm. Both elbow movements are accompanied by scapular adduction and horizontal abduction of the humeri. Scapular adduction contributes to spinal extension. The ATNR seems to be a part of a whole asymmetrical extensor pattern. It is once again important to emphasize that the ATNR is never obligatory in the normal baby.

The ATNR may be used to locate toys visually and subsequently swipe at them. Although the hand may reach and touch the toy, the baby is unable to grasp it voluntarily. This process brings the hand into visual range and enables the initiation of eye-hand regard.

Use of the ATNR to swipe at toys is a step in solving the problem of how to interact with the world physically. The baby who is developing normally uses this scheme along with other schemes. The baby with a movement problem may use this scheme exclusively.

By two months of age, finger extension occurs more frequently. Finger extension is still often associated with elbow extension, and finger flexion with elbow flexion (Vogtle and Albert 1985). The grasp reflex can still be facilitated by deep pressure on the radial side of the palm. According to Erhardt (1984), the grasp reflex continues to be elicited in a 2-month-old when a stimulus is inserted into the radial side of the palm. Stimulation is followed by flexion and adduction of the fingers and thumb and synergistic flexion of the entire arm.

If a rattle is placed in the baby's hand, the baby can briefly retain it but does not pay attention to it (figures 2.3, 2.4). The grasp occurs with forearm pronation and more use of the outside, or ulnar, fingers (figure 2.3). When wrist flexion occurs, there is a resulting tenodesis effect which causes the fingers to extend. The rattle is soon dropped without significant notice by the baby (figure 2.4).

## Lower Extremities

At two months, the lower extremities are quite variable in their positions and kicking patterns. Variability is an important component of normal movement development.

In supine, the lower extremities have not yet gained as much mobility as the upper extremities, but they have gained range in hip extension, external rotation, and knee extension (figure 2.2). Positional abduction and external rotation during quietness has changed very little (figure 2.1). It should be noted that, in the early stages, lower extremity movement development seems to follow the same sequences as that of the upper extremities (that is, external rotation is followed by abduction).

Although the baby frequently assumes a position of bilateral lower extremity flexion (figures 2.3, 2.4), hip and knee flexor tightness has decreased, and the lower extremities have less flexor recoil when passively extended. This decrease in tightness permits the lower extremities to rest in more extension, but even in their most extended position, the hips and knees are still flexed. When the legs are extended, hip abduction and external rotation are reduced (figure 2.2). However, the ankles usually retain a dorsiflexed posture.

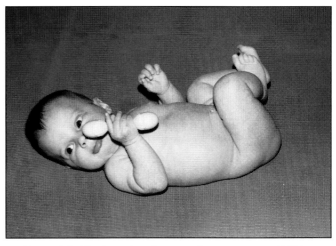

*Figure 2.3.* Head rotation does not always cause an ATNR. The 2-month-old baby will grasp a rattle placed in the hand but will not pay attention to it. Bilateral upper and lower extremity flexion is a common posture.

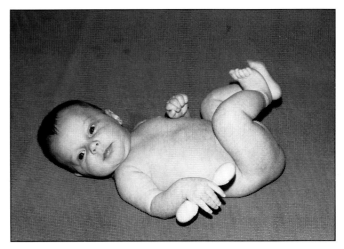

*Figure 2.4.* When the wrist is flexed, the fingers extend as a result of the tenodesis effect, and the baby drops the rattle without notice.

Kicking may be bilateral and symmetrical. During bilateral flexion, the feet come together. During extension, the ankles remain dorsiflexed and seem to be affected very little by the more proximal extensor activity.

The sensory input experienced by the feet coming together is important in developing body awareness and in decreasing tactile sensitivity in preparation for more advanced reactions in the feet. Body-on-body contact and exploration are vital components to the development of body awareness and body image (Quinton 1976, 1977, 1978).

# Prone

Prone continues to be a restricting position for the 2-month-old. Although extension mobility has increased, antigravity extensor control has not increased sufficiently to permit more than head lifting, head bobbing, and head turning in prone (figures 2.5 to 2.7).

### Head

When resting in prone, the baby can rotate the head to the side. Increased cervical spine mobility permits the ear to rest on the supporting surface, contrasted to the cheek for the 1-month-old.

By extending the cervical and thoracic spine, the 2-month-old can momentarily lift the head to 45° (figures 2.5, 2.6). Although lifting continues to be accomplished primarily by unilateral action of the extensor muscles, bilateral control is seen intermittently as the baby tries to sustain the lift. (Unilateral contraction of the extensor muscles will result in slight head rotation, while bilateral symmetrical contraction of the extensors muscles holds the head in midline.) Insufficient sustained contraction of the extensor muscles results in head bobbing. The baby's desire to lift the head and maintain the elevation illustrates the increased effects of the labyrinthine and optical righting systems.

Initiation of head lifting is easier because of increased muscle strength, increased head righting stimulus, and decreased hip flexion, which shifted the weight forward. This decreasing forward weight shift enables a caudal displacement of the weight-bearing fulcrum from the shoulders to the upper chest (figure 2.5). Head lifting, bobbing, and turning provide stimulation to the visual, proprioceptive, kinesthetic, and vestibular systems, which may further enhance or stimulate continued antigravity development.

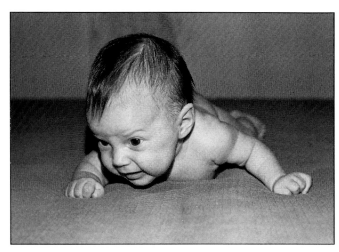

**Figure 2.5.** *By extending the cervical and thoracic spine, the 2-month-old can briefly lift the head to 45° with slight rotation. The upper chest becomes the fulcrum for head lifting.*

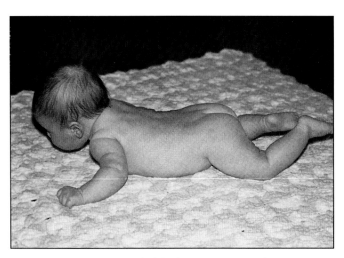

**Figure 2.6.** *The 2-month-old is beginning to use the arms to push up in prone but does not yet assume forearm weight bearing. Weight is borne on the radial side of the hands. Decreased hip flexion allows the weight to be shifted caudally.*

### Upper Extremities

The 2-month-old is beginning to use the arms to push up in prone. However, the baby does not yet have sufficient shoulder girdle control to assume and maintain forearm weight bearing. The shoulders and arms still assume a primitive position, with the elbow behind the shoulder (figures 2.5 to 2.7). When the elbow is behind the shoulder, the humerus assumes a position of abduction, extension, and internal rotation. This arm position continues to be associated with scapular adduction, elevation, downward rotation, and forward tipping.

Bilateral scapular adduction and spinal extension still seem to provide synergistic stability for head and shoulder lifting. Subsequently, the weight is shifted caudally, and the upper chest is pressed into the surface. The upper chest thus becomes the weight-bearing fulcrum for head lifting (figure 2.5).

As the humeri abduct and the elbows extend, the hands move laterally and forward of the shoulders. However, humeral abduction and external rotation are still limited at two months, and the elbows are still behind the shoulders (figures 2.5, 2.6). The hands are loosely flexed.

During head lifting, humeral internal rotation with extension is accompanied by forearm pronation (figures 2.5, 2.6). Subsequently, weight is borne on the radial side of the hand (figure 2.5). The arm posture causes a mechanical increase in wrist extension.

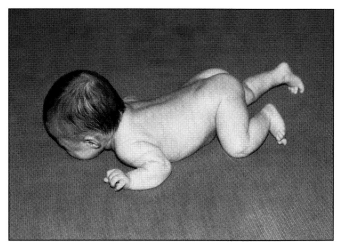

*Figure 2.7.* The shoulders and arms still assume a primitive position, with the elbows behind the shoulders. Head lifting often triggers hip flexion and pelvic elevation, causing a subsequent anterior weight shift. Active hip extensors are vital synergistic muscles for head lifting and head control in prone.

Head lifting often continues to trigger hip flexion and pelvic elevation, causing a subsequent anterior weight shift (figure 2.7), which makes further head lifting and upper extremity weight bearing difficult. However, increased spinal extensor mobility reduces the effect of this weight shift and seems to work with humeral abduction to prevent the shoulders from being pressed into the floor. The hands may be loosely open at the initiation of the movement, but they become fisted as the effort increases. (It will become increasingly obvious that hip extensors are vital synergistic muscles for head lifting and head control in prone.)

Because the hands are bearing some of the weight, head lifting will facilitate proprioceptive feedback into the upper extremities and trunk. Head turning will facilitate asymmetrical feedback. Until approximately five months of age, head turning causes the weight to be shifted to the same side to which the head turns (face-side weight shift). Weight shifting and proprioceptive feedback are important precursors for future forearm weight shifting. The weight shift provides asymmetrical tactile and proprioceptive stimulation which are needed for future development of the body-on-head and body-on-body reactions.

While in prone, the baby can bring the head and mouth to the hand, rather than the hand to the mouth. This is often a method of self calming. Otherwise the baby has minimal functional use of the hands in prone.

## Lower Extremities

Hip flexors have been elongated sufficiently to permit lowering of the pelvis and resting of the anterior aspect of the thigh on the surface (figure 2.6). Hip abduction and external rotation have changed very little, but knee extension has increased. When the baby is relaxed in prone, ankle plantar flexion may occur. The lowered pelvic position reduces the amount of anterior weight shift, and the head and shoulders appear more comfortable in prone.

Although the lower extremities may be extended when the baby is quiet, hip flexion frequently increases as the head is lifted (figure 2.7). Hip flexion subsequently reshifts the weight anteriorly and thus decreases the efficiency of the head lifting.

Although the above response may appear to be the result of the **symmetrical tonic neck reaction** (STNR), the STNR does not appear until six months of age (Barnes, Crutchfield, and Heriza 1978). Such a response in a 2-month-old baby might be attributable to biomechanical factors.

Head lifting and back extension lead to stretching of the anterior trunk muscles (the rectus abdominis and iliopsoas). Because these muscles are not fully elongated at this age, they respond to the stretch by shortening, which subsequently causes hip flexion. There is no resistance from the hip extensors because they are not yet active. Active hip extension, which develops later, is needed to stabilize the pelvis during head lifting. Such stability will enable gradual elongation of the anterior trunk muscles.

Head lifting with concomitant hip flexion is often seen in children with cerebral palsy. The reaction is usually attributed to the STNR; however, there may be other causes which trigger the response.

Therefore, it is imperative, in the developmental sequence, that hip flexion decrease and active hip extension increase so that the hip extensors can provide the synergistic stability to the skeleton for head and trunk extension and further elongation of the abdominals and hip flexors. Even minimal hip flexion in prone will inhibit good head and trunk extension.

# Sitting

In the pull-to-sit test at two months of age (figure 2.8), the increased effect of the developing labyrinthine and optical righting reactions is manifested as fleeting attempts to lift the head. However, insufficient head/neck flexor muscle control results in a head lag. Some 2-month-olds try to reinforce neck stability by visually fixing on the examiner.

The upper extremities are starting to show some response to the pull as passive, unresisted extension is replaced by some active elbow flexion. However, the abdominals and lower extremities still do not participate.

In the sitting position, the 2-month-old's back is flexed, but head lifting is more prevalent (figure 2.9). The closeness of the occiput to the shoulders seems to indicate that much of the mobility for head lifting is occurring between the occiput and the first cervical vertebra. If this is true, then the short and long capital extensor muscles are primarily responsible for the action (Cailliet 1964).

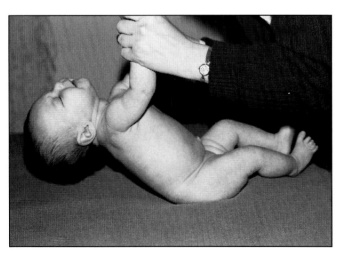

*Figure 2.8. Head lag still occurs in the pull-to-sit test, despite the baby's fleeting attempts to lift the head.*

As back extension increases and the cervical extensors, cervical flexors, and capital flexors become more active and balance each other, neck elongation will occur. The cervical extensors and flexors will stabilize the cervical spine, while the capital flexors tuck the chin (Cailliet 1964; Kapandji 1974). This will reduce head hyperextension by elongating the neck. For these neck muscles to work efficiently, the trunk must be extended to neutral.

Increased effects of the labyrinthine and optical righting reactions plus increased awareness of the environment provide the stimulus for head lifting. However, control of the head in the lifted position is still precarious.

If the baby's hands are held while sitting, the baby often adducts the scapulae and flexes the elbows (figure 2.9). As in prone, this shoulder girdle pattern seems to help provide stability for head lifting and postural stability. This posture may be described as one in which the upper extremities are yoked to the postural system (Gentile 1987).

When the trunk is loosely held, the head and eventually the trunk fall forward (figure 2.10), but not as far forward as at one month. Neither the head nor the chest come to rest on the surface between the legs but are slightly lifted. The hands may rest on the surface, but they do not provide any support.

Lower extremity external rotation has increased but is still limited. Since the lateral sides of the lower extremities do not as yet rest on the surface, the legs still do not provide assistance or postural stability for sitting (figure 2.10).

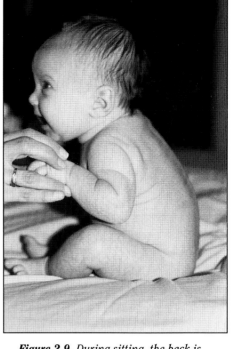

*Figure 2.9. During sitting, the back is still flexed, but head lifting is more prevalent. If the hands are held, the baby often adducts the scapulae and flexes the elbows.*

# Standing

In the upright or standing position (figure 2.11), the 2-month-old has less control than at one month. Primary standing and automatic walking are rarely seen (Touwen 1976). The baby's lack of stepping is called *abasia* (Saint-Anne Dargassies 1972; Barnes, Crutchfield, and Heriza 1978).

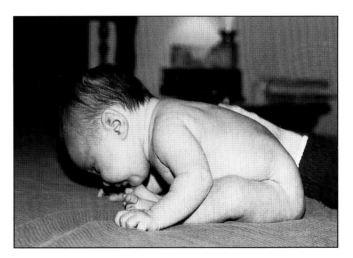

*Figure 2.10. If the trunk is supported only slightly, the head and trunk fall forward, though not as far as at one month. The legs do not provide assistance or postural stability for sitting.*

The baby may or may not take weight on the legs, and the legs may be poorly oriented when weight is borne on the legs. This period of disorientation in standing is called *astasia* (Andre-Thomas, Chesni, and Saint-Anne Dargassies 1960; Barnes, Crutchfield, and Heriza 1978). The astasia-abasia phase is thus characterized by inability to take weight in standing and very poor orientation of the feet when they contact the floor.

In order to stand, the 2-month-old must be securely supported around the chest and under the axillae. Even then, the baby may slip down because of the low tone in the shoulders. When well supported, the baby lifts the head with

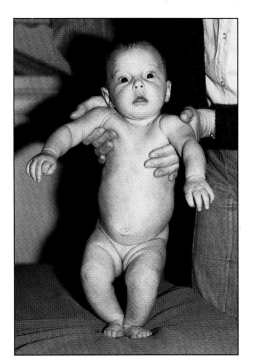

*Figure 2.11.* Primary standing and automatic walking have diminished. Upper extremities show greater extensor activity.

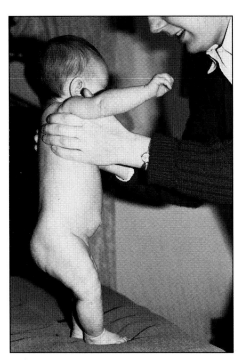

*Figure 2.12.* Hip flexion keeps the hips and pelvic girdle posterior to the shoulder girdle.

hyperextension. Just as at earlier ages, the 2-month-old demonstrates more controlled head lifting in standing than in sitting. The shoulder elevation that occurs when the baby is supported under the axillae may provide some stability for the head lifting.

The developing extensor activity described in other positions is also seen in standing, especially in the upper extremities. Bilateral elbow flexion (figure 1.8) has changed to bilateral elbow extension (figure 2.11). Increased extension is also seen at the wrists and metacarpophalangeal (MP) joints of the hands. Finger interphalangeal (IP) joints are still slightly flexed.

Because of hip flexion, the hips and whole pelvic girdle are still posterior to the shoulder girdle in the vertical position (figure 2.12). Toe curling frequently occurs in standing and may be a response to proprioceptive and tactile stimulation. Toe curling is also used to increase lower extremity stability (fixing), but this is usually seen in older babies who are taking more weight on their legs.

# Indications of Possible Disturbances in Motor Development

The second month of life is a time of asymmetry, hypotonia, astasia, and abasia. Therefore it is usually difficult to discern new, subtle movement problems. On the other hand, babies who have had a significantly troubled birth or postnatal history may present a continuation of obvious problems. These are usually associated with marked hypertonus or marked hypotonus.

# The Third Month

The 3-month-old is alert and aware of the environment. The baby is becoming more adept in visual action (such as following a toy from side to side while in supine) and in interacting visually with the caregivers.

Motorically, symmetry and midline orientation are beginning. The 3-month-old demonstrates a marked increase in bilateral symmetrical activities and antigravity flexor control. However, asymmetry is not uncommon. The head comes into or close to midline, and the upper extremities are becoming more symmetrical in their movements.

The upper and lower extremities are characterized by bilateral abduction and external rotation. Elbow extension has increased, taking the hands further from the body. With increased knee flexion, the lower extremities assume a "frog-legged" position.

Babies at three months can bring their hands to their bodies from widely abducted positions, pulling at their clothes and touching their bodies. The tonic grasp is gone, and the 3-month-old is able to play with the hands or briefly retain a rattle that is placed in the hand.

In prone, improved head and shoulder control, increased spinal extension, and a lowered pelvis enable the 3-month-old to prop on the forearms with sustained head elevation. The baby can rotate the head to each side while it is elevated, which causes subtle weight shifting and sensory feedback to the muscles of the upper trunk and shoulder girdle. However, prone is not yet a functional position for the baby.

When pulled to sit, feedback from the labyrinthine (vestibular) and optical righting systems is more integrated with muscular control. Therefore, there is less head lag in initiation of the movement, and head righting with flexion occurs halfway through the movement. The upper extremities are also becoming more active.

Although the baby must be supported in sitting, increased head control enables sustained head lifting. Cervical and thoracic muscle activity is more obvious, but the spine continues to be flexed. The pelvis remains perpendicular, enabling weight to be maintained on the ischial tuberosities. If unsupported, the baby will fall forward. The trunk and hips offer no resistance to this forward flexion, but the head responds by righting with extension.

The astasia-abasia phase of poor orientation to standing and poor coordination for walking has usually disappeared, and most babies once again accept weight on their lower extremities when supported in standing.

Increased motor ability enables the 3-month-old to interact with the environment more effectively than the 2-month-old. The baby can hold a rattle that is placed in the hand. Although the baby may bring it to the mouth, the baby usually does not attend to the rattle.

The baby continues to swipe at toys, especially those that provide feedback, such as a chime ball (Nash 1991). Babies also like toys they can touch, rattles, dangling toys, and the caretaker's voice and face (Aston 1974).

The baby's increased head control enables increased visual control. The 3-month-old can regard an object in midline and can track 180° with head extension (Inatsuka 1979; Vogtle and Albert 1985). The baby may also regard the hands in midline. Eye-hand regard is a step in the development of body awareness.

# Indications of Possible Disturbances in Motor Development

At three months of age, babies are beginning to organize their movements. Therefore, it is from this month onward that subtle deviations in the normal progress of motor development may be manifested. Slight deviations may be entirely within the range of normal motor development, or they may be the beginning of "soft signs" of abnormal motor development. The interplay of normal and abnormal is especially difficult to discern at this age. Much experience with many typical and atypical babies is needed to discern the quality of the interplay.

However, there are certain specific facets of development which are to be watched closely. These areas will be highlighted under Indications of Possible Disturbances in Motor Development. It must be emphasized that each "problem" discussed may be just a prolonged use of the primitive and may never become abnormal. Once again, experience will enable more accurate judgments to be made as the interplay of all of the baby's movements are observed and evaluated, not just the "problem" areas.

In the 3-month-old, disturbances in motor development may be indicated by the maintenance of strong asymmetry or by the inability to assume and maintain a midline position of the head. Failure to utilize symmetrical extremity movements or to bring each hand, and both hands simultaneously, to the body in supine may indicate poor or delayed development of bilateral symmetrical muscle control.

Ocular motor control is associated with head control. Therefore, if a 3-month-old baby is having difficulty with visual convergence, downward visual gaze, and visual tracking, head control may not be developing normally (specifically head flexion and midline control). Of course, the ocular motor problem may be a separate problem of its own. Both possibilities need to be evaluated further. In the latter case, poor visual control will have a tremendous effect on the development of head control. Therefore, head control and ocular motor/visual control must both be addressed.

In prone, inability or poor ability to abduct and bring both arms forward in line with the shoulders for forearm weight bearing may be indicative of poor or delayed development of the shoulder girdle musculature. Poor ability to weight bear on the forearms in prone will cause the baby to dislike and try to avoid prone. Subsequently the baby will not be able to develop normal antigravity extension control which emerges in prone.

# Supine

In supine, the 3-month-old is characterized by symmetry and midline orientation of the head. The lower extremities frequently assume a position of bilateral flexion, abduction, and external rotation (figure 3.1).

## *Head*

Head movements are more varied at three months than at two months, and symmetry and midline orientation are becoming more dominant. In supine, the baby can rotate the head from side to side with extension. The head can be maintained briefly in midline, and the baby is starting to flex the head and tuck the chin (figure 3.1). The head is brought to and maintained in midline by bilateral contraction of capital (head) and cervical (neck) flexor muscles.

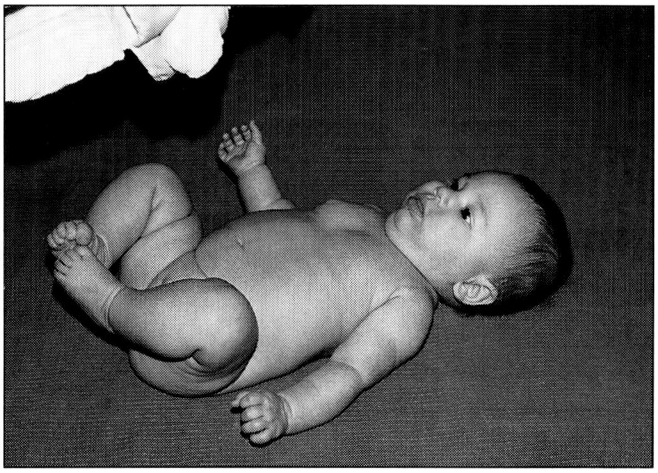

*Figure 3.1.* The 3-month-old is beginning to flex the head and tuck the chin. The head comes into or close to midline, and visual convergence can occur. The baby will try to swipe at an engaging toy.

Full cervical spine mobility is not yet present. Therefore, head rotation can still elicit the neck righting reaction, causing the baby to roll onto the side. For the neck righting reaction to occur at three months, the baby's arms must be close to the body when the head is rotated. Marked extremity abduction, characteristic of the 3-month-old, provides an outrigger effect and thus reduces the occurrence of rolling.

Head and neck flexion occur through a more limited range than extension. There are fewer muscles involved with flexion than with extension. The capital flexors appear to tuck the chin (Cailliet 1964) and serve to elongate the capital and cervical extensors (figure 3.1). The cervical flexors flex the cervical spine (Cailliet 1964; Kapandji 1974).

As bilateral neck flexor muscle control increases, the head is maintained in midline and less frequently rotates to the side. Consequently, the neck receptors for the ATNR are less frequently stimulated, and asymmetrical postures occur less frequently. However, the asymmetrical fencing position may still be observed in the upper extremities during head rotation and even without head rotation. Again, it should be noted that the ATNR is never obligatory.

With the head actively stabilized in midline, visual convergence begins (Nash 1991) (figure 3.1). This control increases the length of time that the baby can regard a toy in midline. Visual attention and interest play an increasingly important role in head movements. Utilizing the increased head and eye control, the supine baby can consistently follow a toy or a face horizontally from side to side (180°) and vertically, if it is within visual range (Inatsuka 1979; Vogtle and Albert 1985) (figures 3.2, 3.3). Downward tracking is inconsistently present (Inatsuka 1979).

The 3-month-old follows best when the head is slightly extended. The capital and cervical extensor muscles seem to have more control than the capital and cervical flexor muscles. The extension is illustrated in figures 3.2 and 3.3 by slight chin lifting. With the development of the capital and cervical flexor muscles, the 3-month-old will become more consistent with downward tracking.

### Indications of Possible Disturbances in Motor Development

At three months of age, symmetry and midline orientation are becoming more dominant. The baby can freely turn the head to each side and can briefly maintain it in midline. Strong obligatory asymmetry or inability to bring and maintain the head in midline may be an indication that bilateral symmetrical muscle control is not developing. This may be due to low muscle tone or unusually active unilateral extensor activity. This may also be indicative of a musculoskeletal problem such as torticollis.

It is very important that 3- and 4-month-old babies develop the ability to actively bring and maintain the head in midline. Failure to do so will interfere with other areas of development such as symmetrical neck, trunk, and extremity movement and control; optical and visual convergence; symmetrical vestibular feedback; and symmetrical weight bearing and proprioceptive feedback.

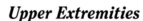

## *Upper Extremities*

The 3-month-old has increased shoulder girdle range in external rotation and abduction. Elbow extension has also increased, and the 3-month-old frequently lies with elbows extended (figure 3.1). The wrists and fingers are also more extended and the hands are usually open.

The upper extremities continue to be responsive to head positions and movements. Midline orientation of the head enables the bilateral symmetrical upper extremity positioning so characteristic of the 3-month-old. However, asymmetrical upper extremity positions and movements are not uncommon (figure 3.2). According to von Hofsten (1990), the 3-month-old begins once again to open the hand when extending the arm, but only when visually fixating on a target. This seems to suggest that there is perception-action coupling of the eyes and hands. It also suggests that the infant is no longer dominated by synchronous synergistic movements. Dissociated movements are beginning to emerge.

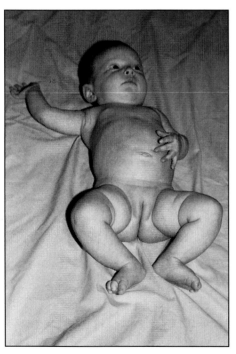

*Figure 3.2. With the increase in head and eye control, the 3-month-old can consistently follow an object horizontally and vertically. The best following occurs when the head is slightly extended. Bilateral upper extremity coordination is beginning to occur, allowing the hands to be brought to the body.*

At three months of age, the baby can actively adduct and internally rotate the shoulders to bring the hands to the body (figure 3.2). Fagard (1990) suggests that this is the beginning of bilateral upper extremity coordination.

By the third month, the palmar grasp reflex is no longer elicited by the traction phase of the reflex. When the 3-month-old's hand is stimulated on the radial side of the palm, the fingers flex, adduct, and hold onto the object (Erhardt 1984). These two steps in the grasp reflex have been described as a "catch phase" (finger flexion and adduction) and a "holding phase" (Halverson 1937, cited in Corbetta and Mounoud 1990).

As 3-month-olds begin to use the hands more, they explore their mouths, bodies, clothing, and caretakers with their hands. These are important steps in the development of body awareness. The hand-on-body and hand-on-clothing incidents provide important tactile experiences which help to reduce the tonic grasp reflex. The hand-on-body, hand-on-clothing experiences may also provide the baby with hand-shaping experiences which may provide the basis for future hand use.

Babies can hold a rattle placed in the hand, but they do not yet seem to know what to do with it, nor do they seem to attend to it (figure 3.4). The rattle is easily dropped if the baby flexes the wrist. (The tenodesis effect of finger extension with wrist flexion causes the fingers to open.) When an exciting toy is presented, the baby initially quiets during visual engagement (figure 3.1), then usually tries to swipe at it with wide shoulder movements.

### Indications of Possible Disturbances in Motor Development

Inability to bring and maintain the head in midline will inhibit the baby's ability to utilize symmetrical upper extremity movements. It will also interfere with the baby's ability to bring the hands to the body. This will lead to consequences such as decreased symmetrical extremity use, decreased body exploration and development of body awareness, and decreased bilateral hand use.

## *Lower Extremities*

Active kicking in supine occurs with symmetrical and reciprocal patterns (figure 3.1). Most kicking occurs in the air. However, some kicking may occur close to or on the supporting surface, and the baby may randomly push against the floor with the foot. Lower extremity pushing may cause spinal extension and lateral weight shifting, but it does not yet cause increased hip extension because the hip flexors are still tight. More frequently, the baby lifts both lower extremities with simultaneous hip and knee flexion and hip external rotation, bringing the feet together (figure 3.1).

The lower extremities rest in symmetrical hip flexion, abduction, external rotation, knee flexion, and ankle dorsiflexion and eversion (figures 3.2 to 3.4). This frog-legged position, characteristic of the 3-month-old baby, enables the feet to come together for foot-on-foot play. This tactile experience contributes to body awareness and reduces tactile sensitivity in the feet.

Active knee extension (quadriceps femoris) initiates changes in the lower extremity components. Knee extension is accompanied by hip extension, hip adduction, and a reduction in hip external rotation.

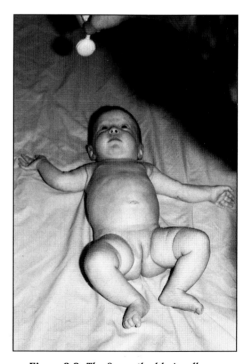

*Figure 3.3.* The 3-month-old visually tracks objects horizontally from side to side and vertically if the object is within visual range. The lower extremities assume the frog-legged position characteristic of three months.

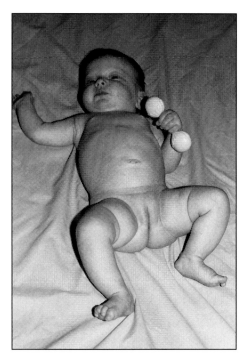

*Figure 3.4. Babies at three months can hold a rattle placed in the hand, but they do not yet seem to know what to do with it, nor do they seem to attend to it.*

When the knee extends, the hamstrings are stretched. This results in hip extension when the hamstrings are tight (as they are in the 3-month-old). Stretch on the medial hamstrings results in increased hip adduction and reduced hip external rotation. Hip adduction and hip internal rotation mobility are still limited by the baby's soft tissue tightness for hip abduction, flexion, and external rotation.

The ankle is also affected by active knee extension. The gastrocnemius muscle crosses the posterior knee joint, and it is stretched when the knee extends, contributing to ankle plantar flexion.

# Prone

By the third month, the baby accepts prone more readily, being able to lift the head more efficiently. Additionally, upper extremity control has improved sufficiently to enable the baby to prop on the forearms occasionally. With the increased neck muscular control and the added stability provided by forearm propping and lumbar extension, the head is steadier when lifted and therefore vision is more functional in prone than it was in previous months. Use of the hands, however, is difficult in the propped position because all of the weight is borne on the forearms. Because visual interest has increased, vision will often direct head movements which will subsequently provide and cause numerous subtle weight-shifting experiences.

## *Head*

Head lifting has improved considerably in range and control. Although increased muscle control is a major contributing factor, there are several other essential components, including (1) increased effect of the labyrinthine and optical righting reactions; (2) increased range in spinal extension, both thoracic and lumbar;

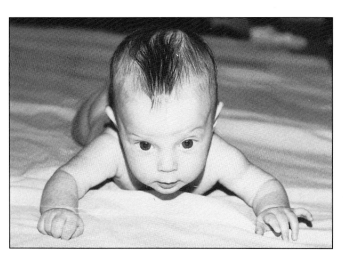

*Figure 3.5. In prone, the head can be held up without bobbing at 45° to 90° in midline. Forearm propping begins to occur. The baby may make scratching movements with the fingers.*

(3) changes in the upper extremity and shoulder girdle positions and improved muscular control; (4) increased synergistic action provided by the lumbar extensors to stabilize the trunk; and (5) increased elongation of the hip flexor muscles and a lowered pelvis.

The 3-month-old can lift the head up to 45° to 90° in midline and maintain it without bobbing (figures 3.5, 3.6). Maintenance in midline is possible because of bilateral contraction of paired extensor muscles. The extended position of the head and neck causes prolonged symmetrical elongation of the head and neck flexor muscles.

The head can be lifted higher because the thoracic and lumbar spine is more extended, suggesting increased and more caudal erector spinae muscle activity. Increased extension is also associated with the lowered pelvis and increased elongation of the hip flexors. The lumbar extensor muscles can provide synergistic action to stabilize the thorax during head lifting.

Once the head is lifted in prone, head flexion movements shift the weight anteriorly and down. Because anterior chest and shoulder girdle muscle control is still not fully developed, the baby usually collapses when the head flexes.

Head rotation from side to side causes lateral weight shifting (figures 3.7, 3.8). As the face turns to one side, the trunk subtly shifts laterally to the same side (face-side weight shift). If the weight shift is sufficient, the baby may roll to the side (figure 3.8).

Because of increased head control, the baby's visual attention in prone has improved. The 3-month-old can track horizontally 180° while in prone (Vogtle and Albert 1985). Because of the head-neck hyperextension, most of the visual attention is with an upward visual gaze.

### Upper Extremities

Forearm propping is possible at three months, suggesting increased and new control of the humeral and scapular muscles in addition to increased spinal extension and increased hip extension. Head lifting no longer causes hip flexion; therefore, when the weight is shifted posteriorly, it is stabilized by active lumbar extension.

At three months, the elbows are in line with or in front of the shoulders, and weight is borne on the elbows and forearms. (At two months, the elbows were behind the shoulders.) Humeral horizontal abduction is modified by increased shoulder flexion, horizontal adduction, and external rotation. This brings the arms forward and back toward the body, which aids in lifting the chest from the surface, enabling forearm propping (figures 3.5, 3.6). Humeral abduction appears to pull the scapula into abduction and slight winging (figure 3.6). Scapular winging suggests that scapular stability from the serratus anterior has not yet emerged.

If the shoulder is markedly flexed and head rotation causes a weight shift, the baby may accidentally roll onto the side (figures 3.7, 3.8). This is not a common occurrence at three months.

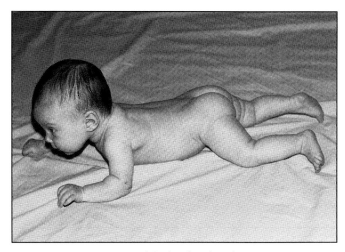

**Figure 3.6.** Extension of the head and neck causes elongation of head and neck flexor muscles. This extension is associated with a lowered pelvis and increased elongation of hip flexors. Elbows are in line with or in front of shoulders for forearm propping. Lower extremities are symmetrical. Scapular winging suggests that scapular stability from the serratus anterior has not yet emerged.

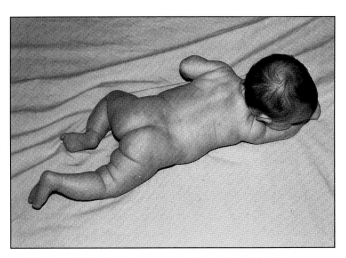

**Figure 3.7.** Head rotation causes the trunk to laterally weight shift to the same side. The lateral weight shift may cause lower extremity dissociation.

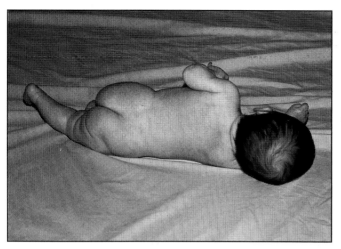

*Figure 3.8. Face-side weight shift: If weight shift is large enough, the baby may roll to the side.*

Elbow flexion and forearm pronation occur during forearm propping. The wrists are slightly extended, and the fingers alternate between being loosely flexed and open. The baby will often make scratching movements with the fingers, especially at the sight of a toy (Vogtle and Albert 1985).

The range of trunk lifting and spinal extension is influenced by the position of the upper and lower extremities. The more abducted the extremities are, the less the trunk is lifted. As shoulder girdle control improves (especially in the cuff muscles, pectoralis major, and serratus anterior), the arms will become more flexed and adducted and raise the chest higher. (This occurs by the fourth month.)

Forearm propping causes a marked posterior weight shift. As a result of this anterior elevation and posterior weight shift, the weight-bearing point (fulcrum for lifting) moves caudally. In the 3-month-old, it appears to be approximately at nipple level.

Forearm weight bearing provides sensory feedback to the upper extremity and shoulder girdle muscles. This feedback is increased by subtle weight shifting which occurs during head movements. Weight is shifted to the same side to which the head turns (face-side weight shift) (figure 3.7).

Forearm propping is the first major step in dynamic weight bearing. The muscles around each joint of both shoulder girdles are involved in simultaneous stability and mobility.

### Indications of Possible Disturbances in Motor Development

The position and control of the shoulder girdles in prone is of prime importance from the third month onward. Inability of the 3-month-old to abduct the arms in prone for forearm weight bearing would indicate a disturbance in motor development. Active humeral abduction indicates that the muscles necessary for scapular stability are developing. Therefore, inability to abduct the humeri would indicate that the scapular muscles and possibly the humeral muscles (all shoulder girdle muscles) are not developing properly.

Poor development of the shoulder girdle muscles results in improper positioning of the arms, head, and neck in prone. This has many far-reaching and rippling effects and can lead to (1) poor shoulder girdle stability; (2) poor dissociation of scapula and humeral movements and poor elongation of the muscles between the two; (3) poor upper extremity weight bearing in prone; (4) poor or abnormal development of neck and trunk extensors and flexors; and (5) poor development of distal upper extremity control.

### Lower Extremities

At three months of age, the lower extremities are usually symmetrical in prone (figure 3.6). Extension is increasing at the hips and knees, and external rotation is decreasing. However, slight hip flexion continues to prevent the pelvis from resting fully on the supporting surface and subsequently still causes a slight anterior weight shift. Hip flexion must continue to decrease to permit caudal displacement of the weight-bearing point into the pelvis and hips, which will enable improved head and trunk lifting. The ankles have started to become more mobile and now fluctuate between dorsiflexion and plantar flexion (figure 3.6).

Some lower extremity movements at three months occur bilaterally and have a hip flexion component (figure 3.9). When bilateral hip flexion occurs, weight is shifted forward. The forward weight shift interferes with head and shoulder girdle alignment, which results in a reversion to a primitive position. The head hyperextends and the shoulders tip forward while the humeri adduct, internally rotate, and hyperextend (figure 3.9).

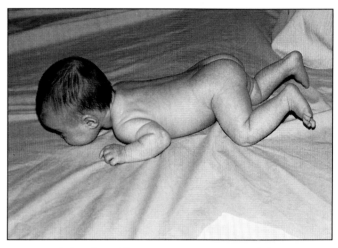

**Figure 3.9.** Bilateral lower extremity activity with hip flexion causes a forward weight shift, which returns the baby to the primitive head and shoulder girdle position.

Occasionally, but rarely, unilateral forward kicking may occur (figure 3.7). The lower extremities may respond with dissociated reactions (figure 3.7) when a major lateral body weight shift occurs. At three months, this is an accidental occurrence rather than a characteristic action.

Near the end of the third month, random antigravity kicking begins, which provides proprioceptive and kinesthetic feedback. This may contribute to the development of more advanced controlled movements in the lower trunk, pelvis, hips, and lower extremities.

# Sitting

Although 3-month-olds can bring their heads to midline in supine, they still do not have antigravity neck flexor control or synergistic stability from the oblique abdominal muscles (Kendall, Kendall, and Wadsworth 1971). When pulled to sit, therefore, midline orientation of the head is lost, and a head lag and shoulder elevation occur. The head lag is most marked at the initiation of the test (figure 3.10). As the baby comes closer to the upright, the head is lifted (figure 3.11). Head lifting occurs without chin tucking. This suggests that the sternocleidomastoid muscles, not the capital flexors, are responsible for the movement (Kendall, Kendall, and Wadsworth 1971).

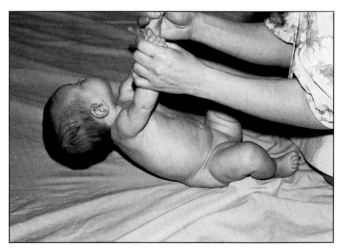

**Figure 3.10.** Head lag still occurs during pull-to-sit, especially in the absence of synergistic abdominal activity. Rotation of the head can trigger asymmetrical responses in the extremities.

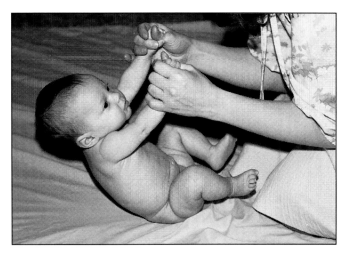

*Figure 3.11.* As the baby comes closer to the upright, the shoulders elevate to stabilize and lift the head. The chin does not tuck because the neck is hyperextended.

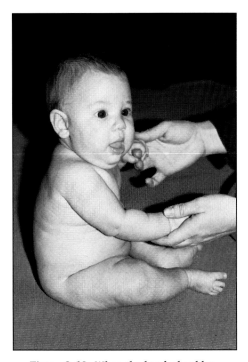

*Figure 3.12.* When the head, shoulder, and pelvis are aligned in supported sitting, the neck is less hyperextended, demonstrating increased antigravity control of head and neck flexors and extensors. Weight is centered on the ischial tuberosities. Head movements do not disturb the baby's balance.

Bilateral symmetrical action of the head (capital) and neck flexors is needed to bring the head to midline and hold it there. In order for the capital and neck flexors to maintain the head position during the pull-to-sit test, the thorax must be stabilized by synergistic contraction of the oblique abdominal muscles (Kendall, Kendall, and Wadsworth 1971). Without this synergistic stability, the thorax and shoulders are elevated in an attempt to stabilize the head. Shoulder elevation subsequently results in neck hyperextension.

The baby's obvious desire to right the head is indicative of the continued maturation of the labyrinthine and optical righting reactions. However, muscular control is not as advanced. The baby uses the visual or optical righting functionally by "fixing" the eyes on the examiner as if to reinforce head stability. This again emphasizes the importance of the optical righting reactions.

The upper extremities resist passive extension, but they are inconsistently active in assisting by pulling into elbow flexion. When elbow flexion does occur, it is usually during the first half of the movement. When the head becomes stable and flexes forward, active elbow flexion decreases.

Abdominal and lower extremity reactions are closely associated with each other and with the head reactions. When the head lag is the strongest, there is little abdominal or lower extremity activity (figure 3.10). When the abdominals and hip flexors are more active, they provide the synergistic stability to the thorax for head lifting (figure 3.11). The lower extremities assume a posture of abduction and external rotation.

During pull-to-sit at three months of age, asymmetrical reactions in the extremities are not uncommon. Although the anterior head and neck muscles and the sternocleidomastoid muscles are strong enough to bring the head to midline while the head is supported in supine, these muscles are not yet strong enough to simultaneously stabilize and lift the head in midline. Consequently, the head may rotate and trigger asymmetrical responses in the extremities.

The increased control demonstrated in prone and supine is observed in sitting (figure 3.12). The antigravity control of the head and neck flexors and extensors is used to sustain head lifting in sitting. The head is less hyperextended. This is probably related to better alignment of the head, shoulders, and pelvis (figure 3.12), as well as increased activity in the head and neck flexors.

The back is more extended in sitting, which may be related to the increase in active trunk extension in prone. The pelvis remains perpendicular to the support, and the baby's weight is maintained on the ischial tuberosities (figure 3.12).

Because head and trunk control have improved, head movements do not disturb the baby's balance, and the baby requires less support while sitting. If a 3-month-old feels insecure with this trunk support, the baby will use bilateral scapular adduction to reinforce trunk stability (figures 3.13, 3.14). Bilateral scapular adduction, or "high guard," is a pattern frequently used to reinforce trunk stability. Gentile (1987) may describe this pattern as the upper extremities being yoked to the postural system.

Scapular adduction pulls the arms and hands away from each other, the body, and the toy. At this early age, this response is needed for postural stability, and stability precedes and precludes hand use. Because the baby's hand control is not developed, the scapular stabilizing action does not interfere with function. This again demonstrates the concept of the upper extremities being yoked to the postural system.

Although the baby cannot reach the hand to a toy that is presented, the 3-month-old can reach visually (figure 3.13). If a rattle is placed in the hand, the baby can hold it but will pay little attention to it.

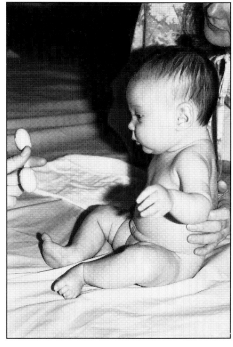

*Figure 3.13.* The 3-month-old uses scapular adduction to reinforce trunk stability. This pulls the arms and hands back, away from a toy.

Trunk control is not yet fully developed. Therefore, the baby will fall forward if left unsupported (figure 3.14). Although there is minimal resistance in the hips, lumbar, or lower thoracic areas for forward bending, the head and upper trunk do respond and resist. The head rights itself by extending. The extension is continued into the upper thoracic area and is seen as scapular adduction and thoracic extension, which lift the trunk. Because of the head righting response and upper trunk extension, neither the head nor the chest come to rest on the floor between the legs.

Although the lower extremities are more externally rotated and abducted than in previous months, they provide only minimal positional stability and no active control for sitting. As hip external rotation and abduction increase, the knees become more flexed. This is due to the stretch being put on the two-joint hip adductor muscles (gracilis, semimembranosus, and semitendinosus). Eventually, full external rotation with abduction, with the lateral sides of the legs resting on the surface, will provide positional stability for sitting. This lower extremity position will prevent lateral weight shifting and thus prevent falling to the side.

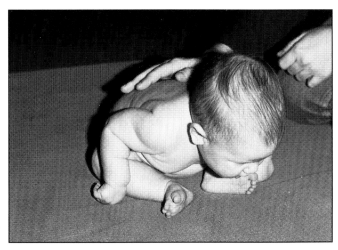

*Figure 3.14.* Although trunk support has increased, it has not fully developed, and the baby will fall forward if left unsupported. The baby responds to the forward movement with head hyperextension and scapular adduction.

# Standing

The astasia-abasia phase introduced at the second month has usually disappeared by the third month. Therefore, when supported upright, the baby once again takes weight on the feet. The amount of weight borne on the legs is often related to the degree of abduction. When the feet are close together, the baby sustains less weight than when the legs are abducted (figure 3.15).

Sustained head lifting is possible with less head hyperextension and less shoulder hiking. The scapulae are adducted, with the arms slightly abducted and flexed forward. This posture again demonstrates the arms being yoked to the postural system in that they are being used to reinforce postural (trunk) stability. When the arms are yoked to the postural system, it is difficult for the baby to use the arms for reaching and the hands for manipulating objects in the environment.

Elbow extension varies. When effort is increased to maintain trunk extension during standing, there is an overflow into increased elbow extension (figure 3.15). When less effort is used, there is less overflow, and elbow extension decreases. Wrist extension is present but less exaggerated than at two months. Metacarpophalangeal (MP) joint extension is now accompanied by increased interphalangeal (IP) joint extension. (Biomechanically, wrist extension increases finger flexion. Therefore decreased wrist extension permits increased efficiency of the MP and IP extensors.)

Hip flexion continues to keep the pelvic girdle behind the shoulder girdle (figure 3.16). Knee extension, not hip extension, seems to provide the extensor tone needed to support the weight.

When the legs are abducted during weight bearing, weight is borne on the medial side of the feet (figure 3.15). Medial weight bearing is usually accompanied by pronation—dorsiflexion, abduction, and eversion of the foot (Root et al. 1971; Root, Orien, and Weed 1977). More pronation is seen in babies with lower tone.

Toe curling occurs frequently during standing. This may be the result of the **plantar grasp reflex** which is elicited when pressure is applied to the ball of the foot (Twitchell 1965; Barnes, Crutchfield, and Heriza 1978). Although toe curling usually occurs as a response to tactile or proprioceptive stimulation, it also seems to occur when the baby is trying to increase stability. This may indicate that toe curling is related to the baby's attempts to increase stability, or to fix to hold on. This fixing seems to reinforce proximal instability through distal-to-proximal synergistic muscle activity.

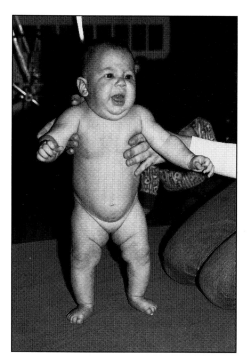

*Figure 3.15. When supported upright, the baby will take weight on the feet. The scapulae and arm position reinforce trunk stability. The upper extremities are yoked to the postural system. When the legs are abducted, weight is borne medially on the feet (pronation). Toe curling may occur to reinforce lower extremity stability.*

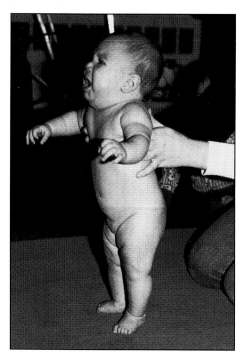

*Figure 3.16. Hip flexion keeps the pelvic girdle behind the shoulder girdle, with knee (rather than hip) extension providing the necessary extensor tone for weight support.*

# The Fourth Month

The milestones of the fourth month mark the beginning of controlled, purposeful movements and the beginning of alternating, coordinated movements. The 4-month-old can easily alternate between extension and flexion in both prone and supine. (These are sagittal plane movements.)

Head and trunk symmetry, midline orientation, and bilateral symmetrical extremity movements are dominant during the fourth month. The alternating bilateral symmetrical activation of extensor and flexor muscles makes possible the strong symmetry and the development of midline orientation. Midline orientation, along with head and trunk symmetry, enable the development of coordination between the two sides of the body.

The 4-month-old is very active visually. Ocular control is becoming more refined as a result of the increased head control. The eyes are now the pathfinders, causing many different head movements which exercise and reinforce the development of various muscles. The eyes are active during reaching for objects, though the upper extremities still lack the coordination and control needed for reaching. Visual "fixing" increases head stability and ensures its proper orientation in space. This is evident during the pull-to-sit test.

The upper extremities demonstrate increasing gross motor control, though fine motor hand control is still limited. During play and exploration, the baby is involved with hand-to-hand, hand-to-mouth, and hand-to-body contact. The 4-month-old continues to use an ulnar grasp to pick up and hold toys but is not yet able to manipulate them. Use of the mouth to explore the hands and toys is a distinguishing characteristic at this age.

The lower extremities also demonstrate more control, but they are relatively quiet. Within this quietness, the baby seems to use the legs in more directed, semipurposeful ways. The 4-month-old's lower extremities often mirror the upper extremities, as if these simultaneous movements reinforce each other. These actions also reinforce the strong symmetry and midline orientation.

The alternating symmetrical movements of the lower extremities and the alternating activation of trunk extensors and flexors facilitate anterior and posterior tilting of the pelvis. These pelvic movements will provide a basis for further normal development of lower extremity movements.

In supine, the 4-month-old maintains the head in midline, tucks the chin, and brings the hands together. The baby is also able to extend the elbows and reach hands to knees when the hips and knees are flexed. The symmetrical flexor activity takes precedence over the asymmetrical activities of the younger babies. Therefore the ATNR is rarely seen.

From the supine hands-to-knees position, the baby can roll to the side. Side lying is a new position of great importance, offering the proprioceptive, tactile, vestibular, and visual feedback needed to stimulate lateral righting or antigravity lateral flexion. The quality of the lateral righting response depends upon the degree of balance between the neck and trunk extensors and flexors.

In prone, the 4-month-old can hold the head up at 90° in midline. Now the baby is also capable of forearm and occasionally extended-arm support because thoracic and lumbar extension (range and muscle action) have increased, and shoulder girdle control is sufficient to maintain the elevated position.

The increasing extensor activity of the 4-month-old is frequently expressed in a "pivot-prone" position with marked scapular adduction. However, the baby can move out of this extension pattern and assume a forearm weight-bearing position. Forearm weight bearing is accomplished with the arms in line with the trunk. Head turning still causes weight shifting to the face-side arm, which limits reaching and may result in the baby rolling (actually falling) to the face side.

When pulled to sit, the 4-month-old's head-righting reactions are strong. Although lacking full head flexion control, the baby can lift and stabilize the head in midline by elevating the shoulders. The baby is beginning to assist with the upper extremities by flexing the elbow. Upper extremity flexion is usually associated with abdominal and lower extremity total flexor activity.

When sitting, the baby uses strong extensor activity to maintain the semierect posture. Mobility in this posture occurs at the hips. The baby's upper extremities are not functional in sitting but remain yoked to the postural system. The typical upper extremity posture is one in which the scapulae are adducted and the arms are abducted. The 4-month-old's lower extremities are starting to be used to assist with positional stability, especially in preventing sideward weight shifting. (Thus, the lower extremities are also yoked to the postural system.)

When placed in standing, the baby takes weight on the extended legs. Control has improved sufficiently so that the baby can be supported by the hands instead of the trunk. Standing is a static position at this age; the 4-month-old cannot shift weight or lift either leg. The upper extremities are still yoked to the postural system and cannot be used functionally for reaching and grasping.

# Indications of Possible Disturbances in Motor Development

Because the fourth month is characterized by symmetrical extremity movements, midline orientation of the head and extremities, and alternating symmetrical extensor and flexor movements of the trunk, failure to achieve these skills indicates a disturbance in motor development which will subsequently lead to poor postural stability (Quinton 1976, 1977, 1978).

Failure to achieve symmetry is often compensated for by overuse of the ATNR, with subsequent poor coordination between the two sides of the body. Failure to achieve symmetry in supine suggests that bilateral symmetrical flexor muscle control has not developed, and this will lead to insufficient flexor muscle activity to balance the extensors. Failure to achieve balance between the flexors and extensors means that the baby will not be able to alternate smoothly between flexion and extension. This will subsequently interfere with the development of lateral flexion.

Inadequate flexor muscle development is manifested in supine by inability to maintain the head in midline with the chin tucked, poor visual convergence and poor downward visual gaze, inadequate head control in pull-to-sit, limited ability to bring the hands together in midline, limited body exploration, inability to flex both hips symmetrically with adduction, failure to achieve the hands-to-knees position, and limited posterior pelvic tilting. In prone, it is manifested by inability to achieve forearm weight bearing with arms close to the body.

Failure to develop symmetrical antigravity extension in prone also demonstrates a motor disturbance which subsequently leads to poor development of postural stability. Inadequate symmetrical extensor activity is manifested as inability to lift and maintain the head in midline, inability to assume the pivot-prone position with extension and bilateral scapular adduction, inability to alternate between pivot-prone and forearm weight bearing, and inability to right (extend) the head and trunk in sitting.

# Supine

In supine, symmetrical actions and midline orientation of the head and hands dominate the 4-month-old's repertoire of positions and movements (figures 4.1 to 4.7).

The marked extremity abduction which characterized the 3-month-old has been changed by increased active flexion with adduction. The baby can bring the hands to midline and to various parts of the body. This contributes to the ability to develop awareness of body parts. The baby can also flex and adduct the hips and knees and bring the legs into line with the trunk. Quinton (1976, 1977, 1978) describes this as a time when babies "re-collect" themselves (figure 4.1) after the abduction of the third month (figures 3.2 to 3.4).

In supine, the 4-month-old has become quite active. Head control now provides a stable base for more coordinated ocular movements and visual pursuit. The upper extremities demonstrate improved coordination for body exploration and for management of lightweight toys. The lower extremities demonstrate increased coordination in kicking and in maintaining antigravity postures.

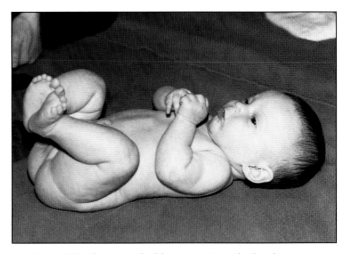

***Figure 4.1.*** *The 4-month-old can maintain the head in midline with the chin tucked. In supine, the lower extremities often mirror the upper extremities, moving symmetrically with each other and in synchrony with the arms. The lumbar spine flattens and the pelvis tilts posteriorly.*

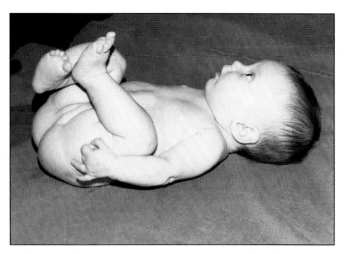

*Figure 4.2.* Eye movements are beginning to dissociate from head movements during visual tracking. Isolated eye movements, rather than combined head and eye movements, are used to track objects.

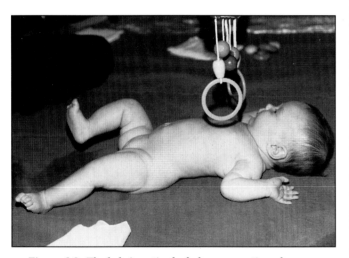

*Figure 4.3.* The baby's entire body becomes active when a toy is held over the chest, and initial reaching attempts usually include reversion to bilateral shoulder abduction and external rotation. There is little isolated movement of independent lower extremity joints: when hips flex, the knees and ankles also flex; when knees extend, the hips extend and feet may plantar flex.

## Head

In supine, the 4-month-old has sufficient muscle control to maintain the head in midline with the chin tucked, using both capital (head) and cervical (neck) flexors (figures 4.1 to 4.7). In addition to increased muscle control, midline orientation of the head suggests increased maturation of the labyrinthine (vestibular) and optical righting systems. At four months, however, the baby cannot yet independently flex and lift the head from the supporting surface. In addition to capital and cervical flexors, head lifting requires synergistic action of the abdominal muscles to stabilize the thorax (Kendall, Kendall, and Wadsworth 1971).

Active chin tucking with posterior neck elongation in supine is a step in the development of postural stability of the cervical spine. According to Kapandji (1974), the longus cervicis straightens the cervical column and holds it rigid. The anterior muscles of the neck (capital flexors, supra-, and infrahyoid muscles) flex the head and cervical column (Kapandji 1974; Cailliet 1964).

The muscles of the tongue and jaw (suprahyoid muscles) need a stable synergistic base for their normal development and normal use. The cervical spine and the shoulder girdle (attachment for the infrahyoid muscles) is the base from which these muscles work (Kapandji 1974). Without proper stability of the cervical spine, the muscles of the tongue and jaw do not have a stable base from which to contract and therefore may not develop normally. Without this proximal stability, a risk exists for developing problems with oral motor control.

Improved head control enables improved ocular control. The 4-month-old can visually track an object without turning the head (Inatsuka 1979). The emerging ability to flex the head is coupled with the ability to gaze downward. The eyes are beginning to develop a downward gaze in conjunction with head flexion (Vogtle and Albert 1985) (figures 4.5, 4.6), which enables babies to inspect their bodies.

Active head rotation occurs freely in each direction, usually in response to visual or auditory stimulation. However, the neck righting reaction can still be elicited at four months. When the head rotates, the body follows (or rolls) as a unit (Barnes, Crutchfield, and Heriza 1978). Because of limited spinal rotational mobility, the neck righting reaction becomes a primary means by which the 4-month-old rolls from supine to side lying.

Rolling to side lying usually occurs when the head rotates while it is flexed (figures 4.9 to 4.11). Head rotation with extension may also occur (figure 4.12), but it is a more primitive pattern than rotation with flexion, and it increases spinal extension. The latter is observed more frequently in premature babies. As described below, its biomechanical effects are different from those of rotation with flexion.

When the baby rotates the head with slight flexion (figures 4.9 to 4.11), a neutral position of the spine and trunk is stimulated. When the baby rotates the head with extension (figure 4.12), extension in the spine and trunk is stimulated. The use of flexion or extension will influence visual gaze and vestibular stimulation and feedback. Head rotation with flexion is usually accompanied by downward visual gaze, while head rotation with extension is accompanied by upward visual gaze.

When head rotation with flexion initiates rolling from supine to the side, lateral flexion of the head occurs in side lying. (Lateral flexion, pure frontal plane movement, is the combined action of unilateral flexors and extensors working together. See discussion under Side Lying.) When rolling from supine is initiated with head rotation with extension, lateral flexion of the head in side lying does not occur. As will be discussed later, rolling to side lying is an important step in development, and how the baby rolls will influence other areas of development.

Although the 4-month-old can actively rotate the head from side to side in supine, the baby is beginning to dissociate eye movements from head movements during visual tracking. When an object is moved in front of the supine 4-month-old, the baby uses isolated eye movements, rather than combined head and eye movements, to track (Inatsuka 1979) (figure 4.2). This indicates increased ocular muscle control with synergistic postural stability from the head and neck muscles. The head and neck muscles thus provide the postural stability for the eye movements. Babies who do not develop normal head control have difficulty developing dissociated eye movements, and thus continue to move head and eyes together (Nash 1991).

In addition to dissociation, the eyes have become more specific in their reaching and "holding," and they are more capable of sustained midline convergence (Nash 1991). Visual tracking, optical righting, and visual fixing are very influential components in the development of head control and head righting reactions.

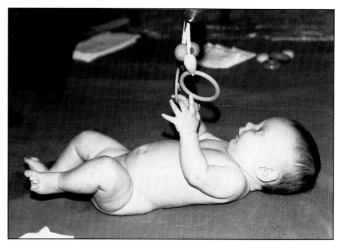

*Figure 4.4.* The 4-month-old reaches for toys in supine with forearm pronation and wrist and finger extension. Reaching skills are not yet accurate and the baby frequently misses the toy in early reaching.

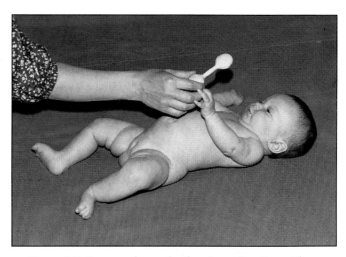

*Figure 4.5.* Downward gaze develops in conjunction with head flexion. Although the 4-month-old uses a bilateral reaching pattern, one arm usually reaches the object first.

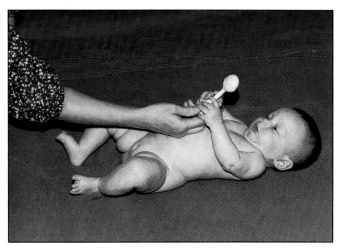

**Figure 4.6.** *Once the baby's left hand touches the mother's hand, the right arm comes forward with increased accuracy. The frog-leg position is still evident.*

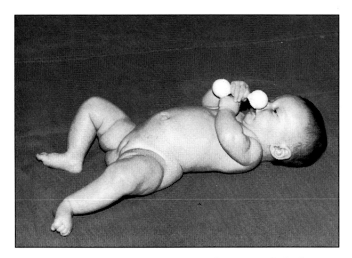

**Figure 4.7.** *The 4-month-old does not have controlled release and cannot transfer an object from one hand to the other.*

Although an ATNR can be elicited, it is rarely observed at four months due to the increased bilateral symmetrical control of the capital and cervical flexor muscles and the baby's developing ability to use the hands in midline and look downward.

From four months onward, balance of antigravity extension and flexion (sagittal plane movements) will be incorporated into the development of antigravity lateral flexion (frontal plane movement). At four months, the combined action of the cervical extensors and flexors is demonstrated as lateral head righting when the baby is in side lying. (See discussion under Side Lying.)

### Indications of Possible Disturbances in Motor Development

If antigravity capital and cervical flexion do not develop normally, significant motor problems may be generated, including (1) lack of midline orientation of the head and trunk, (2) lack of symmetry of the head and trunk, (3) poor visual tracking, (4) continued stimulation for trunk extension and asymmetry, (5) oral-motor dysfunction, and (6) inability to actively laterally flex in side lying.

## Trunk

At four months, the trunk in supine is symmetrical, moving primarily as a whole unit into either slight flexion or extension (sagittal plane movements). The abdominals and lumbar extensors demonstrate reciprocal activity as the baby alternates between flexion (figure 4.1) and extension (figures 4.7, 4.8). The baby is beginning to use the trunk flexors actively in supine. Controlled lateral (frontal plane) and rotational (transverse plane) movements of the trunk are not seen at this age.

Active anterior and posterior tilting of the pelvis is an obvious indication of sagittal plane trunk activity. Posterior tilting occurs during contraction of the hip flexors and the abdominals, particularly the rectus abdominis, which lifts the pubis (figure 4.1) (Kendall, Kendall, and Wadsworth 1971). Anterior tilting of the pelvis is due both to active muscle contraction (lumbar extensors and iliopsoas) and biomechanical muscle stretching (iliopsoas) during hip extension (figures 4.3, 4.5, 4.8). Anterior-posterior (sagittal plane) pelvic mobility is an important step in the normal development of pelvic movements and a precursor of normal development of lower extremity movements.

## Indications of Possible Disturbances in Motor Development

Failure to achieve the basic postural stability of alternate flexion and extension and bilateral symmetrical muscle activation interferes with normal development. Symmetrical muscle action is important for proper midline orientation and trunk stability. The ability to alternate between flexion and extension seems to be associated with the baby's expression of emerging control on the sagittal plane. Sagittal plane control is utilized in the development of frontal and transverse plane movements of the trunk.

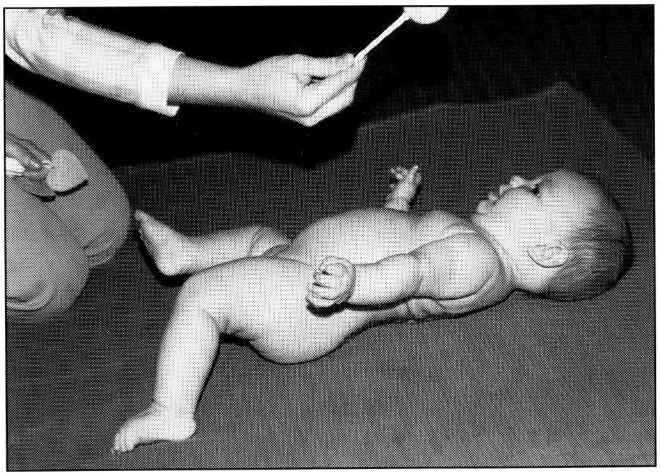

*Figure 4.8.* Anterior tilting of the pelvis occurs with contraction of lumbar extensors and biomechanical stretching of the iliopsoas during hip extension. Lower extremity asymmetry occurs when the baby pushes with the feet and arches the back.

The balance between anterior and posterior pelvic tilting is an important step in the development of trunk synergistic activity for lower extremity movements. Therefore, if the baby practices one movement (such as anterior pelvic tilting) without balancing it with the other (posterior pelvic tilting), lower trunk control would be inadequate to stabilize the pelvis dynamically for controlled femoral movements. Subsequently, the pelvis and femur would move as a unit rather than with dissociation.

Problems in the trunk may be manifested as overuse of flexors, excessive low tone, or excessive high tone with pushing into extension. If a baby maintains or overuses a flexed posture, the abdominal muscles and hip flexors may fail to become elongated. Failure to elongate these anterior trunk and hip muscles will cause difficulty in developing skills in the prone position.

Babies with excessive low tone may maintain a frog-legged position, which causes the pelvis to tilt anteriorly. These babies often have difficulty developing abdominal control in supine. Without abdominal control, synergistic control for head, arm, and leg lifting will be missing (Kendall, Kendall, and Wadsworth 1971). Therefore the baby will experience difficulty with skills related to movement of these parts in supine (for example, head lifting, arm reaching, and leg kicking). This difficulty may extend into other positions, such as sitting and standing.

Babies with excessive high tone often push into extension. If this extension is never balanced with flexion, the extensor muscles become tight while the flexor muscles are stretched and weakened. Excessive extension interferes with normal development in the areas of head control, oral-motor control, visual control and tracking, eye-hand coordination, arm and hand movements, and lower extremity movements and control.

## *Upper Extremities*

The 4-month-old baby is beginning to demonstrate active control of the shoulders in supine. During quiet times, the positions of the arms vary from shoulder adduction with internal rotation (figure 4.1) to abduction with external rotation (figure 4.3). As the control of the muscles around the shoulder girdle increases, the scapular muscles can provide dynamic stability for an increased variety of humeral and elbow movements. The arms can now flex, abduct, adduct, and internally and externally rotate. Elbow positions vary between flexion and extension.

Although arm control is still limited, the 4-month-old can now reach with arms as well as eyes. The baby uses this increased motor and visual control to reach more body parts. The baby can bring hands to the face, bring hands together above the chest (figure 4.1), reach hands to hips (figure 4.2), and reach hands to flexed knees.

These shoulder and elbow movements enable the baby's hands to engage in many new tactile and exploratory experiences which are important for continued development of body awareness, hand shaping, and hand use, as well as continued development of arm movements. Infants develop "control of arm and hand movements based on visual and tactile information related to extrinsic properties of objects—contact, direction, distance" (Corbetta and Mounoud 1990, 206).

Midline eye-hand regard has improved (Corbetta and Mounoud 1990) because of the baby's increased ability for head flexion in midline with chin tucking, downward visual gazing with visual convergence, and shoulder flexion. The baby can then direct vision to the hands. When the hands are together or on the knees and vision is directed to these areas, awareness of body parts is reinforced. As the 4-month-old's interest is captured in these hand and eye activities, the baby repeats them over and over, thus increasing motor control for reaching and grasping.

Von Hofsten (1990) reports that 4-month-olds can use vision to adjust the final path of their reaching. With this increased eye-hand coordination, the baby is more successful in reaching for toys that are on or near the chest. However, coordinated reaching out into space over the chest and abdomen is more difficult, and the baby has not yet developed the motor control to accomplish this (figure 4.4). At four months, the lower extremities may mirror the upper extremities during reaching. This may reinforce trunk stability.

At four months, babies in supine usually reach for toys with forearm pronation and wrist extension (figure 4.4). The fingers are usually slightly flexed at the metacarpophalangeal (MP) joints and loosely flexed or extended at the proximal interphalangeal (PIP) and distal interphalangeal (DIP) joints. Grasping occurs as a primitive ulnar grasping and squeezing pattern (Erhardt 1984; Nash 1991). The grasping may be aided by the tenodesis effect of wrist extension which facilitates finger flexion.

When a toy is held over the baby's chest, the baby's entire body becomes active and excited. Initial reaching attempts usually include reversion to a more primitive position of bilateral shoulder abduction and external rotation (figure 4.3). This is followed by active bilateral shoulder adduction, slight internal rotation and flexion, forearm pronation, and wrist and finger extension (figure 4.4). The baby's reaching skills are not yet accurate and the baby frequently misses the toy in early reaching. However, most babies continue to persevere and try to problem solve how to reach the toy. This problem-solving phase is critical for motor learning and skill development.

Although the 4-month-old uses a bilateral reaching pattern, one arm usually reaches the object first (Fagard 1990). The sequence in figures 4.5 and 4.6 shows that, once the baby's left hand contacted her mother's hand, the right arm came forward with increased accuracy. It may be that the baby's left hand on the mother's hand provided some postural stability or a point of reference that enabled the right arm and hand to reach with increased accuracy.

The baby's reaching in supine also appears to become more coordinated and successful when the toy or the hand of the caregiver touches the baby's abdomen (figure 4.6). This pressure, although light, may provide proprioceptive feedback which gives a point of reference for the reaching pattern. The pressure may provide some trunk (abdominal) stability or increased proprioceptive awareness which enhances or facilitates forward flexion of the upper extremities. In other words, the pressure may provide the trunk stability needed for the pectoralis major to contract more efficiently (Kendall, Kendall, and Wadsworth 1971). (This concept of touch or pressure to reinforce reaching is frequently used in treatment sessions to enhance a baby's reaching pattern.)

Once the ring or rattle has been contacted, the baby can grasp it if it is positioned so that the ulnar side of the baby's hand and fingers can flex around it without the baby's having to move the forearm. (The 4-month-old cannot yet control forearm supination and pronation.) Once the object has been grasped, the baby can bring the other hand to it (figure 4.6). However, the 4-month-old cannot yet transfer it to the other hand (figure 4.7) or manipulate it. At this age, the baby does not have controlled release. At four months, release is usually accomplished by flexing the wrist, causing the fingers to extend.

Once the toy has been grasped, the baby's ability to interact with it is limited. The baby can shake or bang it with flexion-extension movements of the elbows. These movements often result in total body participation. Using forearm pronation and elbow flexion, the baby can also bring the toy to the mouth for mouth exploration (figure 4.7). Because the baby cannot manipulate toys with the hands, mouthing of toys is important for early development of perceptual awareness of shapes, sizes, and textures. Mouthing is also an important process for decreasing tongue and mouth sensitivity.

## Indications of Possible Disturbances in Motor Development

Bilateral symmetrical upper extremity use is dominant at four months. These movements require bilateral activation of scapula and shoulder girdle muscles (serratus anterior, pectoralis major, cuff muscles, and deltoids) with synergistic rib cage stability from the abdominals. Failure to achieve symmetrical upper extremity use may indicate poor development of these shoulder girdle muscles, poor coordination of their use, and/or poor synergistic stability from the abdominals. Further normal development and upper extremity use will be impaired. Development of body awareness and body scheme will also be impaired because of the baby's limited ability to explore the body. Poor reaching skills may also affect the baby's development of hand use and grasping patterns. Reaching positions the hand for grasping.

Continued use of the ATNR suggests poor development of bilateral symmetrical flexor muscle action in the head, neck, shoulders, and trunk. Persistent asymmetry will have serious biomechanical and musculoskeletal consequences throughout the body. Persistent asymmetry inhibits bilateral hand use which subsequently affects manipulation and tactile exploration of objects and transfer of objects from hand to hand.

## Lower Extremities

At four months, the lower extremities are rarely as quiet as they were at three months, but their movements are more specific than the earlier random movements. In supine, the lower extremities frequently mirror the upper extremities. The legs move symmetrically with each other and often in synchrony with the arms (figure 4.1). Although dissociated lower extremity movements do occur (figure 4.3), bilateral symmetrical movements of the lower extremities dominate the 4-month-old's repertoire.

The 4-month-old actively engages in bilateral symmetrical flexion and extension. The lower extremity movements are total synergistic movements, with little isolated movement of independent joints. When the hips flex, the knees and ankles also flex (figure 4.1). When the knees extend, the hips extend and the ankles may plantar flex slightly (figure 4.3), or they may still remain dorsiflexed.

In supine, mobility into hip extension is increasing, permitting the thighs to come closer to the floor. However, hip flexion is still a major component. Although hip abduction and external rotation (the frog-legged position) are still present (figures 4.5 to 4.7), this position is beginning to be modified by increasing activity of the hip adductors (figure 4.9).

The most obvious lower extremity change in supine is the increased range in knee extension (figure 4.3) that develops as the baby practices kicking. As the baby extends the knee with the quadriceps, the hamstrings, gastrocnemius, and other soft tissue around the knee are elongated. Although the ankles are still usually dorsiflexed at this age, slight plantar flexion may be observed when the knees extend. This initial ankle plantar flexion may be due to proximal elongation of the gastrocnemius muscle as the knee is extended. (The gastrocnemius is a two-joint muscle; therefore when the proximal end is stretched, movement occurs at the distal end.)

Ankle inversion and eversion with dorsiflexion also occur in supine. Eversion seems to be the stronger component at this age. At four months, toe flexion occurs frequently, usually when increased effort is exerted by other body parts (figures 4.5 to 4.8). Toe flexion may also occur during foot-on-foot contact. Foot-on-foot play decreases foot tactile sensitivity in preparation for standing and increases body awareness.

Alternating flexion and extension patterns of the lower extremities have a marked and important effect on the pelvis and its anterior-posterior mobility. When the lower extremities strongly extend (within their limited range), anterior tilting of the pelvis and concomitant spinal extension occur (figures 4.3, 4.5). When the lower extremities flex (figures 4.1, 4.2), there is flattening of the lumbar spine and posterior tilting of the pelvis. This is usually accomplished by simultaneous abdominal contraction.

These pelvic movements are critical for the further development of lower extremity movements. By alternating flexion and extension, the trunk muscles (especially the lumbar extensors and abdominals) can develop sagittal plane balance. These muscles subsequently can provide stability to the pelvis. Because all of the femoral muscles attach to the pelvis, the pelvis must be dynamically stabilized for the femur to move efficiently. Therefore, synergistic activity of the muscles around the pelvis dynamically stabilizes the pelvis so that the pelvic-femoral muscles can move the femur and the lower extremities can move with dissociation.

Although the fourth month is the age of strong symmetry, spontaneous asymmetrical extremity movements also occur. Lower extremity asymmetry occurs most frequently in supine when the baby pushes with the feet (figure 4.8). As the baby presses the foot into the surface, the back arches, resulting in spinal extension, anterior tilting of the pelvis, semiextension of the pushing hip, and lateral weight shifting of the whole body (figure 4.8). Pushing with the feet provides the baby with new proprioceptive weight-bearing experiences in the lower extremities. Weight bearing through the heel (calcaneus) seems to further influence the development of lower extremity extension.

When the baby pushes with the lower extremity and lifts the hip away from the surface, hip extension is not seen (figure 4.8). At this age, extension occurs at the lumbar spine (anterior pelvic tilt) rather than at the hip. Soft tissue mobility is still limited at the hips, and the hip extensors are just beginning to become active.

Other dissociated lower extremity movements also occur (figures 4.3, 4.9). In supine, one foot may come to rest on the opposite knee (figure 4.9), causing the weight to shift laterally. If the shift is subtle, the oblique abdominals may be able to bring the baby back to midline. On the other hand, the weight shift may cause the baby to roll to the side. This action results in asymmetrical tactile and proprioceptive feedback, which may be used in future weight-shifting activities.

## Indications of Possible Disturbances in Motor Development

Anterior-posterior tilting, or movement on the sagittal plane, is the first controlled movement of the pelvis. If it does not occur, further lumbar-pelvic and pelvic-femoral dissociated movements will not develop normally.

It is also important that the baby achieve symmetrical hip flexion with adduction in supine around four months of age. This action demonstrates antigravity flexor control in the leg muscles.

Prolonged maintenance of the frog-legged position observed at three months demonstrates poor development of hip flexor and hip adductor muscles. Failure to develop antigravity hip flexion in supine is usually accompanied by poor development of the abdominal activity. Conversely, the failure to develop active hip flexion with adduction (iliopsoas action rather than sartorius action) has an effect on further normal development of the trunk. Without active hip flexion with adduction, the pelvis will not be posteriorly tilted and the lumbar extensors will not be elongated in supine. Alternate anterior/posterior tilting of the pelvis will not occur. The baby will not be able to achieve the normal hands-to-knees position and will subsequently not be able to explore the body with the eyes and hands. This will limit the development of body awareness.

Active hip flexion without hip adduction does not have the same biomechanical effect. Hip flexion with abduction occurs as a result of contraction of the sartorius muscle (Kendall, Kendall, and Wadsworth 1971). Hip flexion with the sartorius has a minimal effect on the pelvis. Anterior tilting of the pelvis is often maintained, rather than the posterior pelvic tilting that accompanies hip flexion with the iliopsoas. If the pelvis remains in an anterior tilt during hip flexion, the lumbar extensors are not elongated and the abdominals are not activated.

If the hips cannot be flexed with adduction, the baby will not be able to bring hands to knees or cross the midline. Instead, the baby will be able to reach the right hand to the right knee only and the left hand to the left knee only. This may lead to problems in integration of the two sides of the body.

### Rolling to Side Lying

At four months, the baby can roll from supine to side lying (figures 4.9 to 4.11). This usually occurs from a flexed posture, with the hips and knees flexed and the hands together or on the knees. Rolling is often initiated by head rotation which, due to the neck righting response, causes the trunk to follow as a unit to the side. Rolling may also be initiated by asymmetrical positions of the lower extremities (figure 4.9), which cause a lateral weight shift.

At this age, symmetrical flexion is the dominant component of rolling. The baby starts with symmetrical flexion in supine and maintains that symmetrical flexion while rolling to side lying. In side lying, both lower extremities are flexed at the hips and knees (figure 4.11). This symmetrical lower extremity flexion posture in side lying precedes lower extremity dissociation, which starts at five months.

Side lying is an important position for the baby. It contributes to rib cage shaping, both by the weight-bearing experience and by the pull of gravity. (Rib contouring also occurs as a result of the pull of the oblique abdominal muscles.) Babies who always lie on their backs and do not have active oblique abdominal muscles have noticeably flat chests.

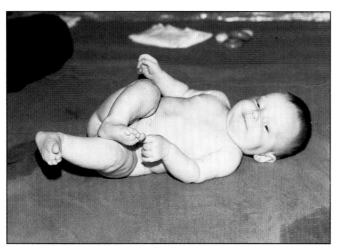

**Figure 4.9.** *At 4 months, rolling to side lying usually occurs from a flexed posture. It is initiated by head rotation. Rolling may also be initiated by asymmetrical positions of the lower extremities, which cause a lateral weight shift.*

Side lying also provides a new visual orientation, a new vestibular orientation, and asymmetrical tactile and proprioceptive feedback to the weight-bearing side. These stimuli work together to provide sensory feedback which will help facilitate the development of antigravity lateral flexion. This will be observed first in lateral head righting.

Some babies roll from supine to side lying by using marked head and neck extension (figure 4.12). This method of rolling is often brought about by toy placement which stimulates visual following.

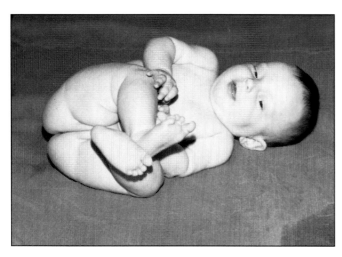

**Figure 4.10.** *Moving from supine to side lying usually occurs from a flexed posture, with hips and knees flexed and hands together or on the knees.*

Although this is still considered within normal limits, it is a more primitive method of rolling because extension, not flexion, is the primary controlling component. This method of rolling results in the baby being in a different side-lying position, one that exaggerates extension (compare figures 4.11 and 4.12). Consequently, proprioceptive (neck-spine extension), visual (upward visual gazing), and vestibular (head extension) feedback reinforces further extension. This exaggerated extensor feedback does not aid the development of antigravity lateral flexion. Because lateral flexion in side lying is an important step in development, rolling with flexion is more favorable than rolling with extension.

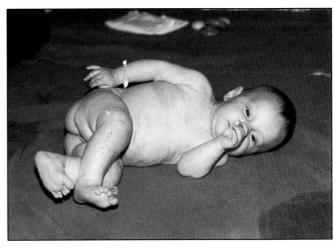
***Figure 4.11.*** *In rolling from supine to side lying, symmetrical flexion is the dominant component of rolling. Both lower extremities are flexed at the hips and knees.*

### Indications of Possible Disturbances in Motor Development

Rolling with head extension rather than head flexion facilitates increased development of extensor muscles but not flexor muscles. Occasional use of this method of rolling is normal. However, frequent or sole use of head extension to roll to side lying may indicate a problem in flexor muscle development. If flexor muscles do not develop sufficiently to balance extensor muscles, antigravity lateral flexion will not develop. Visual, labyrinthine, and neck proprioceptive feedback will then be abnormal, and subsequent motor development may also become abnormal.

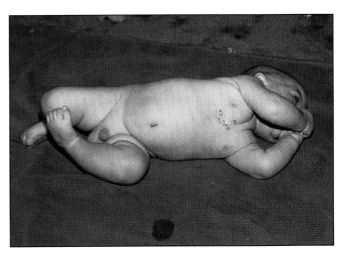
***Figure 4.12.*** *Rolling to side lying may occur with head and neck extension. This method of rolling uses different kinesiological components from rolling with flexion and provides different feedback.*

# Prone

At four months of age, symmetry and increased extension are dominant in prone. Head and neck extension (head righting), spinal extension, and hip extension range have increased markedly during the preceding month. These extension components, in combination with increased shoulder girdle control, enable chest lifting, low back arching, forearm support, and occasional extended-arm weight bearing in prone (figures 4.13, 4.14). Although the 4-month-old can move from forearm weight bearing to the prone-extension pattern (figure 4.15) and rock in an anterior-posterior (sagittal) plane (figure 4.15), the baby cannot yet use the hands or functionally reach out in prone.

Rood described the prone extension pattern as the "pivot-prone" position (Stockmeyer 1967; Ayres 1972). This pattern coincides with the beginning of the **Landau reaction,** which reaches maturity at five to six months (Barnes, Crutchfield, and Heriza 1978).

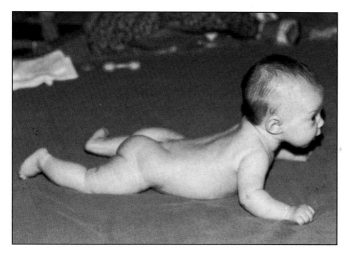

*Figure 4.13. At four months, head and neck extension, spinal extension, and hip extension range have increased. These combine with increased shoulder girdle control to enable chest lifting, low back arching, and forearm support. The head can be held indefinitely at a 90° angle in midline. Shoulders are flexed and horizontally adducted, bringing the arms nearly in line with the body. Forearms are pronated, wrists are slightly extended, fingers are loosely flexed.*

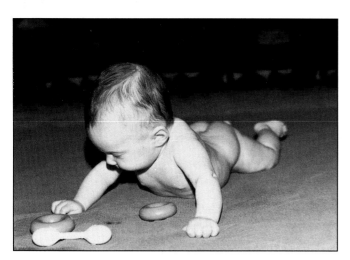

*Figure 4.14. At four months, symmetry and extension are dominant in prone. Extended-arm weight bearing occurs occasionally. The baby is able to maintain the propped position during head flexion.*

While forearm propping, the baby is beginning to experience weight shifting concurrent with head rotation (figure 4.16). Head rotation causes the weight to be shifted to the same side to which the face rotates. Therefore the face-side arm becomes the weight-bearing arm. This early weight shifting is primitive in that the weight is shifted to the face-side arm and thus does not permit this upper extremity to reach. This weight shift usually results in the shoulder girdle collapsing and the baby falling to the side.

## Head

The 4-month-old can hold the head up indefinitely at a 90° angle in midline (figure 4.13). Head, neck, and spinal extension development have been strongly influenced by the maturing vestibular system and the labyrinthine righting reactions which facilitate extension. Labyrinthine and optical righting provide the desire (internal stimulus) to lift (right) the head. When the head is actively extended, the labyrinths activate spinal extensors, which increases trunk extension; when the head is flexed, activity in the back extensors decreases (Cupps, Plescia, and Houser 1976).

Head lifting and extension cause a posterior (caudal) weight shift. Increased range and strength in extensors enable the weight to shift to the lower ribs and abdomen. Upper extremity weight bearing and low back extensors help to maintain the posterior weight shift and anterior elevation.

Controlled head flexion during forearm weight bearing is a new accomplishment for the baby (figure 4.14). At three months, the baby collapsed when the head flexed during prone propping; the extensor activity was lost, illustrating the findings that head flexion in prone produces a decrease in back extensor activity (Cupps, Plescia, and Houser 1976). Therefore the 4-month-old's ability to maintain the propped position during head flexion seems to be related, at least in part, to increased shoulder girdle and upper extremity stability.

Head flexion with neck extension contributes to the baby's development of a visible neck. The head and neck extensors, upper trapezius, and erector spinae muscles contract bilaterally and symmetrically to lift and maintain the head in midline. The upper trapezius muscles assist with head and neck extension, and they also elevate the scapulae (Kendall, Kendall, and Wadsworth 1971). Scapular elevation may cause the appearance of a posterior "neck roll" (figure 4.13) during forearm weight bearing. As the scapulae depressors (lower trapezius) become active around five months of age, this roll disappears.

Head rotation has been practiced in each of the preceding months. It continues to contribute to spinal rotational mobility and to trunk lateral weight shifting. The spinal vertebral bodies rotate in the same direction as the baby's face and cause the weight to be shifted to the face side of the trunk (figure 4.16).

Asymmetrical head rotation (such as occurs with a torticollis) will lead to asymmetrical spinal rotation, asymmetrical weight shifting, and asymmetrical trunk muscle development. This illustrates the direct anatomical effect of head control (mobility, antigravity activity) on the subsequent normal development of trunk and extremity control.

As head-neck stability and active mobility improve, there is a concomitant increase in ocular muscle control and mobility. Ocular muscle control is intricately related to head control through the vestibular system. Ocular control both contributes to and depends upon head control. Optical righting stimulates head righting. Visual interest facilitates head and eye movements, which subsequently exercise the developing muscles. Eye movements and vision lead the head first into extension and rotation and then into flexion. To reinforce and exercise these eye movements, the head and eyes must be able to move.

At four months, vision is the baby's primary means of reaching and holding onto objects in prone (Quinton 1976, 1977, 1978). The 4-month-old cannot yet accomplish reaching and holding with the upper extremities.

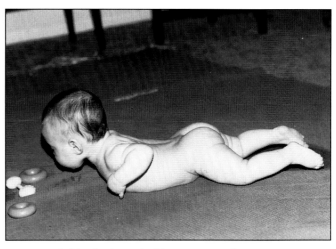

*Figure 4.15.* *The 4-month-old can move to the prone-extension pattern and rock in an anterior-posterior plane, using the abdomen as a pivot. Hips are more adducted and less externally rotated than at three months.*

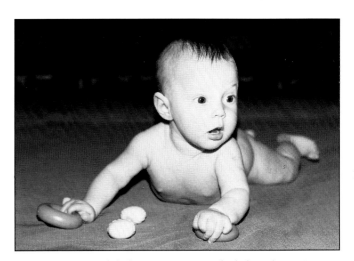

*Figure 4.16.* *While forearm propping, the baby is beginning to experience weight shifting concurrent with head rotation. The weight shifts to the same side to which the face turns, producing lateral flexion of the trunk on the face side. The unweighted shoulder abducts with slight internal rotation and forearm pronation, simultaneously shifting the weight to the radial side of the hand. The fingers are loosely open during nonstressful upper extremity weight bearing.*

The Landau reaction begins during the third and fourth months and coincides with the use of the pivot-prone position (figure 4.15) (Barnes, Crutchfield, and Heriza 1978). When the baby is held in prone horizontal suspension, the labyrinthine righting reaction and the optical righting reaction cause lifting (extension) of the head and subsequent back extension (Cupps, Plescia, and Houser 1976; Barnes, Crutchfield, and Heriza 1978). In this early phase of the reaction, bilateral scapular adduction may reinforce thoracic spine extension.

## Trunk

At four months of age, it is difficult to separate head and trunk movement. The head, through the cervical spine, vestibular, and proprioceptive systems, has a major effect on trunk muscle activation, mobility, and subsequent development. The Landau righting reaction illustrates this well.

In prone, bilateral symmetrical muscle action, stimulated by the midline orientation of the head and aided by bilateral symmetrical extremity movements, keeps the trunk essentially symmetrical, even in the active state. Trunk movement to and from forearm weight bearing and pivot-prone extension are also characteristically symmetrical. Asymmetrical trunk movements may also occur as a result of head rotation in prone, which causes subtle lateral weight shifting and subtle lateral flexion of the trunk on the face side (figures 4.16, 4.17).

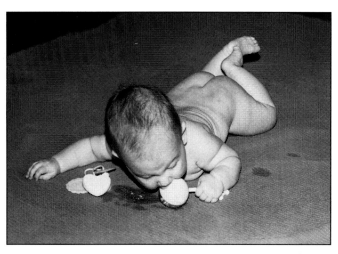

*Figure 4.17. Head rotation in prone causes subtle lateral weight shifting and lateral flexion of the trunk on the face side. Because the baby cannot lift the toy and bring it to the mouth, the baby will bring the mouth to the toy.*

In the pivot-prone position at four months, the baby can rock in an anterior-posterior (sagittal) plane (figure 4.15), using the abdomen as a pivot. This rocking further increases the extensor activity by exercising the extensor muscles and by stimulating the vestibular system.

Head extension in midline activates symmetrical erector spinae action (Landau reaction). Bilateral scapular adduction, a component of the Landau reaction, may also contribute to reinforcement of thoracic extension. (Bilateral scapular adduction is often a coincident component of spinal extension in developmentally new active positions in space: prone, sitting, standing, and walking.) Although back extension is strongest when the head is extended, some extensor muscles may still be active when the head is flexed.

As the erector spinae muscles become more active, the thoracic kyphosis will be reduced and the lumbar lordosis will increase. As the erector spinae muscles extend the spine, they also act on the ribs and may work with the oblique abdominal muscles to help angle them down from their original horizontal position. Angulation of the ribs is important for respiration, phonation, and trunk and rib cage mobility. Changes in rib angulation seem to occur concurrently with the beginning of lateral and rotational movements in the thoracic spine. The horizontal position of the ribs seems to limit the mobility of the thorax. In addition to erector spinae action, thoracic and rib cage mobility depends upon development of the diaphragm, external and internal oblique abdominals, and the intercostal muscles (Kapandji 1974).

Lumbar spine extension facilitates anterior tilting of the pelvis. The degree of anterior pelvic tilting and concurrent lumbar extension is strongly influenced by the position of the lower extremities. (This is discussed further under Lower Extremities.)

Trunk extension in prone elongates the abdominal muscles and the hip flexors. As described earlier, increased spinal extension and increased anterior trunk elevation cause caudal displacement in the fulcrum from which, and on which, the extension occurs. At four months, the abdomen is the fulcrum.

Activation of the trunk flexor muscles in prone is very subtle and is initially limited to active muscle contraction in the upper trunk (pectoralis major). The activation of trunk flexors in prone depends on active humeral flexion and horizontal adduction (by the pectoralis major muscles) during forearm weight bearing. This initial activation of flexors in prone contributes to (a) further development of the abdominals in prone through synergistic activation, (b) the assumption of the quadruped position, and (c) the development of equilibrium reactions in prone and quadruped.

It is important to note that these trunk flexors are activated on an extended trunk. The trunk does not actually flex, but the flexors work on the trunk to balance the action of the extensors. If the activity of the extensors is not balanced, the baby assumes an abnormal position of marked hyperextension.

When the head is flexed in prone, the weight is shifted anteriorly and down into the supporting surface. Because of this weight shift and the decreased activity in the back spinal extensors (Cupps, Plescia, and Houser 1976), the pectoralis major muscles must increase their contraction power to maintain the humeri in horizontal adduction for forearm propping. When the pectoralis major muscles contract strongly, there is simultaneous synergistic facilitation of the oblique abdominal muscles (Brunnstrom 1979). According to Daniels, Williams, and Worthingham (1964), the external oblique muscles provide fixation for strong horizontal adduction of the humeri.

The development of shoulder girdle control appears to be instrumental in subsequent trunk development. Strong active contraction of the pectoralis major muscles during forearm weight bearing appears to contribute significantly to the development of the oblique abdominals musculature. Conversely, if the baby does not experience controlled upper extremity weight bearing in prone, interference with oblique abdominal development may occur.

If forearm weight bearing is not practiced in prone, the baby may not develop head flexion in prone. If, instead, head extension is used consistently, the back extensors become increasingly stronger, inhibiting the abdominals from developing normally. Lack of normal development of the abdominals has serious consequences (lack of thoracic cage and pelvic girdle stability and lack of balance to the trunk extensors), which lead to the development of many compensations and often to abnormal motor development.

Active trunk rotation is not yet possible. However, active head rotation is the precursor of spinal and trunk rotation and trunk lateral flexion. Spinal rotational mobility is necessary for the development of trunk lateral righting reactions and for equilibrium reactions.

Spinal rotation and lateral weight shifting of the trunk accompany head rotation during forearm weight bearing in prone. Weight shifts toward the face side and, as the head rotates further, lateral flexion of the trunk on the face side occurs (figure 4.16). This weight shift and lateral flexion are considered primitive because they result in lateral flexion on the weight-bearing side. This will be modified by the fifth month as active shoulder and trunk control increases and the weight-bearing side becomes the elongated side.

### Indications of Possible Disturbances in Motor Development

The most obvious problems may be cited as the 4-month-old's poor ability or inability to extend the head and trunk in prone, and a limited ability to achieve forearm weight bearing. A decline in a baby's ability to extend in prone may be an early sign of a motor problem (Cupps, Plescia, and Houser 1976).

Because early head, spine, and hip extension seem to be related, lack of head and/or spinal extension may contribute to poor hip extension. Lower extremity activity has been reported to be a component of ventral suspension (Cupps, Plescia, and Houser 1976). Thus a paucity of kicking or rigid extension of the legs may indicate an abnormal extensor pattern.

## *Upper Extremities*

By the age of four months, the baby can assume forearm weight bearing with shoulders flexed and horizontally adducted so that the arms are nearly in line with the body (figure 4.13). The changes from the third to the fourth month suggest increased strength and coordination in the shoulder girdle musculature (cuff muscles, serratus anterior, and pectoralis major). As the arms achieve more adduction, they help to lift the chest from the floor and shift the weight posteriorly (compare figure 4.16 with figure 3.5).

Increased trunk extensor activity enables the 4-month-old to actively alternate the upper extremity/shoulder girdle position between forearm weight bearing (figure 4.13) and retraction in the pivot-prone position (figure 4.15). The transition between the two positions is an example of alternating interaction between the flexors and extensors and the abductors and adductors of the shoulder girdle. Alternating interaction among the various scapular-humeral positions is essential to develop a balance between muscle activation and elongation.

Forearm propping is the first major step in dynamic weight bearing. The muscles involved in forearm weight bearing represent dynamic and synergistic muscle action. Trunk spinal extensors are active in trunk elevation; shoulder flexors are active in bringing the scapulae and arms forward and under the shoulders.

Clinical observations suggest that the specific muscles involved in simultaneous stability and mobility include (1) the shoulder cuff muscles (to stabilize and externally rotate the head of the humerus), (2) the middle deltoid (to abduct the humerus), (3) the anterior deltoid and clavicular portion of the pectoralis major (to adduct and flex the humerus), (4) the serratus anterior (to stabilize, abduct, and upwardly rotate the scapula), and (5) the spinal extensors (to extend the spine and lift the trunk) (Kendall, Kendall, and Wadsworth 1971; Cailliet 1964; Kapandji 1970a; Brunnstrom 1979; Lehmkuhl and Smith 1983).

If elbow extension occurs, the triceps brachii are also recruited. Isolated action and strength of these muscles is not enough. They must work in coordination and in synergy with each other.

## Forearm Weight Bearing

The position of the upper extremities during forearm weight bearing depends on shoulder muscle control and activation. At four months, the humeri—and thus the elbows—are horizontal to the shoulders or slightly forward of them, with neutral rotation. The hands are in front of and in line with the shoulders (figure 4.13). Weight is borne on the forearms and through the humeri to the shoulders.

At four months, the baby has sufficient shoulder girdle strength and control to maintain forearm propping and trunk elevation when the head is flexed. The baby also has sufficient control to sustain the lateral weight shifting and asymmetrical weight bearing which occur when the head rotates (figure 4.16). However, the 4-month-old does not yet have the control or the coordination to maintain weight on one arm in order to reach with the other, nor does the baby have the control to lift one arm forward for reaching (figure 4.17).

During forearm weight bearing, the forearms are pronated, the wrists slightly extended, and the fingers loosely flexed (figure 4.13). This position continues to provide proprioceptive and kinesthetic feedback to the upper extremities, shoulders, and shoulder girdle.

Distal upper extremity control in prone is less developed than proximal control. It is difficult for the baby to use the arms and hands when bearing weight on them. The fingers may be loosely open during nonstressful upper extremity weight bearing (figure 4.16). However, the stress of seeing a toy but being unable to reach for it often results in increased flexor activity in the fingers.

## Indications of Possible Disturbances in Motor Development

Inability or poor ability to achieve forearm weight bearing by four months of age indicates poor development of shoulder girdle flexor musculature (Quinton 1976, 1977, 1978). It may also indicate poor interaction of extensors of the head and trunk with flexors of the shoulders.

Failure to achieve forearm weight bearing may have the following consequences: (1) continued inadequate development of the shoulder girdle muscles, (2) decreased proprioceptive feedback to the shoulders and upper extremities, (3) poor development of scapular stability on the trunk (serratus anterior), which will lead to (4) lack of elongation of the muscles between the scapula and humerus, which subsequently (5) will limit the development of dissociated movements of the scapula and humerus.

Without dynamic scapula-shoulder girdle control, the baby will have difficulty with reaching skills and will have to develop compensatory reaching patterns. Reaching patterns influence hand placement and thus grasping patterns. Therefore compensatory reaching patterns may lead to compensatory hand-grasp patterns.

Some of the long-range and ensuing consequences include (1) inability to bear weight on extended arms, with long-term effects of poor transitional skills in such areas as prone to sit, (2) no upper extremity protective extension reactions, (3) inability to weight shift on upper extremities, with subsequent lack of stimulation (and lack of control) to produce lateral righting of head and trunk in prone, (4) inability to develop weight shift with the shoulder to achieve face-side reaching, and (5) failure to develop the normal sequence of elongation on the weight-bearing side and lateral flexion on the unweighted side.

### Pivot-Prone

Pivot-prone is the initial phase of the Landau reaction (figure 4.15). It is characterized by bilateral symmetrical adduction of the scapulae during head and back extension. This position is often assumed when the baby is trying to reach for a toy in the visual field. The position, however, does not enable the baby to reach the toy.

Although the pivot-prone extension pattern is strong due to frequent reinforcement by head extension, the normal 4-month-old can easily make a transition from pivot-prone to forearm weight bearing. The baby's ability to alternate smoothly between two opposing patterns of movement demonstrates the maturing process. For example, scapular adduction with downward rotation alternates with abduction and upward rotation; humeral hyperextension, adduction, and internal rotation alternate with flexion, horizontal adduction, and external rotation; and elbow flexion and pronation alternate with extension and pronation. (Compare figures 4.13 and 4.15.)

Babies who have not developed normal shoulder girdle control will collapse when coming out of the pivot-prone position. These babies may go on to develop increasing extensor activity while avoiding weight-bearing activities. This is not normal motor development and subsequently will cause disturbances (some very subtle) in normal movements and balance.

It is extremely important that scapular adduction (where the arms are used as part of the postural system) be counterbalanced with scapular abduction and forward humeral flexion for reaching. Failure to develop this balance may disrupt the baby's normal reaching patterns. It must be noted that active spinal extension activity is also necessary for this alternating transition.

### Extended-Arm Weight Bearing

Although forearm weight bearing is common at four months, the baby may also bear weight on extended arms (figure 4.14). This is usually accomplished without full elbow extension. If present, full elbow extension may indicate elbow locking and lack of graded triceps control, or it may be due to low muscle tone. The arms are abducted to provide a wide, stable base of support (positional stability), which may compensate for lack of good muscle control.

The wrists are biomechanically extended when the elbows extend. This puts a stretch on the wrist and finger flexors. Consequently, the fingers are often flexed during initial acts of extended-arm weight bearing. As range is gained in the finger flexors, the baby will be able to bear weight on extended wrists and extended fingers or open hands.

Although the upper extremities are active in prone, their function is limited primarily to weight bearing. Upper trunk weight shifting is primitive (to the face side) and, therefore, upper extremity reaching is not yet possible. The changes in upper extremity control are best demonstrated during weight shifting.

### Weight Shifting

Weight shifting onto one upper extremity occurs as a result of head rotation. How well the baby manages this shift is a measure of shoulder girdle development and control. At three months of age, head rotation and concurrent weight shift caused collapse of the shoulders because the scapular-humeral muscles could not contract sufficiently to stabilize the shoulder girdles when even subtle asymmetrical movement was imposed on them (figures 3.7, 3.8).

At four months, shoulder girdle control has increased. When the weight shifts to the face side (figures 4.16, 4.20), the arm on the face side adducts and the arm on the skull side abducts. As the face side accepts more weight, the pectorals, serratus anterior, and cuff muscles must work with more strength and coordination to maintain this asymmetrical weight-bearing position.

Head turning affects the position of the shoulders, which subsequently affect the position of the forearms. When head rotation shifts the weight to the face-side shoulder, the shoulder adducts and subtly rotates externally. Concurrent with this, the forearm subtly supinates so that the weight is shifted to the ulnar side of the arm. The unweighted shoulder abducts and internally rotates with subsequent forearm pronation, simultaneously shifting the weight to the radial side of the forearm (figures 4.16, 4.20). These weight shifts are precursors to active forearm pronation and supination.

Although shoulder control has increased markedly, it is not yet sufficient at four months to support the unilateral weight bearing needed for reaching in prone. Reaching is further inhibited by this primitive weight shifting because the weight is shifted to the face-side arm, subsequently preventing coordinated eye-hand reaching. Therefore, reaching in prone is still limited to visual reaching.

Although the 4-month-old cannot weight shift, lift the arm, and reach during forearm weight bearing, the baby can still obtain toys which are on the surface near the hands. The baby does this by "crawling" with the fingers and thus pulling the arms until the toy is obtained (Nash 1991). Although the toy can be grasped, the baby cannot lift it and bring it to the mouth. Consequently, the 4-month-old brings the mouth to the toy (figure 4.17). Mouthing is the primary means of toy exploration in prone.

Mature reaching in prone with the face-side arm begins at five months. It involves shoulder and trunk weight shifting to the skull side of the head, elongation of the weight-bearing side, trunk antigravity lateral righting, shoulder girdle dissociation, arm lifting, and eye-hand coordination.

Shoulder girdle/upper trunk weight shifting at four months frequently results in the baby's rolling (falling) from prone to side lying or even to supine. (This is discussed under Rolling.)

## Lower Extremities

In prone at four months, the lower extremities are symmetrically extended at the hips, knees, and ankles. None of these joints, however, has full range of extension. The increased range in hip extension and lowering of the pelvis onto the surface have contributed markedly to the increase in anterior trunk elevation. In addition to increased extension, the hips are more adducted and less externally rotated than they were at three months. (Compare figures 3.6 and 4.15.) These new components bring the legs more into line with the trunk. This is similar to the alignment occurring in the upper extremities.

Increased hip extension develops concomitant with elongation of the hip flexors (especially the iliopsoas) which is now occurring in both prone and supine. Because the iliopsoas still lacks full mobility, its elongation during hip extension causes anterior tilting of the pelvis, which further exaggerates the lumbar extension. The hip extensors still appear relatively inactive in the quiet state.

Hip adductors (adductor magnus, adductor longus, adductor brevis, pectineus, and gracilis), which were elongated proximally by marked abduction and external rotation, are now beginning to adduct the legs on the frontal plane. Note the similarity of the developmental process for the lower and upper extremities (horizontal abduction followed by horizontal adduction).

Knee extension has increased markedly from the previous month, suggesting increased activity in the quadriceps muscles and increased mobility in the hamstring muscles. Elongation of the rectus femoris by hip extension may also contribute to increased knee extension (a two-joint biomechanical effect). Elongation of the hamstrings at the knee during knee extension may contribute to the increase in hip extension range. (This is also a two-joint biomechanical effect.) Knee extension also elongates the gastrocnemius muscle, which may contribute to ankle plantar flexion (another two-joint effect).

Active antigravity knee flexion is not usually seen, suggesting that the 4-month-old lacks antigravity hamstring function and full quadriceps mobility. Consequently, knee flexion in prone is accomplished as part of a total pattern of lower extremity flexion-abduction-external rotation (figures 4.13, 4.16). This flexion is not against gravity.

At four months, the baby frequently alternates between patterns of total lower extremity flexion and total lower extremity extension. These are total synergies which work together. These total patterns may also be related to muscle biomechanics and present mobility. Hip flexion stretches the hamstrings at their origin, causing movement at the insertions (knee flexion). Knee flexion reduces the stretch on the gastrocnemius and allows resumption of ankle dorsiflexion. Knee extension stretches the hamstrings at the knees and causes movement at the origin (hip extension). Knee extension also stretches the gastrocnemius at the knee and causes movement at its insertion (ankle plantar flexion).

The lower extremities are not always quiet and predictable. The 4-month-old's desire to move—without the control to do so—often results in random lower extremity movements. These movements provide proprioceptive and kinesthetic input to the low back and pelvic girdle. The movements may occur as unilateral or bilateral lower extremity kicking.

### Indications of Possible Disturbances in Motor Development

Low-tone babies may maintain a frog-legged position into the fourth month. This becomes a problem if they cannot also extend and adduct their legs. Failure of the 4-month-old to develop normal hip adduction and extension with neutral rotation in prone may indicate a subtle problem in motor development which may have far-reaching effects if normal lumbar-pelvic-hip movements cannot develop.

If the lower extremities maintain the frog-legged position, the following consequences are likely to occur:

- Lumbar spinal extension and anterior pelvic tilting will be exaggerated in prone extension with concomitant abdominal inhibition.

- Normal hip extension cannot develop. This will interfere with more upright positions.

- Hip flexors will not be elongated. This will also interfere with upright positions.

- Lateral weight shifted with elongation on the weight-bearing side and lateral flexion on the unweighted side will be blocked. Normal transitional movements will be blocked.

- Therefore normal prone righting reactions cannot develop.

- Asymmetrical lower extremity movements cannot occur. This will interfere with locomotion skills such as crawling and walking.

- Isolated antigravity knee flexion cannot be initiated, leading to poor control of the hamstrings as knee flexors.

Babies with increased extensor activity may assume a position of marked hip extension with adduction. This pattern is abnormal if the baby cannot break out of it, and if it is always assumed with excessive head and trunk extension. This pattern also leads to consequences in lumbar-pelvic and pelvic-femoral development. Normal joint mobility is often compromised when there is increased muscle tone around the joint. This can lead to poor weight-shifting and poor transitional skills, decreased development of the righting reactions in the head and trunk, and poor lower extremity dissociation, which will interfere with locomotion skills such as crawling and walking.

# Rolling

At four months, the baby may roll from prone to side lying, occasionally even rolling completely to supine. However, this is more common during the fifth month. Rolling from supine to prone requires greater motor control and coordination and occurs at six months.

Initial rolling experiences usually occur accidentally when the baby is elevated on the forearms and shifts weight to one arm. The shoulders do not yet have sufficient control to support the weight shift. Therefore, the arm adducts under the body and the baby rolls to the side (figures 4.18, 4.19).

The position of the lower extremities influences the effect of the weight shift. Legs that are abducted and externally rotated will provide a positional block to the weight shift, preventing the baby from rolling. If, however, the lower extremities are adducted and extended with neutral rotation, the baby will roll to the side or to the back when the shoulder collapses (figures 3.7 and 3.8 at three months of age).

In figures 4.18 and 4.19, a 3½-month-old (Baby A) has shifted her weight over the left upper extremity, but because her shoulder control is not sufficient to support the weight shift, her arm collapses in adduction under her chest. As she attempts

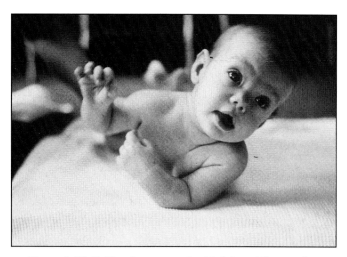

*Figure 4.18. Rolling from prone to side lying at three and a half months is usually accidental. The head and trunk respond to the weight shift with increased extensor activity. The shoulders do not have sufficient control to support a weight shift, the baby's arm adducts under the body, and the baby rolls to the side.* (photo by Joan Mohr)

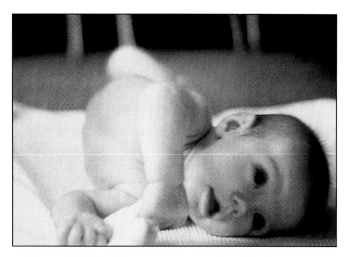

*Figure 4.19. The baby may try to stop the roll by bringing hands together to increase flexion and counterbalance extension, but the baby falls onto the side.* (photo by Joan Mohr)

to regain her balance, extension becomes stronger because it is more active than flexion in prone. Scapular adduction occurs and retracts the arm as well as the shoulder girdle. This increases the extension and lateral weight shift to the left. The baby may try to stop the fall by bringing her hands together to increase flexion and counterbalance extension, but she falls onto her side (figure 4.19). The extended position of the head prevents her from rolling to prone. This position also demonstrates the strong extension reaction.

In figures 4.20 through 4.22, a 4½-month-old (Baby B) has shifted her weight to her left shoulder. She also demonstrates inadequate shoulder stability to support her weight. However, her head and trunk react with more advanced control than the younger Baby A. Because Baby B has better balance between her neck flexors and extensors, attempts to regain her balance result in lateral head righting rather than in neck extension. (Compare the head positions in figures 4.18 and 4.20.) As discussed under Side Lying, below, lateral head righting is a result of synchronous action of unilateral neck extensors and neck flexors on the same side of the spine. This synchronous action neutralizes the opposing rotational effects and combines the lateral flexing effects. In figure 4.18, the neck extensors are obviously stronger than the flexors.

As Baby B continues to fall, the trunk responds to the neck lateral righting reaction and also laterally flexes. This produces an equilibrium reaction in the trunk and right lower extremity (figure 4.21). Lateral trunk righting and equilibrium responses are rare occurrences at this age. They become more predictable at five and six months. However, it is important to be aware of the variable rate of development in each baby.

In figure 4.22, Baby B falls or rolls to supine as a consequence of the unstable weight shift. Rolling to supine instead of to side lying occurs because of improved head control. The neck flexors balance the neck extensors from the beginning of the movement, putting the head in the proper position to roll to supine. In figure 4.19, head extension prevents Baby A from rolling all the way to supine. The stimulation and integration of coordination for Baby B's rolling response may have occurred through the vestibular, visual, and tactile systems, but it was made possible by appropriate control and coordination of her muscles.

# Side Lying

Side lying on each side is very important for the baby because of the tactile, proprioceptive, visual, and vestibular feedback it provides, and because antigravity lateral flexion control (frontal plane control) develops from this position. Antigravity lateral flexion is a more complex, integrated movement than antigravity flexion or extension. Movement in the frontal plane requires equal, simultaneous contraction of the flexors and extensors on the same side of the head, trunk, and spine. Unilateral contraction of the head and trunk flexors or the extensors alone usually produces rotation rather than lateral flexion (Cailliet 1964; Kapandji 1974; Kendall, Kendall, and Wadsworth 1971). Therefore, pure lateral flexion occurs when the neck and trunk flexors and extensors are balanced and neutralize the rotational components of each other during the lateral flexion action.

Antigravity lateral flexion occurs first in the neck. Lateral neck flexion requires unilateral contraction of the cervical extensors and the cervical flexors. If one muscle group is stronger than the other, rotation of the head, rather than lateral flexion, will occur in the direction of the stronger muscle group. For example, if the extensors are stronger (as is usually the case), attempts to laterally flex the head in side lying will result in extension and rotation of the head backwards. This causes the baby to roll onto the back (because of the neck righting reaction) rather than to remain on the side.

For the neck to laterally flex in side lying, the cervical extensors must be balanced by the cervical flexors as they contract unilaterally, and the oblique abdominals must synergistically stabilize the thorax (Kendall, Kendall, and Wadsworth 1971). This produces pure lateral flexion, and the face remains perpendicular to the surface as the head is lifted. If the oblique abdominals do not contract synergistically, the thorax is not stabilized and the cervical muscles do not have a stable base from which to move.

At four months, lateral lifting of the head is minimal if it occurs at all. The oblique abdominals have not yet developed control. The side-lying position is new and the muscles must discover how to work together. Their first coordinated act is maintaining the neutral position of the head during side lying. As coordination, synergistic stability, dynamic co-contraction, and muscle strength increase, the head will be lifted laterally. Lateral movements of the head affect the cervical spine and

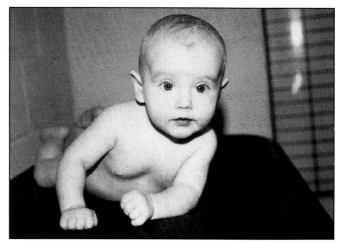

*Figure 4.20.* During the weight shift, the face-side shoulder adducts and subtly externally rotates and the forearm subtly supinates so that weight is shifted to the ulnar side of the hand. At 4½ months, there is still inadequate shoulder stability to support the weight, but the baby's head and trunk react with more advanced lateral righting control.

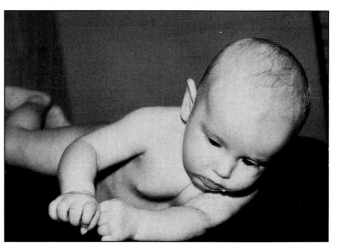

*Figure 4.21.* As the baby continues to fall, the trunk responds to the neck lateral righting reaction and laterally flexes, producing an equilibrium reaction in the trunk and right lower extremity.

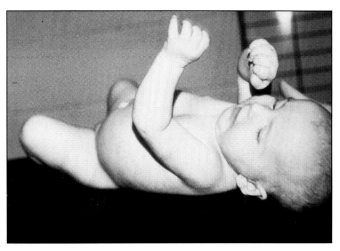

*Figure 4.22. The baby rolls to supine due to the unstable weight shift.*

subsequently the whole spine, causing it to flex laterally. Controlled antigravity lateral flexion of the spine is a valuable precursor to further normal development of the trunk, especially its righting and equilibrium reactions.

### Indications of Possible Disturbances in Motor Development

Babies who cannot achieve or maintain a symmetrical side-lying position by four months may be demonstrating poor balance between antigravity flexor and extensor muscle development. A 4-month-old who thrusts backward or constantly rolls onto the back when placed in side lying is also demonstrating poor balance between flexor and extensor muscle development.

Inability to maintain the side-lying position will interfere with development of antigravity lateral flexion. Visual and labyrinthine righting from the lateral position will not develop normally. The baby will not receive proprioceptive and tactile stimulation to the lateral side of the body, and the rib cage will not receive the lateral pull and shaping caused by gravity. These combined factors interfere with the process of normal motor development. Inability to maintain side lying may also interfere with the baby's eye-hand use.

# Pulled to Sit

The baby's desire to right the head in supine (flex against gravity) is strong because of the increasing maturation of the labyrinthine and optical righting systems. Optical righting is especially strong at four months and the baby tries to reinforce the head-righting ability and stability by visually "fixing" on the examiner when pulled to sit.

When pulled to sit at four months, the baby exhibits increased symmetrical antigravity flexor muscle control and antigravity righting. The baby organizes the movement with increased anticipatory flexor activity. The baby grasps with finger flexion and flexes the elbows, legs, and head, and tucks the chin prior to the movement (figure 4.23). This initial flexor postural control is lost as the baby moves up against gravity, suggesting that the antigravity flexor strength is not fully developed. However, a head lag does not occur and symmetry is maintained throughout the movement.

The baby's anticipation of the pull-to-sit is a significant occurrence. This suggests that the baby is beginning to anticipate the consequence of having a head lag and thus makes postural adjustments prior to the lift. Postural adjustments that are made prior to or in synchrony with movements are a result of "feedforward" information (Kelso 1982). This illustrates the baby's beginning ability to advance from feedback to feedforward postural adjustments.

The baby anticipates the transition to sitting with chin tucking, which is achieved by action of the capital and cervical flexors. After initiation of the movement, chin tucking is lost, but the head is stabilized and lifted in midline (figure 4.24). This stability is reinforced by shoulder elevation, which causes head and neck hyperextension. Head lifting and head flexion are not synonymous.

The sternocleidomastoid muscles are responsible for lifting the head and keeping it in midline, thus preventing a head lag. But when the sternocleidomastoid muscles contract without chin tucking, subtle head and neck hyperextension with shoulder elevation occurs (figure 4.24) (Kapandji 1974; Kendall, Kendall, and Wadsworth 1971). Head lifting without head flexion (chin tucking) is characterized by an open mouth and jutted chin (figure 4.24).

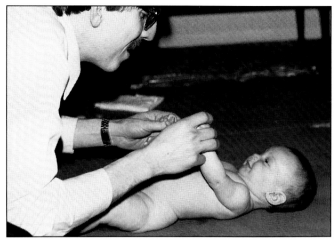

*Figure 4.23.* Anticipating the pull-to-sit, the baby organizes the movement with increased flexor activity, grasping with finger flexion, flexing elbows, legs, and head, and tucking the chin.

Within the following month, bilateral contraction of the sternocleidomastoids will cause cervical flexion during head lifting. This occurs when the head flexors and abdominals have sufficient coordination to contract synergistically with the sternocleidomastoids and sufficient strength to stabilize the flexed posture (Kendall, Kendall, and Wadsworth 1971; Kapandji 1974). In other words, bilateral contraction of the sternocleidomastoid muscles flexes the head when there is synergistic support from the capital flexors and abdominals. On the other hand, bilateral contraction of the sternocleidomastoid muscles extends the head and neck when the synergistic support from the capital flexors and abdominals is missing.

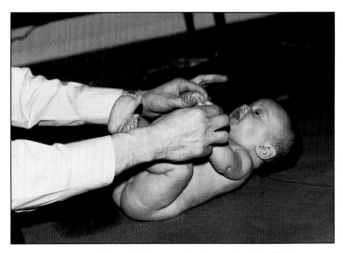

*Figure 4.24.* When pulled to sit, the 4-month-old exhibits increased symmetrical antigravity flexor muscle control and antigravity righting. The head stabilizes and lifts in midline, the stability reinforced by shoulder elevation which causes head and neck hyperextension.

The upper extremities are becoming more active when the baby is being pulled to sit. The humeri adduct and flex slightly. Having grasped the examiner's fingers, the baby flexes the elbows and initiates pulling the body forward (figure 4.24). Upper extremity pulling and elbow flexion are usually lost when the baby is halfway up.

Strong upper extremity adduction and flexion occur in synergy with trunk and lower extremity flexion (figure 4.24). When the abdominals contract, stability is achieved in the trunk for the entire movement. Total flexion of the lower extremities (hip flexion, knee flexion, and ankle dorsiflexion) also occurs.

The baby stabilizes the sitting posture after passing through the erect vertical position. The baby stops the forward momentum of the pull-to-sit when the shoulders are in front of the pelvis. This enables the baby to right the head and body and maintain the posture with the head and trunk spinal extensors (figure 4.25).

## Indications of Possible Disturbances in Motor Development

The pull-to-sit test is often used to evaluate a baby's developing motor control. Because this test is a measure of the baby's active ability, the baby must be interested in coming to sit. This is easily seen in the baby's visual interest. Therefore it is important to capture the baby's visual attention when pulling the baby up to sit.

Babies with visual problems may initially have difficulty organizing the movement, but once the movement is understood and initiated, they should be able to use vestibular and proprioceptive feedback to organize the movement.

The pull-to-sit test should also be used to evaluate the baby's feedforward control. Babies who do not anticipate the consequences of the pull-to-sit do not organize their flexor posture and thus have a head lag. Such a lack of anticipation in this early movement activity may suggest problems in feedforward postural adjustment in other positions.

Babies who cannot right their heads during pull-to-sit may be demonstrating a problem in motor development. This may be a motor control problem and/or a sensory feedback problem. A motor control problem may be caused by very low muscle tone which makes it difficult for the baby to move against gravity. Another motor control problem may be strong head/neck extensor tone which resists flexion activity.

Evaluation of the sensory components is also important. If sensory changes in the head position are not being perceived, the baby has no feedback to indicate a change in head position. As the baby becomes older, this inability to use feedback information to organize head lifting may lead to a feedforward problem. (In other words, the baby cannot anticipate postural needs.)

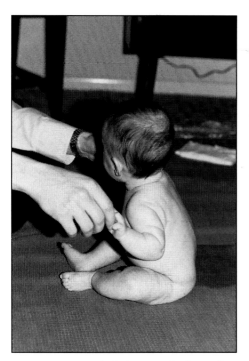

*Figure 4.25.* The baby stops the forward momentum of the pull-to-sit when the shoulders are in front of the pelvis. Sitting is precariously stable. The baby stabilizes the sitting posture and maintains it with the trunk spinal extensors.

# Sitting

At this age, sitting is precariously stable and barely functional. However, the 4-month-old can sit unsupported for several seconds. The baby stabilizes the head and trunk posture by leaning forward from the hips (figures 4.25, 4.26). When the shoulders are in front of the pelvis, the trunk extensors contract to stabilize the head and trunk in an upright position.

The baby enjoys supported sitting. Gesell and Amatruda (1947) describe this experience as a "widening of the horizon," a new social orientation. McGraw (1945) attributes the baby's desire to sit as an innate drive for the upright posture.

## Head

Though the head is stable in midline, the capital extensors are still more active than the capital flexors. Therefore the chin is not tucked and the neck is not fully elongated (figure 4.26). The 4-month-old does not flex the head in the unsupported sitting position, possibly due to the forward position of the shoulders and trunk. When the shoulders are in front of the hips, the head automatically rights itself with extension. Flexion could throw the baby off balance.

Head rotation initiates a weight shift toward the side to which the head turns. When the baby is unsupported, head rotation causes the baby to fall. Thus, for the baby to use active head rotation while sitting, the trunk must be supported (figures 4.25, 4.28).

The 4-month-old does not yet use lateral head flexion in sitting. The head/neck flexors and extensors are not yet balanced in this position. The lack of balance is illustrated by neck hyperextension and chin jutting instead of chin tucking (figure 4.26). Because of the lack of lateral control, the head wobbles when the baby's trunk is swayed.

The baby's ocular control in sitting depends upon head control, which is limited to extension and rotation. Therefore, ocular movements are similarly limited. Downward visual gazing, although possible in supported sitting, is not yet possible in unsupported sitting.

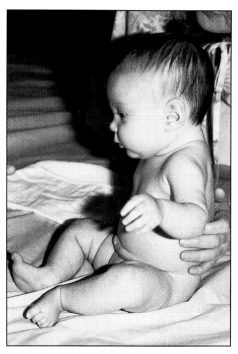

*Figure 4.26.* The 4-month-old stabilizes the sitting posture with scapulae adduction while leaning forward from the hips.

## *Trunk*

The 4-month-old maintains a semierect sitting posture with erector spinae extensor activity in the neck and trunk while leaning forward from the hips (figure 4.26). Extensor activity will help to reduce spinal flexion, especially the thoracic kyphosis. Lumbar extension is also increasing (figure 4.26). The increased spinal extensor postural control provides a more stable base on which the head can move.

## *Upper Extremities*

Although spinal extensors are the primary postural muscles used in sitting, the 4-month-old reinforces this stability with scapular adduction (figures 4.25, 4.26). When scapular adduction is used as part of the postural system, upper extremity function is very limited. Scapular adduction extends the humeri, preventing forward flexion and reaching. This posture is also accompanied by elbow flexion. The hands are usually loosely open, indicating lack of effort.

Occasionally the 4-month-old can lightly prop on flexed or extended arms when leaning forward and the arms have been placed in position. This is another example of the upper extremities being part of the postural system as they provide some positional stability.

When stabilized or supported in sitting, the baby does not have to reinforce postural stability; therefore the bilateral scapular adduction is relaxed (figure 4.27). When supported, the baby can flex the arms and bring the hands together or to the mouth. The hand-to-mouth position is very common at four months; it is performed with elbow flexion and forearm pronation.

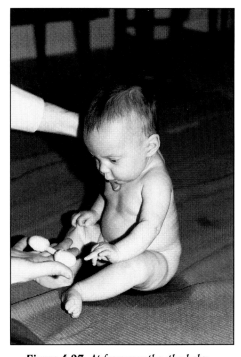

*Figure 4.27.* At four months, the baby does not need to reinforce postural stability when stabilized or supported in sitting and can relax bilateral scapular adduction. The baby cannot yet coordinate arm movements to reach for a toy.

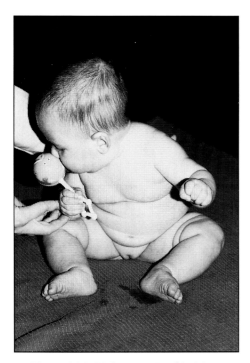

**Figure 4.28.** *With increasing hip joint mobility, the legs come closer to resting on the supporting surface. Ring sitting provides a wide base of support for sitting. Because the 4-month-old cannot yet bring a grasped toy to the mouth, the baby will bring the mouth to the toy.*

When presented with a toy, the 4-month-old can fixate on it visually but is unable to coordinate arm movements to reach the toy (figure 4.27). If the toy is placed in the hand when the baby is sitting, the baby may grasp it but will usually drop it quickly. When grasp is maintained on the toy, the baby tries to bring it to the mouth. However, upper extremity coordination is limited; therefore the baby usually brings the mouth to the toy (figure 4.28). The upper extremities often mirror each other during these activities. Fagard (1990) reports that bimanual reaches are the most common responses to all presentation at 4 to 4½ months.

### Lower Extremities

The 4-month-old has increased mobility in the lower extremities for hip external rotation, abduction, and flexion during sitting. The marked stretch on the hip adductor muscles continues to facilitate knee flexion. Ankle dorsiflexion is still present. The lower extremities function as part of the postural system and provide positional stability; therefore their position does not vary during sitting.

As hip joint mobility increases, the legs come closer to resting on the supporting surface and become more effective in providing positional stability for sitting. The wide base of support provided by ring sitting guards against lateral weight shifting and sideward falling (figure 4.28).

### Indications of Possible Disturbances in Motor Development

Babies who cannot sit at four months should be further evaluated. Poor sitting is usually not the only problem.

Poor sitting control may be due to low muscle tone and poor ability to right against gravity. This may be indicative of other postural problems, especially those related to antigravity extension.

Poor sitting control may also be due to strong extensor tone. In this case, the baby's strong extensor activity may throw the body backward. This extension is most often initiated in the head and shoulder girdle at four months. Soon it may also be initiated at the hips. This problem can be especially troubling because it may indicate that the baby is also not developing antigravity flexor control.

# Standing

When supported in standing, the 4-month-old takes weight on extended legs (figure 4.29). The legs are more adducted than they were at three months, and the baby takes more control of the weight. The baby can now maintain standing when only the hands are held (figure 4.30).

The 4-month-old seems to adjust better to the fully erect position than to the sitting position. This may be due to standing's total extensor pattern, as opposed to the combined action of extension and flexion needed in sitting. However, the total extensor activity makes standing a very static posture for the 4-month-old.

## Head

Head control is better in standing than in sitting, possibly because the trunk is more stable due to the increased extension. Head extension is still the most dominant movement (figure 4.29), but head flexion with slight chin tucking is possible (figure 4.30). This action of the capital flexor muscles helps to elongate the posterior neck.

## Trunk

The trunk is symmetrically extended with a slight lumbar lordosis (figure 4.30) and increased range in hip extension. The hips, although flexed, are nearly in line with the shoulders. Increased hip extension is due to increased activity in the hip extensor muscles (gluteus maximus) and the increased but limited mobility of the iliopsoas muscles. As the hips become more extended, the iliopsoas is elongated, extending the lumbar spine and tilting the pelvis forward, thus contributing to the lumbar lordosis.

The trunk is very static in standing, with extension being the only component observed. Trunk rotation and trunk flexion are not seen at four months.

## Upper Extremities

The 4-month-old's shoulder girdles and arms are coupled with the postural system in standing. When the baby's trunk is supported, the scapulae adduct and the humeri abduct, reinforcing trunk extension (figure 4.29). When the baby's hands are held, slight scapular adduction is maintained even when the humeri begin to flex (figure 4.30).

The elbows are usually extended when the baby is supported at the trunk (figure 4.29). When the baby's hands are held, elbow flexion increases (figure 4.30). The wrists are slightly extended and the fingers loosely flexed.

When the hands are held, the 4-month-old reacts with a voluntary grasp. The grasp seems to increase the flexor activity in the entire upper extremity. According to EMG studies reported by Brunnstrom (1979), the biceps contract automatically when a strong fist is made. The baby's increased ability to flex the elbow enables the hand to be brought to the mouth while the baby is standing (figure 4.30), rather than the mouth to the hand.

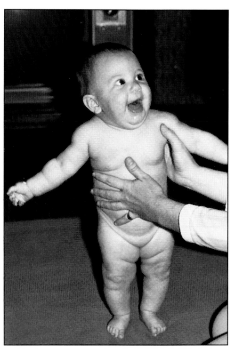

*Figure 4.29.* The 4-month-old bears weight on extended legs when supported in standing. The scapulae adduct and the humeri abduct to reinforce trunk extension; elbows are usually extended. Head extension is still dominant.

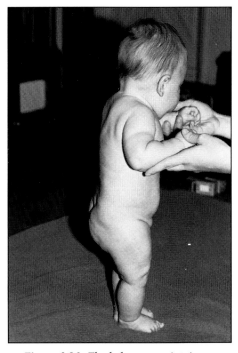

*Figure 4.30.* The baby can maintain a standing posture when being held only by the hands. The trunk is symmetrically extended with a slight lumbar lordosis.

## Lower Extremities

Lower extremity extension is achieved primarily through strong contraction of the quadriceps. Mobility in hip extension has increased, and active contraction of the hip extensors (gluteus maximus) may be beginning. The feet are flat on the floor; the ankles are dorsiflexed.

Increased hip extension contributes to the lumbar lordosis because the iliopsoas is stretched. The hips are more adducted than they were at three months, but external rotation is still present. In addition to the soft tissue tightness for external rotation, contraction of the gluteus maximus may contribute to hip external rotation.

Knee extension is active, but it seems to be a total (almost locked) response. When knees are not fully extended, the baby collapses into flexion. This indicates an "all or none" response by the quadriceps, or biomechanical locking of the knee in extension, rather than graded quadriceps action.

The ankles remain dorsiflexed with the feet flat on the floor. The feet are pronated (dorsiflexed, abducted, everted). Toe curling, which may be a response to the tactile and proprioceptive stimulation, is usually observed. Toe curling may also be the baby's attempt to reinforce muscle stability in the lower extremities. It is accompanied by synergistic activity in other lower extremity muscles. This distal stability may help to compensate for the lack of proximal stability in the trunk and hips.

# The Fifth Month

During the fifth month, the baby uses the symmetry, midline orientation, and coordination of the two sides of the body developed during the fourth month to produce voluntary, asymmetrical, dissociated, and reciprocal movements. The baby uses proximal stability to weight shift on upper extremities and reach in prone.

Antigravity extension control continues to increase in the trunk and hips (pivot-prone), and antigravity flexor control continues to increase in the head and trunk (feet to mouth). These sagittal plane movements are thus balancing each other. The increased balance on the sagittal plane enables development of antigravity lateral flexion (frontal plane) in the head, neck, and trunk. This muscle activation facilitates additional mobility in the spine and provides the basis for body righting reactions, equilibrium reactions, and diagonal movements (transverse plane).

Head control and head righting have improved significantly. The 5-month-old can right the head in prone with extension, in supine with flexion when the hands are held, and momentarily in side lying with lateral flexion. These reactions illustrate development of control in the head, neck, and trunk muscles and maturing of the vestibular and optical righting reactions.

Mobility in the cervical and thoracic spine is increasing; therefore, head movements have a more subtle effect on the body and on weight shifting than in previous months. Head movements are more dissociated from trunk movements, a precursor of full, normal head control.

Increased proximal (trunk and shoulder) control enables better use and control of distal joints in space. The baby can now visually direct reaching in supine, prone, and supported sitting. Reaching is fairly coordinated, and the baby can use a palmar grasp on toys. Manipulation and transfer of a toy is an occasional occurrence. The baby can explore a toy with the eyes and bring it to the mouth for mouthing.

The lower extremities are becoming more active and mobile. Active hip flexion and hip extension have both increased, but the 5-month-old cannot yet alternate smoothly between the two. Isolated knee flexion and extension have both increased in their antigravity control, but again, the baby cannot yet smoothly alternate between the two.

The lower extremities can now actively assume dissociated or asymmetrical positions in supine and prone. These positions cause and/or are caused by lateral and rotational movements in the pelvis, and they stimulate oblique abdominal muscle activity.

In supine, increased use of antigravity flexion is noticeable. The 5-month-old actively brings the feet to the mouth and reaches with both hands to one foot when the foot is close to the chest. Flexion elongates the capital, spinal, and hip extensors. The 5-month-old can also flex the head and lift it from supine when grasping the examiner's hands. Shoulder flexion with adduction and elbow extension enable the baby to reach up from supine for toys or toward a person in anticipation of being picked up.

The 5-month-old can actively roll from supine to side lying. The action is initiated with symmetrical total flexion, similar to that of the 4-month-old, but when the baby reaches side lying, symmetry changes to asymmetry. The lower leg extends while the top leg remains flexed, and the baby momentarily laterally rights the head (laterally flexing against gravity). The baby may then rest the head on the supporting surface but maintains the asymmetrical leg positioning.

In prone, the 5-month-old uses extensors and flexors to raise the body and bear weight on extended arms. The baby also uses the increased proximal control to weight shift on forearms and functionally reach for a toy. This more mature weight shifting is initiated in the shoulder girdle and occurs prior to reaching, thus freeing the face-side hand for reaching. The weight shift stimulates a reaction at the head. Earlier, the head movement caused the weight shift.

If the responses in the head and trunk are marked, the pelvis will also laterally flex on the unweighted side, and asymmetrical reactions in the lower extremities will follow. Although lower extremity dissociation may occur as a part of this sequence, it can also occur independently and facilitate the pelvic and lumbar spine reactions.

At five months, the baby can combine extensor components and upper extremity weight shifting to roll from prone to supine. Initially, the rolling is a loss of control rather than an act of control. It usually frightens the baby and, therefore, is not voluntarily practiced.

When pulled to sit, the 5-month-old can actively flex and lift the head while holding the examiner's hands. The elbow flexors, not scapular adductors, now assist in the pulling. The abdominals contract to stabilize the thorax and pelvis, while the lower extremities flex at the hips, knees, and ankles. Knee extension with hip flexion is occasionally seen during the pull-to-sit, indicating a more mature reaction.

The 5-month-old uses positional stability to sit independently. The ring position of the lower extremities provides a wide, stable base of support for the pelvis and spine. The baby may be able to sit unaided momentarily by leaning forward from the hips and adducting the scapulae. Leaning forward enables the baby to use the extensors to right the body and stabilize the trunk. The baby may add more positional stability by propping forward on extended arms. Scapular adduction and extended-arm propping are both methods in which the arms are used as part of the postural system.

When supported in sitting, the baby can free the arms from the postural system and use them more functionally. The 5-month-old can reach for and grasp a toy using a palmar grasp and bring it to the mouth, rather than bringing the mouth to the toy, as at four months.

The 5-month-old takes almost the full weight on the legs when placed in standing. Head and trunk control have improved, and the legs are more in line with the body. The upper extremities are freed from the postural system as trunk control increases. The arms are starting to become more functional during standing. However, standing is still a static posture.

At five months of age, the baby is more successful in attempting to interact with the environment. Increased hand control enables the child to hold a small toy or rattle and shake or bang it. The baby also likes squeeze toys that fit into the hand and that can be brought to the mouth. Arm control is still poorly developed; therefore toys that provide cause-effect but do not move away provide the most enjoyment.

The baby's play schemes consist primarily of grabbing, mouthing, banging, and shaking. The baby will repeat the movements of an enjoyable activity and practice problem-solving strategies of how to best interact with and explore the toy. This experimentation contributes to the baby's development of goal-directed movements. Examples of toys for this age include rattles, squeeze toys, suction toys, and chime balls (Aston 1974; Fritts 1990).

# Supine

In supine, the 5-month-old has markedly improved antigravity control of head, neck, shoulder, abdominal, and hip flexors, and elbow and knee extensors. Symmetry is still possible, but it is intermingled with voluntary asymmetrical activities. Upper extremity control has increased sufficiently to enable the beginning of more functional interaction of the arms and hands with the environment. The lower extremities have more mobility and control than they did at four months. The 5-month-old can bring the feet to the mouth and the hands to the feet, using upper and lower extremity control (figure 5.1). This enables the baby to continue to develop body awareness through body exploration and tactile stimulation.

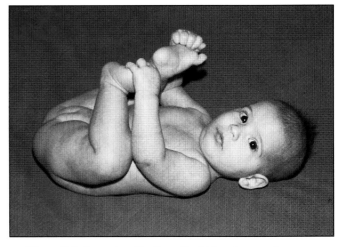

## *Head*

When the baby engages in flexion in supine, the head flexes. This uses capital and cervical flexors, which thus elongates the capital and cervical extensors (figure 5.3). Elongation of the extensors is exaggerated as hip flexion and buttocks lifting increases (figure 5.1). The baby can still rotate and extend the head even from this very flexed position.

*Figure 5.1. In supine, the 5-month-old has improved antigravity control of head, neck, shoulder, abdominal, and hip flexors, and elbow and knee extensors. The baby can bring the feet to the mouth and the hands to the feet, rotating the forearm while doing so. The extensors are elongated as the hips flex and the buttocks are lifted.*

Ocular control has improved due to better head control. Eye movements are becoming dissociated from the head movements. The eyes can track an object without the head moving (Inatsuka 1979). The eyes usually track with the hands during body exploration, enhancing body awareness. Eye-hand coordination has improved and vision is now used to guide the final phase of reaching and grasping (von Hofsten 1990).

## Trunk

During flexion (figure 5.1), the abdominals give stability to the pelvis and actively tilt it posteriorly. When the pelvis is stabilized, the hip flexors can contract more efficiently. The strength of the abdominals has increased since the fourth month, causing the buttocks to be lifted further from the surface during hand-to-foot play. As the rectus abdominis becomes stronger and pulls the pubis closer to the sternum, the spinal extensors are concurrently elongated. It is important to note that in this flexed position, the back (especially the thoracic spine) is not kyphotic but remains extended (figure 5.1).

The oblique abdominals are activated in supine as the baby brings hands and feet together over the chest and as the flexed legs sway from side to side. The obliques bring the legs back to midline and help to maintain them there. The trunk no longer moves symmetrically as a whole unit. (According to Kendall, Kendall, and Wadsworth [1971], the oblique abdominals activate synergistically with the pectoralis major.)

## Upper Extremities

### Reaching

Reaching in supine is more refined and demonstrates increased eye-hand coordination. Von Hofsten (1990) reports that 5-month-old infants use vision to make crude preparatory adjustments for hand orientation. This preparation is made prior to or early in the reach. Von Hofsten also reports that some 5-month-olds adjust the orientation of the hand during the approach. However, this is more common at six months.

These findings continue to suggest that vision influences and guides the reaching and grasping patterns from the neonatal period. Vision may originally operate in a feedback mode by providing a target for the hand and by guiding adjustments of the hand once it is in the visual field. Vision is also beginning to operate in a feedforward mode (for example, prompting adjustment of the hand before the reach has begun or while it is occurring).

The baby uses a bilateral symmetrical upper extremity approach (figures 5.2, 5.3). The most predictable, coordinated bilateral upper extremity reaching occurs when the baby reaches to the caretaker in anticipation of being picked up. This reaction is further stimulated when the caretaker offers hands to the baby.

The 5-month-old can reach to the knees, lower legs, and feet, regardless of whether they are abducted or adducted during supine flexion. Shoulder flexion and adduction occur through a greater range and with more control. Elbow extension during shoulder flexion has also increased. Increased shoulder adduction enables the baby to reach over the midline. The 5-month-old still uses forearm pronation, wrist extension, and finger extension during reaching, but the forearm is beginning to rotate when the baby is holding the foot or leg (figure 5.1).

Rotation of the forearm (figure 5.1) is facilitated, at least in part, by the use and position of the baby's hand. Corbetta and Mounoud (1990) report that infants use tactile and visual information about objects to develop control of their arms and hands. Between three and six months, infants orient their hands in the direction of the source of tactile stimulation. Therefore, when the 5-month-old reaches the hands to the feet, tactile and visual information is being used to adjust the arm and hand for the grasp. These adjustments reinforce a distal-to-proximal developmental process. Subsequently, the baby's desire to place a hand on the feet or legs influences the proximal shoulder girdle adjustment.

The 5-month-old also employs the increased shoulder girdle and upper extremity muscle control and eye-hand coordination to reach and grasp toys (figures 5.2 to 5.4). During each of these activities, the baby may attempt to reinforce total body stability by crossing the ankles or legs (figure 5.4) or by pressing the feet together. The lower extremities no longer mirror the upper extremities during reaching, as they did at four months.

The baby's control of antigravity elbow extension has increased markedly since the fourth month. The triceps appear to work in synergy with the other shoulder girdle muscles. Forearm pronation is still dominant. Neutral rotation of the forearm, observed when the elbow is extended (figure 5.2) may be attributed to shoulder external rotation rather than active supination. The shoulder and elbow control developed and utilized in supine reaching is also used in prone extended-arm weight bearing.

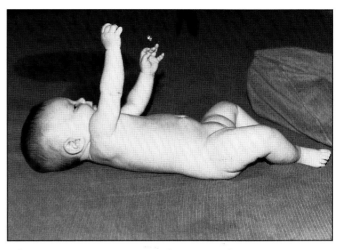

*Figure 5.2.* Shoulder girdle protraction with scapular abduction enables humeral flexion and adduction to occur through a greater range and with greater control. Elbow extension during shoulder flexion also increases.

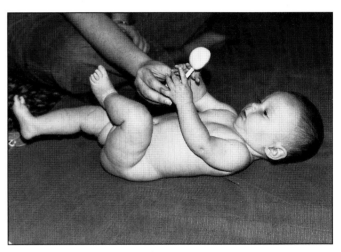

*Figure 5.3.* As the baby's hands come closer to the toy, the wrists flex (right hand) or extend (left hand) and the fingers extend in preparation for the grasp. The 5-month-old can actively flex one leg while extending the other leg.

The wrists extend during reaching. The fingers extend at the MP joint but remain loosely flexed more distally (figure 5.2). Wrist extension may still have a subtle tenodesis effect on the finger flexors. As the hands come closer to the toy, the fingers extend in preparation for the grasp (figure 5.3, right hand). Wrist flexion often accompanies (and may contribute to) this finger extension through the tenodesis effect.

Bilateral upper extremity reaching is the most common approach at five months, but unilateral reaching can also take place. Unilateral reaching may occur when an object is presented at the baby's side. Unilateral reaching across the body (figure 5.7) may cause the baby to roll to the side.

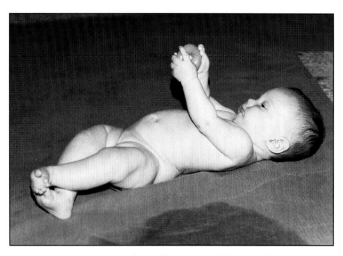

**Figure 5.4.** *Crossing the ankles or legs helps reinforce total body stability. The baby can actively maintain lower extremity extension while flexing the upper extremities.*

When reaching up with one arm while in supine (figure 5.2), the baby uses shoulder girdle protraction with scapular abduction. This forward reaching utilizes spinal rotation which increases segmental spinal mobility. Segmental spinal mobility is needed for the baby to change log rolling to segmental rolling and for further development of reciprocal extremity movements.

### Grasp

At five months, the grasping act is tactually and visually controlled (von Hofsten 1990; Corbetta and Mounoud 1990). Preparatory adjustments of the hand prior to grasp are visually controlled. Tactual adjustments are made after contact. Therefore the visual adjustments can be considered to operate on a feedforward mode, while the tactual adjustments operate on a feedback mode.

According to Corbetta and Mounoud (1990), a 5-month-old tactually explores an object before grasping it. This tactile information is used to adjust the hand for grasping. However, the 5-month-old also uses vision to orient the hand before or during the reaching phase, before the object is touched (von Hofsten 1990). Von Hofsten (1990) also reports that the hand is usually open during the approach.

In previous months, the supine baby used a primitive squeeze (ulnar grasp) to hold objects momentarily that were placed in the hand. Now, at five months, the baby has developed the ability to combine a visually directed approach (reaching) with a voluntary palmar grasp (Erhardt 1984). The 5-month-old is developing coordination of the proximal (shoulder control) and distal (finger movement) functions. In the palmar grasp, the fingers hold the object firmly in the center of the palm (Erhardt 1984). In this grip, the hand is used as a whole and depends on movement at the wrist, arm, or shoulder (Elliott and Connolly 1984).

The wrists may flex just prior to grasp (figure 5.3, right hand) in a reverse tenodesis effect which aids finger extension. However, finger extension may also occur with the wrist extended (figure 5.3, left hand), enabling crude finger flexion on the object. Finger flexion is often reinforced by wrist extension. The thumb abducts during pregrasp but does not participate functionally in the grasp (Erhardt 1984).

The 5-month-old baby can hold a bottle when feeding. This grasp must be coordinated with strong shoulder adduction (pectoralis major). Because of the bottle's shape and weight, the baby needs assistance to keep the bottle in proper position.

### Manipulation

It is difficult for the 5-month-old to manipulate toys with the hands when in supine. Visual inspection usually substitutes for hand manipulation. The baby can flex the shoulders to bring the toy into the visual field, but the 5-month-old lacks the dynamic stability in the shoulder girdles and upper extremities to simultaneously maintain the position and use dissociated finger movements to move the toy.

Small toy manipulation in supine is usually accomplished with the mouth and tongue. Once the toy has been grasped and explored visually, the baby brings it to the mouth for further exploration of texture, size, shape, and other characteristics. In supine, mouthing is still the most functional means of manipulation.

### *Lower Extremities*

In the fifth month, the lower extremities no longer mirror the upper extremities during reaching in supine, as they did at four months. Leg movements are now less predictable. The lower extremities may move with symmetrical flexion (figure 5.1) or extension (figure 5.4). In addition, asymmetrical positions and movements of the lower extremities are also used frequently (figure 5.3). Lower extremity fixing postures may be used to reinforce stability during attempts at upper extremity manipulation (figure 5.4).

By the fifth month, hip flexion range has increased greatly and reaches nearly 180° (figure 5.1). However, the baby still frequently flexes the legs to 90° with adduction and knee flexion. Marked hip flexion combined with knee extension (even slight) enables the 5-month-old to bring the feet within reach of the hands and into the visual field (figure 5.1) and subsequently to bring the feet to the mouth. The eyes-hands-feet and feet-hands-mouth contact and play enhance the baby's body awareness. These also provide tactile stimulation to the feet, decreasing their sensitivity in preparation for standing (Quinton 1976, 1977, 1978).

Although both legs may be flexed simultaneously, the baby may play with both hands on one foot. This enhances movement into and through midline with the hands and/or leg. This also enhances the development of diagonal muscle action in the trunk and causes asymmetrical weight shifting in the pelvis. The off-centered position of the pelvis necessitates and facilitates increased oblique abdominal activation.

Although antigravity flexor control has improved, the 5-month-old is not always flexed in supine. The range of hip extension (by elongation of the iliopsoas and abdominals) continues to increase slowly. This increased elongation of the abdominals and iliopsoas muscles is demonstrated by a slight decrease in the degree of anterior pelvic tilting during hip extension (figure 5.4).

Active hip adduction and knee extension are also increasing (figure 5.4). Hip external rotation is decreasing, but the 5-month-old does not internally rotate the hips. Increased strength in the hip adductor muscles enables closer alignment of the legs with the body. The adductor muscles also contribute to hip extension and hip-pelvic stability.

The 5-month-old is beginning to demonstrate active lower extremity dissociated movements and dissociation of the upper extremities from the lower extremities. This is a significant step. The baby can now actively flex one leg while extending the other leg (figure 5.3) and can actively maintain lower extremity extension while flexing the upper extremities (figure 5.4).

Each of these actions demonstrates the baby's beginning ability to inhibit one movement selectively in preference to another, which means that the baby is no longer dominated by symmetrical mirroring of extremity activities. Thus the upper extremities are becoming dissociated from the lower extremities, and the lower extremities are becoming dissociated from each other. These dissociated movements are particularly dependent upon the proper synergistic trunk control and dynamic muscle stability. The dissociated movements become more controlled when the baby practices them frequently.

Active range of knee extension is nearly complete. Contraction of the quadriceps is strong and the baby can actively press the legs to the floor (figure 5.4). However, in most situations, the baby seems to maintain a loosely flexed knee (figure 5.2).

Ankle positions fluctuate very little. Dorsiflexion is still the most dominant position. Ankle dorsiflexion with eversion seems to occur most strongly when the hips are simultaneously externally rotated (figures 5.2, 5.4). Active plantar flexion is not usually seen in supine, although it may occur. When it is seen, it is usually part of a total lower extremity extension pattern. Toe flexion may be seen during periods of effort and may contribute to plantar flexion.

### Indications of Possible Disturbances in Motor Development

Supine antigravity flexion is a critical component in normal development. At five months of age, the baby should have sufficient flexor muscle control and extensor muscle mobility in supine to bring the feet to the mouth and the hands to the feet flexed onto the chest. Inability to do so may indicate a disturbance in motor development.

The problem may be a result of tight back extensors and/or insufficient abdominal activity, both of which contribute to the development of significant problems. Abdominal activity is necessary for the baby to achieve the flexed position and for dynamic stability of the anterior trunk. Flexion is also necessary for the elongation of all of the extensor muscles from the head to the hips.

If the back extensors are not elongated by counterbalancing flexor activity, they will develop abnormal strength and shortness. This will further inhibit normal antigravity flexor activity and will prevent reciprocal and coordinated activation of the flexor and extensor muscle groups. Lack of trunk control and coordination will lead to problems in the development of combined and integrated trunk movements, such as lateral flexion, righting reactions, and equilibrium reactions.

Overactive spinal extensor muscles and underactive abdominal muscles lead to poor trunk control, poor pelvic control, and poor rib cage stability. Each of these problems generates its own subsequent problems. Poor trunk control leads to problems in all movements and movement sequences.

Poor pelvic control will lead to compensatory pelvic movements in all planes: sagittal (anterior-posterior), frontal (lateral), and transverse (rotation). The pelvis will continue to move with the femur, and pelvic-femoral dissociation will not develop. This will necessitate compensatory movements in the hips and the lower extremities. Consequently, the baby (and later, the child) will have problems during ambulation which may range from poor coordination to inability to walk.

Poor rib cage stability (due to weak abdominal muscle activity) leads to problems with respiration, phonation, upper extremity use, trunk mobility, and head control. The abdominals are needed to provide dynamic stability to the rib cage during each of these activities. When the oblique abdominals are not active, the ribs develop a flared position from the pull of the diaphragm without stability from the obliques (Kapandji 1974).

The development of supine antigravity flexion of the arms and legs is also critical and should be strongly demonstrated in the fifth month. Antigravity shoulder flexion with adduction and elbow extension is needed for the baby to reach out into the environment, explore it, and have an effect upon it. Antigravity shoulder flexion also enables the baby to explore the body and develop an awareness of the body scheme. Thus, if the appropriate muscle action does not develop, these adjunct areas of development will be compromised.

Lack of active hip flexion and mobility will lead to abnormal motor development in the lower extremities. The development of more distal leg muscles is affected by the mobility and stability in the hip muscles. Also, if the feet are not explored by the hands and mouth, they will not be properly desensitized in preparation for weight bearing.

# Rolling: Supine to Side Lying

Increased muscle control, more stimulation, and greater motivation enable the 5-month-old to move out of supine by rolling actively to side lying. Neck righting still contributes to the baby's rolling to the side (figure 5.5). However, upper extremity reaching across the chest (figure 5.7) or lower extremity pushing (figure 5.10) may now also cause the lateral weight shifting which leads to rolling.

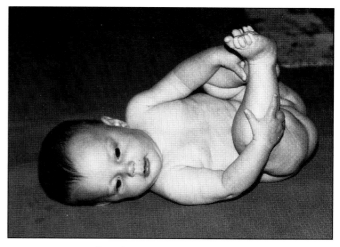

*Figure 5.5.* Rolling from supine to side lying is usually initiated from a symmetrically flexed position, with neck righting still contributing to the rolling.

Rolling from supine to side lying is usually initiated from a symmetrically flexed position (figure 5.5), as it was at four months. As the baby rotates the head to the side, usually because of visual interest, the rest of the body follows as a whole symmetrical unit (figure 5.6). Once in side lying, symmetry gives way to asymmetry (figure 5.7) as the baby actively extends the lower leg while the top leg stays flexed. This initiates the process of elongation on the weight-bearing side, which enables antigravity lateral flexion, or shortening, on the nonweight-bearing side (figure 5.8).

Elongation on the weight-bearing side with lateral flexion on the unweighted side is the first phase of antigravity lateral flexion, which is movement on the frontal plane. Separation of the legs, with one flexed and one extended, also indicates that the baby is no longer dominated by "total" movement patterns. In the developmental sequence, frontal plane muscle activation seems to lead to dissociated extremity movements.

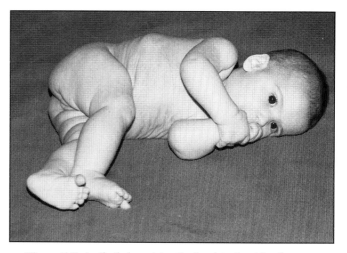

*Figure 5.6.* As the baby rotates the head to the side, the rest of the body follows as a whole symmetrical unit.

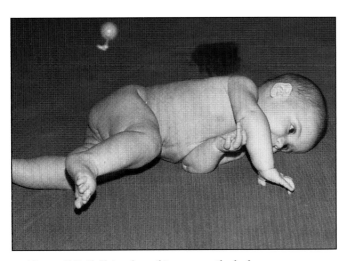

*Figure 5.7. Unilateral reaching across the body may cause the baby to roll to the side. Once the 5-month-old is in side lying, symmetry is replaced with asymmetry: the lower leg actively extends while the top leg stays flexed. The bottom arm is in a weight-bearing position, functioning as part of the postural system. The top arm can reach forward and interact with the environment. With the head resting on the surface, the baby can easily play.*

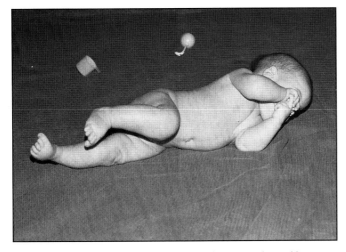

*Figure 5.8. Elongation on the weight-bearing side enables antigravity lateral flexion on the nonweight-bearing side.*

Lateral flexion is usually initiated in a cephalo-caudal direction; lateral head righting facilitates spinal lateral flexion. Lateral flexion can also be initiated in a caudal-cephalic direction by lower extremity dissociation with extension of the bottom leg. Lower extremity dissociation causes lateral flexion and rotation of the pelvis and, subsequently, lateral flexion of the lumbar spine.

Although the baby may initially respond to the side-lying position with active antigravity lateral flexion (figure 5.8), the position is not maintained because of insufficient muscle power. Therefore, in the typical side-lying position at 5 months, the lower extremities are dissociated and the head rests on the surface (figure 5.7). In this position, the baby can easily play.

The new side-lying position demonstrates the 5-month-old's increasing trunk/spinal mobility, pelvic mobility, and lower extremity mobility for dissociated positioning. The new position provides feedback from all of the systems—vestibular, visual, proprioceptive, and tactile—which will influence subsequent motor development.

Ability to assume the asymmetrical side-lying position is a precursor of continuous rolling from supine to prone, which occurs at six months. If the lower leg does not extend, rolling to prone is blocked (figure 5.9).

At times, the 5-month-old may roll from supine to side lying by pushing with one lower extremity, hyperextending both the lower back and the head (figure 5.10). Although side lying may be achieved, the sensory feedback from this method is very different from that of the previous method of rolling. Here, extension is continually reinforced, and lateral flexion and lower extremity dissociation are not practiced. Although this method is normal, it should not be encouraged, and babies who use this method exclusively for rolling should be evaluated to be sure they are also capable of balanced flexion activities.

## Head

The head rotates to the side, usually from a slightly flexed position. Once in side lying, simultaneous unilateral (top side) action of the cervical extensors and flexors lift the head laterally due to vestibular and optical stimulation and the developing body righting reaction on the head. (This is discussed further under Prone and Forearm Weight Bearing.)

## Trunk

The trunk initially responds as a total unit, the spine rotating with the head. In side lying, head lateral flexion has a ripple effect into trunk lateral flexion. At five months, trunk mobility and muscle control are very limited and, therefore, lateral flexion is brief. Regardless of how brief the contraction is, the oblique abdominal muscles must contract to stabilize the thorax for the head to right laterally (Kendall, Kendall, and Wadsworth 1971). Lumbar lateral flexion is also facilitated by the lower extremity dissociation, and the oblique abdominals are needed to stabilize the pelvis for lower extremity dissociation.

## Upper Extremities

Upper extremity dissociation is also seen at five months. The bottom arm is in a weight-bearing position and, therefore, functions as part of the postural system. The top arm can reach forward and interact with the environment (figure 5.7). Forward reaching of the arm requires contraction of the serratus anterior to abduct the scapula as the cuff muscles, deltoid, and pectoralis major control the humerus (Brunnstrom 1979). Scapular abduction and shoulder girdle protraction facilitate spinal rotation and lateral weight shift to side lying.

Upon reaching side lying, the baby can bring the hands together as well as bring the hands to the knees and feet. This enhances the ability to explore the body and develop body awareness. In side lying, the baby also has increased ability to reach for and interact with toys. Because of their feedback, cause-effect toys (such as chime balls) encourage the baby to practice rolling and reaching. Motivation and practice are important components for further motor development.

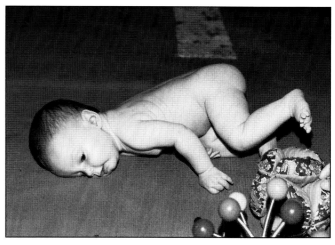

*Figure 5.9. The ability to assume the asymmetrical side-lying position is a precursor of continuous rolling from supine to prone. If the lower leg does not extend, rolling to prone is blocked.*

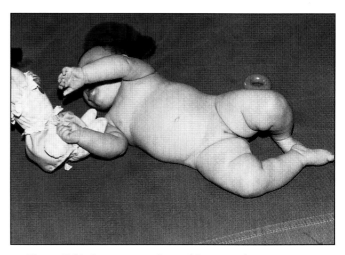

*Figure 5.10. Lower extremity pushing may also cause lateral weight shifting, leading to rolling. Extension is reinforced throughout the movement, and lateral flexion or lower extremity dissociation will not occur.*

If the shoulder girdle remains retracted in supine and the serratus anterior is not activated (as often occurs in prolonged use of the ATNR), the baby will find it difficult or impossible to roll to side lying and will miss the sensory, kinesiological, and motivational feedback provided by this position.

## Lower Extremities

The change from lower extremity symmetry to lower extremity dissociation is a major step in the 5-month-old baby's developing motor control. Rolling is initiated with hip and knee flexion (figure 5.5), which is maintained into side lying. Once in side lying, the knees extend as the quadriceps contract, elongating the hamstrings. Subsequently the bottom hip extends and elongates the entire weight-bearing side (figure 5.7).

Hip extension may be facilitated in part by elongation of the hamstrings when the knee extends. The top leg is maintained in abduction and flexion. The pelvis must be stabilized by synergistic activity of the oblique abdominals for the top leg to abduct (Kendall, Kendall, and Wadsworth 1971). The oblique abdominals thus contribute to the baby's development of lower extremity dissociation by stabilizing the pelvis during femoral movements.

The pelvic movements (tilting, rotation, and lateral flexion) which accompany the changing lower extremity movements require lumbar spine mobility and bilateral hip joint mobility. Without complementary mobility in each joint, pelvic movements will be impaired. Concurrent with mobility, muscles around each of these joints must work synergistically to control the movements.

### Indications of Possible Disturbances in Motor Development

Control in the side-lying position is very important for development of balance and interplay between the head and trunk flexors and extensors. In side lying, the baby can alternate between flexor and extensor components. When the baby rolls forward from side lying, extensor muscles are activated; when rolling backward from side lying, flexor muscles are activated. However, if the baby does not develop a balance between the flexors and extensors, lateral flexion does not occur and transitions in movement become difficult.

Babies who initiate rolling to side lying from supine by using extensor components have no need to laterally flex in side lying. These babies often continue to roll to prone rather than play in side lying. As noted above, this extensor method (figure 5.10) may be used occasionally by babies who are developing normally, but it is used more frequently by babies who are having difficulty developing antigravity flexion. Their desire to move and change positions is strong; therefore, they substitute this more primitive pattern of extension for better-quality movement and normal sensory feedback. Because the pattern works for them in achieving their goal (reaching a toy), they repeat it over and over again, and this pattern for rolling soon becomes a habit pattern.

Constant use of the extension method further impairs normal motor development because extension is constantly reinforced and flexion is constantly inhibited. Therefore, the baby will not develop the normal balancing flexor components necessary in higher functioning activities. The baby also will not develop the antigravity lateral components needed for smooth, efficient transitions in movement and dissociated extremity movements.

The extension method of rolling also encourages upward visual gazing. Therefore the rolling pattern may contribute to visual problems (poor control of downward visual gaze and poor visual convergence).

# Prone

By the fifth month, prone is a functional position for the baby. Extension is strong, but it is balanced by flexor components. The baby uses this interplay of extensor and flexor components during forearm weight bearing, extended-arm weight bearing, and forearm weight shifting. The infant uses primarily extensor components for pivot-prone "swimming."

The 5-month-old is very active in prone. The baby can make swimming movements in the pivot-prone position, reach with both arms or weight shift and reach with one arm, weight shift in the pelvis and lower extremities, and dissociate the lower extremities. The baby can also roll (fall) from prone to supine.

At five months, the body righting reaction on the head is especially useful in prone when the baby shifts weight laterally. The asymmetrical tactile stimulation which occurs during the lateral weight shift causes the head to adjust (right) by laterally flexing away from the supporting side (Twitchell 1965; O'Connell and Gardner 1972; Barnes, Crutchfield, and Heriza 1978). This helps to prevent the baby from falling backwards. At five months, equilibrium reactions are starting to occur in prone.

# Extended-Arm Weight Bearing

Extensor activity continues to increase in prone, enhanced by continued maturation of the labyrinthine righting, optical righting, and Landau reactions. The result is improved head control, increased strength and range in back extension, and increased hip extensor activity. The prone extensor activity is complemented by increased shoulder girdle and upper extremity control, which enables the 5-month-old to push up into and maintain extended-arm, open-hand weight bearing (figure 5.11).

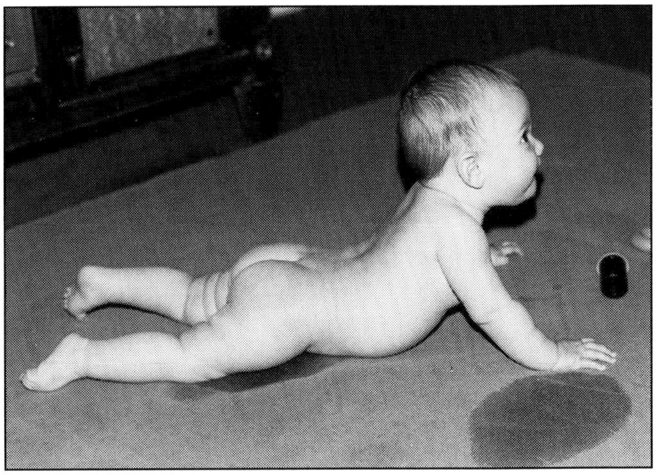

*Figure 5.11.* Improved head control, increased strength and range in back extension, and increased hip extensor activity, along with increased shoulder girdle and upper extremity control, enable the 5-month-old to push up into and maintain extended-arm, open-hand weight bearing in prone.

## *Head*

At five months, head control in prone is nearly fully developed. The baby can extend, rotate, flex, and laterally flex the head in prone. Most of the time the baby uses shoulder girdle stability as the base for these head movements. Shoulder girdle and upper extremity stability help to neutralize the effects of head movements on the trunk. Head and trunk movements are becoming dissociated.

Head and neck (capital and cervical) extension and hyperextension are possible at will, in midline or out of midline. At five months, the baby frequently combines cervical extension with capital flexion. This usually results in elongation of the neck and tucking of the chin (figure 5.15). Increased control in head flexion and neck extension enhances downward visual gazing and enables the baby to visually regard objects near the chest and between or in the hands during forearm weight bearing (figure 5.15).

The baby can rotate the head to either side. Although subtle weight shifting does occur, the increased shoulder girdle control helps to counterbalance the lateral movement (figure 5.12).

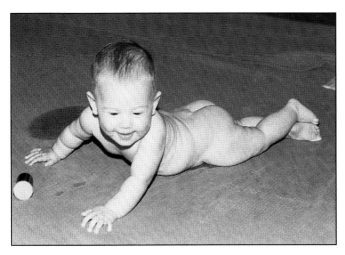

*Figure 5.12. Although subtle weight shifts occur with head rotation, increased shoulder girdle control helps to counteract the lateral movement.*

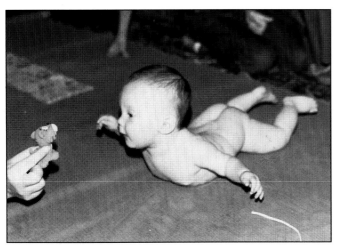

*Figure 5.13. The 5-month-old still uses the pivot-prone position, appearing to "swim" because of the rocking movement and the alternation between scapular adduction and abduction during extension. The marked shoulder girdle retraction often precedes forward reaching.*

The increased repertoire of head movements enables the baby to increase the visual field and visual awareness of the environment. Visual interest, pursuit, and tracking still provide the greatest stimulus to head movement and thus exercise the baby's developing muscle control.

## Trunk

Spinal extensor activity is stronger, and range in spinal extension has increased from the fourth month. The lower abdomen, pelvis, and hips are now the fulcrum for elevation of the trunk and for extended-arm weight bearing (figure 5.11). Extension in the lumbar area may be exaggerated because of increased activation of the lumbar extensor muscles. The anterior pelvic tilt is reduced by increased lower extremity adduction, increased length in the hip flexors, and subtle abdominal contraction. The hips now contribute to the range into extension.

At five months, the baby still uses the pivot-prone position (figure 5.13), a component of the Landau reaction in which head extension activates back extensors through the labyrinthine (vestibular) system (Cupps, Plescia, and Houser 1976). The extensor reaction is stronger in the neck, back, and elbows at five months than at four months, and it is combined with more activity. (Compare figures 5.13 and 4.15).

At five months, the pivot-prone position is described as "swimming" because of the rocking movement and the alternation between scapular adduction and abduction during extension (figure 5.13). Increased scapular mobility during spinal extension suggests increased strength in the erector spinae muscles. Scapular adduction is no longer needed to reinforce thoracic extension in prone. The added trunk strength and control enable the upper extremities to be freed from the postural system.

This swimming motion causes the baby to rock on the abdomen, which exercises the extensor muscles and stimulates the vestibular system, further increasing extension. The rocking also provides additional tactile, proprioceptive, and kinesthetic input. Increased extension is demonstrated in elbow, wrist, and finger extension. (Compare figures 5.13 and 4.15). Humeral abduction has also increased.

Although symmetrical extension and shoulder retraction are strong (figure 5.13), the 5-month-old can move out of this position into upper extremity weight bearing or forward reaching with both arms (figure 5.14).

According to Kapandji (1970a), bilateral forward flexion of the upper extremities causes an increase in the lumbar lordosis and activates the spinal muscles. The lordosis is most marked during shoulder flexion beyond 150°. Forward flexion of the arms also elongates the latissimus dorsi, which subsequently mechanically extends the spine (Kapandji 1970a). Because the latissimus dorsi attaches from T-7 through the remaining thoracic and lumbar vertebrae, the thoracic and lumbar spines extend synchronously when the latissimus dorsi is stretched.

## *Upper Extremities*

Greater shoulder girdle and elbow control enables the 5-month-old to push up onto extended arms. This involves the integrated action of many different

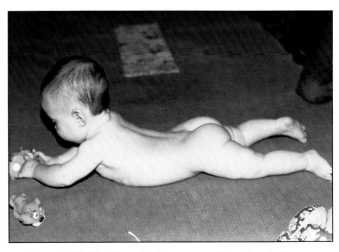

*Figure 5.14. The 5-month-old can move from the pivot-prone position into forward reaching with both arms, playing with a toy between the hands.*

movement components. The erector spinae muscles extend the back and lift the chest while the pectoralis majors (clavicular portions) adduct the humeri in synergy with other scapulo-humeral muscles (the serratus anterior, upper and lower trapezius, anterior deltoid, and cuff muscles) (Kendall, Kendall, and Wadsworth 1971; Brunnstrom 1979). The pectorals work in synergy with the abdominals.

The triceps contract to extend the elbow while the wrists are biomechanically extended. Wrist and finger flexors have been elongated through wrist extension during prior weight bearing. Therefore the fingers are open and extended during weight bearing.

When the baby rotates and laterally flexes the head during extended-arm weight bearing, a weight shift occurs (figure 5.12). The weight is shifted to the same side to which the face turns (face-side weight shift). Concurrent with the weight shift, the face-side arm is subtly rotated externally and the weight is shifted to the ulnar side of the hand, freeing the radial fingers for grasp. The skull-side shoulder internally rotates and weight is shifted to the radial side of the hand, elongating the thenar muscles. This weight shift with alternating elongation and weight bearing may contribute to the development of grasp in which the ulnar fingers are quiet and the radial fingers are active.

While in prone, the 5-month-old can reach forward for toys (figure 5.14). Forward reaching often seems to be preceded by marked shoulder girdle retraction (the Landau reaction) (figure 5.13). This may elongate the anterior shoulder muscles in preparation for efficient contraction. (According to Brunnstrom [1979], elongation of a muscle almost always occurs before a sudden burst of tension in the muscle is needed.) In addition to anterior muscle elongation, the Landau (pivot-prone) position strongly activates the extensor muscles of the trunk and the upper extremities in preparation for use as stabilizers. The head stays in midline and the trunk is symmetrically extended.

In the retracted position (figure 5.13), the scapulae are adducted and neutrally rotated (middle trapezius). The humeri are abducted and neutrally rotated (cuff muscles, posterior and middle deltoid). The elbows are extended (triceps brachii), and the wrists and fingers are loosely extended (extensor carpi radialis longus and brevis and extensor carpi ulnaris). The head and spinal extensor muscles are strongly activated bilaterally and symmetrically.

From the retracted posture, the baby reaches forward with both arms, flexing and adducting them together into or near midline (figure 5.14). This requires movement of the scapulae from adduction to abduction with upward rotation, and movement of the humeri from horizontal abduction to forward flexion with adduction and slight internal rotation. At five months of age, because the baby has increased muscle strength as well as increased scapulo-humeral mobility, the arms can be flexed farther forward than at four months.

The lower trapezius and serratus anterior play an important role in forward shoulder flexion because of the dynamic stability they provide the scapula for upward rotation. In addition, the serratus anterior abducts the scapula and the lower trapezius depresses the scapula (Kendall, Kendall, and Wadsworth 1971; Brunnstrom 1979). The lower trapezius also plays an important role in aiding thoracic spine extension.

With arms flexed forward, the baby can play with a toy between the hands (figure 5.14). The baby can also shift weight onto one arm and lift and reach forward with the other arm (figure 5.17).

## Indications of Possible Disturbances in Motor Development

Extended-arm weight bearing is an important step in motor development. Therefore babies who do not like prone or who cannot bear weight on their arms in prone by five months of age should be evaluated further. Prone extension activities may contribute to the baby's development of postural control in the upright position, and upper extremity weight bearing may contribute to dynamic stability of the shoulder girdle.

Extended-arm weight bearing also contributes to activation of the triceps and elongation of the wrist and finger extensors. Weight shifting on extended arms reinforces elongation of the intrinsic muscles of the hand and the thenar muscles. Babies who do not push up into extended-arm weight bearing do not receive reinforcement of any of these kinesiological components.

Constant use of shoulder girdle retraction in prone without equal, balancing forward actions suggests lack of development of proper balancing muscle control in the trunk and shoulder girdle. Without forward movement of the arms, upper extremity weight bearing and weight shifting are inhibited.

Upper extremity forward flexion and weight bearing contribute to the development of the serratus anterior and lower trapezius. Therefore the development of these muscles is impaired if the baby does not reach forward or does not bear weight in prone.

The serratus anterior is especially important in providing dynamic scapular stability. It stabilizes the scapula during humeral movements, thus assisting with scapulo-humeral dissociation and elongation of the muscles between the scapula and humerus. It also functions in most reaching patterns.

If the muscles between the scapula and humerus are not elongated and scapulo-humeral dissociation does not develop, the scapula and humerus continue to move as a total unit rather than with the normal scapulo-humeral rhythm (Quinton 1976, 1977, 1978). Reaching skills are impaired, and the baby often learns compensatory arm and trunk movements to substitute for poor shoulder-arm control. When reaching skills are impaired, compensatory movements are needed for grasp and manipulation skills.

The lower trapezius contributes to upward rotation and depression of the scapula during shoulder flexion, and because of its attachment onto the thoracic vertebrae, it also contributes to thoracic spine extension (Kendall, Kendall, and Wadsworth 1971). Lack of activity or weakness in this muscle will contribute to poor shoulder flexion and a thoracic kyphosis.

Lack of bilateral forward flexion also interferes with normal elongation of the latissimus dorsi and its effect on trunk extension. When the shoulders are flexed and the latissimus dorsi contracts bilaterally, it assists with extension of the spine (Kendall, Kendall, and Wadsworth 1971; Kapandji 1970a). Therefore babies who cannot flex their shoulders above 90° will miss out on elongation of the latissimus dorsi, which contributes to spinal extension. The result may be an increased thoracic kyphosis.

## *Lower Extremities*

The lower extremities play a role in upper extremity reaching. Strong trunk extension and forward reaching of both arms depends on strong hip extension to anchor the pelvis and thus the trunk (figures 5.11, 5.14).

Although the lower extremities are less active than the upper extremities, quiet and important changes are occurring. Subtle extension activation continues into the hips, knees, and ankles, which is enhanced by pushing up with extended arms, maturation of the Landau reaction, and rocking in prone. Extension combined with abdominal activation helps to reduce hip abduction and anterior tilting of the pelvis. The hip adductors bring the legs closer together and into line with the body.

There are five primary hip extensor muscles. Although all produce hip extension, they have different rotational effects. The gluteus maximus and biceps femoris extend the hip with external rotation (Brunnstrom 1979) (figure 5.11). The semitendinosus, semimembranosus, and adductor magnus (posterior portion) extend the hip with internal rotation (Brunnstrom 1979). Hip extension with internal rotation is rarely seen at five months of age. This may be due to the original soft tissue tightness of hip flexion, abduction, and external rotation. If hip internal rotation is observed at this early age, further observations of the baby should be conducted.

Hip extension at this age is due, at least in part, to contraction of the gluteus maximus. The hamstrings may also contribute to this extension, especially through a mechanical effect. During active knee extension by the quadriceps, the hamstrings are stretched. Because the hamstrings are a two-joint muscle, stretching at the knee during knee extension causes movement at the hip, namely hip extension. As the hamstrings become elongated, this two-joint effect will be reduced.

The 5-month-old is beginning to flex the knees against gravity when the hips are extended in prone (figure 5.16). This dissociated sagittal plane movement can occur when the thigh is stabilized in extension and neutral rotation and the hamstrings have sufficient strength to lift the leg. In addition, isolated active antigravity knee flexion in prone requires and provides elongation of the quadriceps muscles (especially the rectus femoris). Tightness in the rectus femoris will cause hip flexion when the knee flexes. Prior to this, knee flexion occurred as part of a total lower extremity flexion pattern.

The ankles are beginning to alternate more between dorsiflexion and plantar flexion. This alternation seems to be strongly affected by action in the hip. Plantar flexion usually occurs with active hip extension (figure 5.11), and dorsiflexion with active hip or knee flexion (figure 5.18). These ankle responses may be part of a total muscle synergy and/or a result of biomechanical stretch on the muscle. (Knee extension stretches the gastrocnemius, which responds with plantar flexion.)

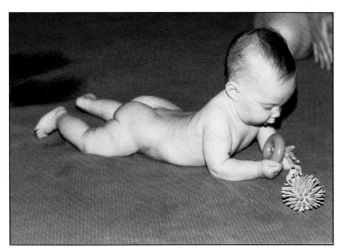

*Figure 5.15.* Forearm weight bearing is usually the preferred position at five months of age. With more weight being borne through the humeri than the forearms, hand movements are freer.

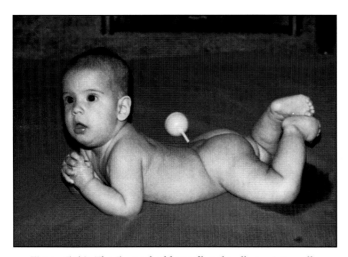

*Figure 5.16.* The 5-month-old can flex the elbows, internally rotate the shoulders, and bring the hands together while in forearm weight bearing. The baby is also beginning to flex the knees against gravity with the hips extended in prone.

# Forearm Weight Bearing

Forearm weight bearing is usually the preferred position at five months of age (figure 5.15). From this position the baby can weight shift in the shoulder girdle and reach for toys with the face-side arm (figure 5.17). This reinforces eye-hand coordination and upper extremity-hand use in prone.

During forearm weight bearing there is increased scapular depression, which helps to eliminate the neck roll seen at four months. This suggests that the lower trapezius may be active.

The 5-month-old seems to bear weight more through the humeri than through the forearms. As a result, the hand movements are freer (figure 5.15). In addition, the baby can flex the elbows, internally rotate the shoulders, and bring the hands together while in forearm weight bearing (figure 5.16). The baby uses this movement to collect or corral toys (Erhardt 1984).

In addition to symmetrical weight bearing on forearms, the 5-month-old can shift weight and assume a more asymmetrical posture. This enables the baby to reach for and play with toys. Asymmetrical weight bearing also encourages dissociated movements of the upper and lower extremities. One side is used for weight bearing while the other is free to reach and interact with the environment. One side continues to be yoked to the postural system as the other is freed from the postural system. Because of these dissociated activities, it is important for the baby to weight shift to both sides.

The 5-month-old's method of weight shifting is different from that of the 4-month-old. At four months of age, the baby shifted weight by rotating the head. This resulted in the weight being shifted to the same side to which the head turned (figure 4.16). With the weight on the face-side arm, eye-hand coordination was inhibited. At five months, the baby can weight shift at the shoulders and free the face-side hand for reaching with eye-hand coordination (figure 5.17).

The 5-month-old adjusts the posture away from the face-side arm prior to head turning and arm lifting. This suggests that the baby is beginning to anticipate the consequences of the head rotation (such as the weight shift to the face-side arm) and thus makes postural adjustments prior to the weight shift. This illustrates the baby's beginning

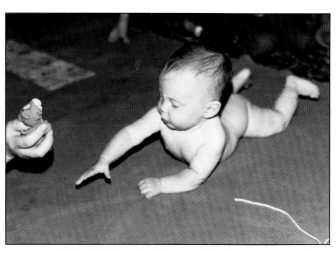

*Figure 5.17.* The 5-month-old can use feedforward postural adjustments to shift weight in the shoulder girdle and free the face-side arm for reaching.

ability to make feedforward postural adjustments. Postural adjustments that are made prior to or in synchrony with movements are a result of feedforward information (Kelso 1982). This ability to make automatic postural adjustments for weight shifting prior to movement enables the baby to reach in many different directions.

For the 5-month-old to achieve this milestone, there must be sufficient strength and control in the shoulder girdle to stabilize the weight while the baby lifts the other arm. As weight is shifted onto the arm, shoulder external rotation and forearm supination are biomechanically facilitated (figure 5.17).

Lifting of the unweighted arm for reaching seems to be accomplished with the lower trapezius and serratus anterior. As more shoulder control is developed, the baby reaches higher, causing more lateral weight shifting. This leads to increased head tilting, which requires lateral head righting to bring the head back into the proper position against gravity (figure 5.17). If the weight-bearing shoulder stability is insufficient or if lateral head righting does not occur, the weight will shift too far and the baby will collapse or roll over (figure 5.20).

In addition to reaching for toys while in forearm weight bearing, the baby can corral toys and begin to explore them (Erhardt 1984). The 5-month-old is beginning to use isolated active wrist extension with active finger extension during forearm weight bearing (figure 5.18). Weight on the forearms may provide the stability from which the wrist extensors can contract. Until this time, wrist extension in prone was produced primarily biomechanically by weight bearing on extended arms.

Once the 5-month-old has reached the toy, it can usually be grasped with a palmar grasp. As the toy is held with one hand, the baby can finger the toy with the other hand (figure 5.15). The baby is also becoming more efficient at scratching and raking finger movements while prone.

Manipulation skills are still very limited. The baby can finger large objects or press smaller ones between the hands when stable in weight bearing. The baby uses forearm movements to move a grasped toy. At three months in supine, large toys were manipulated using bilateral shoulder movements; now the baby has increased distal control. Elliott and Connolly (1984) describe this type of manipulation as

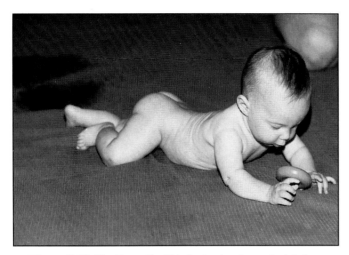

*Figure 5.18.* The 5-month-old is beginning to use isolated active wrist extension with active finger extension during forearm weight bearing. Lower extremity dissociation is occurring more frequently.

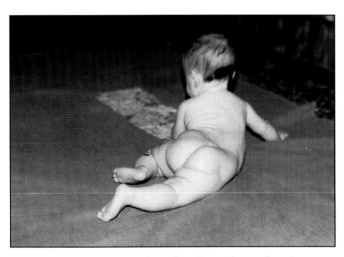

*Figure 5.19.* During unilateral reaching, the trunk and head respond with elongation on the weight-bearing side and lateral righting on the unweighted side. Lower extremity dissociation occurs as a component of this frontal-plane activity.

"extrinsic hand movement": the hand is used as a whole by moving the wrist, arm, or shoulder. Digital manipulation is described as "intrinsic hand movement."

## Head and Trunk

As the baby practices unilateral reaching, head and trunk asymmetry emerge (figures 5.17, 5.19). This asymmetry is due in part to the presence of the body righting reaction on the head. This reaction facilitates the more mature weight shift which includes elongation on the weight-bearing side, lateral righting (lateral flexion) on the unweighted side, and face-side reaching.

The body righting reaction on the head occurs as a result of asymmetrical tactile stimulation to the body (such as the prone weight shifting described above). This stimulation causes the head to right itself with the horizon (Twitchell 1965; O'Connell and Gardner 1972; Barnes, Crutchfield, and Heriza 1978). Labyrinthine and optical righting reactions also contribute to the head-righting response (Barnes, Crutchfield, and Heriza 1978).

Therefore, during unilateral reaching in prone, the lateral weight shift and asymmetrical tactile stimulation should produce lateral head righting with the head slightly laterally flexed and rotated away from the supporting side (figures 5.17, 5.19). The head movement, therefore, is a balancing reaction rather than an initiating action. As a result, the skull side becomes the weight-bearing and elongated side. The face side becomes the unweighted and laterally flexed side (figure 5.19). This promotes eye-hand-coordinated or visually directed reaching.

Achievement of this more advanced response is critical for further normal development of the body righting actions, equilibrium reactions, and dissociated movements between the upper extremities and between the lower extremities. This weight-shifting response is the basis of all normal reciprocal locomotion, including crawling, creeping, climbing, and walking.

The head and trunk movements may initially occur as a response to the sensory feedback. That is, the sensory feedback elicited by the weight shift causes the head and trunk to right themselves for balance. In a short time, the head and trunk movements will occur as a part of feedforward control. In this case, the head and trunk righting will actually occur prior to the weight shift in anticipation of the changing posture.

Contraction of the head and neck extensor and flexor muscles must be balanced to produce lateral flexion. These muscles each cause lateral flexion and rotation when they contract unilaterally (Kapandji 1974; Cailliet 1964). For pure frontal-plane lateral flexion to occur, the rotational components of the flexors must counterbalance the rotational components of the extensors. When rotation is neutralized, pure lateral flexion occurs (figure 4.20).

If the extensors are stronger (which is often the case in early development), lateral flexion will not occur, but extension will increase and throw the baby backward (figure 5.20), as it did at four months (figures 4.18, 4.19). Spinal movements depend on head movements; therefore, if the head reacts with extension, the spine will also extend. The head-neck response is facilitated through the vestibular, ocular, and neck proprioceptive systems.

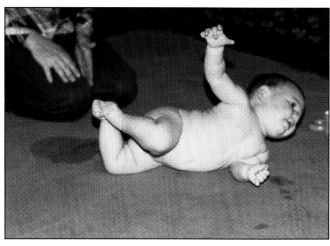

*Figure 5.20. If stability in the weight-bearing shoulder is insufficient or if lateral head righting does not occur, the baby's weight will shift too far and the baby will collapse or roll over.*

Trunk lateral flexion occurs in synchrony with head and neck lateral flexion if the baby has sufficient strength in the trunk muscles and sufficient joint mobility. This mobility should have been practiced in previous months and through earlier motor activities. Elongation of the latissimus dorsi bilaterally by forward flexion of both arms and unilaterally by forward flexion of one arm prepares the trunk and spine for the proper lateral and rotational response.

### Indications of Possible Disturbances in Motor Development

Forearm weight bearing with lateral weight shifting to free the face-side hand for reaching is a critical step in normal motor development. Failure to achieve this milestone may indicate the need for further evaluation of the baby. It may suggest that the baby cannot make feedforward postural adjustments.

If forearm weight bearing does not develop, the baby will have difficulty using face-side reaching in prone. The baby will also have difficulty playing in prone and may roll out of prone to supine. Poor ability to weight shift in prone will also affect the baby's further development of head and trunk lateral righting. Subsequently, if the baby does not practice lateral righting in prone, lower extremity dissociation will not develop.

Babies who do not develop the body righting reaction on the head are demonstrating problems in motor development. Babies who from five months onward constantly weight shift to the face side and rarely weight shift away from the face side receive abnormal sensory and kinesiological feedback for their age. Constant repetition of the pattern leads to increased lateral flexion of the trunk and muscle shortening on the weight-bearing side. This trunk response is the opposite of the response needed for trunk righting and equilibrium reactions.

The ability to weight shift away from the reaching arm demonstrates the emergence of feedforward postural control and may be the basis on which further postural control is developed. Anticipatory postural adjustments are needed for all reaching and transitional movements. If the baby cannot make normal anticipatory postural adjustments in the head and trunk, abnormal compensatory movements to prevent the weight shift will develop. Poor control in weight shifting leads to abnormal motor development.

### *Lower Extremities*

The baby's early attempts at using more advanced upper extremity control and weight shifting are accomplished by fixing the lower extremities in a position of hip flexion, abduction, and external rotation, and ankle dorsiflexion with eversion (figure 5.17). This posture provides positional stability which prevents or controls lateral weight shifting.

### Indications of Possible Disturbances in Motor Development

Although use of positional stability is normal throughout the course of motor development, its overuse or unmodified use indicates a lack of development or use of normal trunk stability. The abdominals and hip muscles are needed to stabilize the pelvis, which in turn stabilizes the rest of the trunk. If the abdominal and hip muscles do not develop normally, the lower extremities are kept in wide abduction to provide positional stability. Widely abducted or externally rotated legs inhibit lower trunk weight shifting and lower extremity dissociation. Therefore its overuse will interfere with total body weight shifting, upper extremity weight shifting, and further development of lateral righting control.

## Lower Extremity Weight Shifting

Lower extremity weight shifting and dissociated positioning may occur as part of the body righting reaction on the head, or it may occur independently. These movements indicate the development of muscle control and joint mobility in the lumbar spine, pelvis, and lower extremities. The lower extremity dissociated positions are precursors of crawling, creeping, climbing, and walking.

Increased active pelvic mobility is a prerequisite for dissociated lower extremity movements. At four months, the baby started playing with anterior and posterior tilting of the pelvis (sagittal plane movement) in association with other body movements. The pelvis was being moved and mobilized on the lumbar spine and over the femoral heads. Anterior-posterior tilting of the pelvis has a symmetrical effect on the spine and lower extremities.

At five months, the baby is developing lateral (frontal plane) and rotational (transverse plane) pelvic movements in addition to the anterior and posterior tilting. Pelvic hiking (lateral flexion) occurs conjointly with lumbar spine lateral flexion as a result of unilateral contraction of the quadratus lumborum and with assistance from the internal and external obliques on the same side (Kapandji 1974). These new movements contribute to spinal lateral flexion and rotation and to hip (femoral) rotation and lower extremity dissociated movements.

The pelvic movements may occur as a ripple effect of the body righting reaction on the head. After the weight shift, the head laterally flexes and rotates away from the supporting side. This prompts a similar reaction in the spine, which stimulates the pelvis to flex laterally (move on the frontal plane) and rotate away from the supporting surface. These spinal-pelvic reactions facilitate lower extremity dissociated positions (figure 5.19).

The weight-bearing lower extremity moves into hip extension, adduction and neutral rotation, knee extension, and ankle plantar flexion. The unweighted leg flexes, abducts with external rotation at the hip, flexes at the knee, and dorsiflexes at the ankle. The lower extremities are in opposite positions, facilitated by the head and spinal movements.

At five months, the baby can also assume a dissociated lower extremity position without stimulating a body righting reaction (figure 5.18). This requires active isolated hip flexion on one side, with active hip extension on the other side. These components of weight shifting and weight bearing on the elongated side with lateral righting on the nonweight-bearing side are essential components in all phases and positions of normal weight shifting and weight bearing.

### Indications of Possible Disturbances in Motor Development

Lack of development of lower extremity dissociation may indicate disturbances in motor development. It may reflect prolonged use of bilateral symmetrical back extensors without reciprocal interaction of the abdominals, and resulting lack of development of antigravity lateral flexion, including lack of pelvic hiking which normally accompanies spinal lateral flexion.

Absence of lower extremity dissociation and maintenance of lower extremity symmetrical positioning will cause problems in weight shifting. The baby will not be able to elongate on the weight-bearing side and will instead maintain the primitive pattern of weight shift to the face side which causes lateral flexion on the weight-bearing side. Thus lack of lower extremity dissociation will generate the development of abnormal components for weight bearing and weight shifting, such as upper trunk weight shifting without lower trunk weight shifting, and lateral flexion instead of elongation on the weight-bearing side.

# Rolling

At five months, the baby can roll (actually fall) from prone to supine. Spinal and head extension, scapular adduction, and the ability to weight shift on forearms all contribute to the rolling. Rolling from prone to supine uses extension as its primary component; therefore, it occurs before rolling from supine to prone, which uses flexion as its primary component. Again, note that extension activities are a little ahead of flexion activities.

Rolling from prone to supine is initially accidental because the baby does not yet have full shoulder control. If the weight is shifted too far or too fast, or if the arm is not in a position for controlled weight bearing, the baby cannot sustain the weight shift and falls onto the back (figures 5.20, 5.21). The baby may attempt to recover balance with lateral head righting (figure 5.20), but the extensor components are too strong, and the infant continues to roll to supine (figure 5.21).

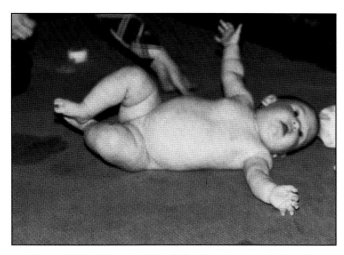

**Figure 5.21.** *If the weight is shifted too far or too fast, or if the arm is not in a position for controlled weight-bearing, the baby cannot sustain the weight shift and will fall onto the back.*

As shown in figures 5.20 and 5.21, rolling from prone to supine is a frightening experience for the baby. At this early age, it represents a loss of control and is therefore rarely performed voluntarily. For this reason, even though the milestone of rolling from prone to supine is achievable at five months of age, it is rarely practiced until the baby is older and has more control in weight shifting.

### Equilibrium Reactions

At five months of age, the baby does not yet have equilibrium reactions in prone. However, the baby's attempts to counterbalance the roll from prone to supine are precursors of body righting and equilibrium reactions in prone. In the 5-month-old, antigravity neck and trunk extensors are still stronger than progravity neck and trunk flexors; therefore, extension takes over and the baby falls backwards. When the flexors balance the extensors in prone, increased lateral flexion of the head and trunk will occur, enabling the baby to right the body before a significant weight shift occurs.

At five months, the bases for these components are emerging but not fully developed. Therefore, the baby does not yet have equilibrium reactions in prone. These will be seen in the sixth month after the baby practices lateral weight shifting.

# Pulled to Sit

When the 5-month-old is pulled to sit, the baby uses the antigravity flexor control that has been developing in supine. This control is obvious in the head, upper extremities, trunk, and lower extremities. Once in sitting, the increasing balance of extensors and flexors becomes obvious.

### Head

Although head righting in supine (flexion) is stronger because of the maturing labyrinthine and optical righting reactions, it is still incomplete. The 5-month-old continues to use visual fixing to reinforce head stability and still cannot independently lift the head in supine. However, the baby can flex the head and lift it when actively grasping the examiner's fingers (figure 5.22). Finger flexion seems to help reinforce upper extremity flexion (Brunnstrom 1979), which provides stability for head flexion. The baby now has no head lag when pulled to sit but may still elevate the shoulders slightly to help stabilize the head.

Head flexion and lifting are achieved with symmetry, through bilateral symmetrical contraction of the capital flexors, anterior neck flexors, the sternocleidomastoid muscles, and the abdominals which provide synergistic stability to the rib cage. The capital flexors contract first to flex the head and maintain the chin tuck, while the sternocleidomastoids contract to flex the cervical spine and lift the head. (At four months, the baby did not have sufficient muscle control to maintain the tucked chin. Therefore, contraction of the sternocleidomastoids extended the cervical spine while lifting the head.) The abdominals contract as part of the synergy to stabilize the rib cage in a lowered position while the head is flexed and lifted. Slight shoulder elevation and rib cage elevation illustrate the lack of full abdominal stabilizing control.

### Trunk

The abdominals (rectus abdominis, external obliques, and internal obliques) contract strongly during pull-to-sit. While stabilizing the rib cage in a lowered position, they also stabilize and posteriorly tilt the pelvis, facilitating hip flexion. The abdominals contract in synergy with the pectoralis majors (Brunnstrom 1979), helping to provide stability for upper extremity flexion and pulling.

### Upper Extremities

At five months, the baby can actively reach out with both upper extremities (shoulder flexion-adduction and elbow extension) in anticipation of being picked up. The baby can actively grasp the examiner's fingers and flex the elbows in an attempt to pull up. (According to Brunnstrom [1979], the biceps contract strongly and automatically when a fist is made.)

Bilateral scapular adduction usually does not occur during the early phases of pull-to-sit. The elbow muscles, not the scapular muscles, do the work. Bilateral scapular adduction, however, may occur at the end of the movement.

### Lower Extremities

The lower extremities flex bilaterally when the abdominals contract strongly. Total lower extremity flexion occurs—hip flexion, knee flexion, and ankle dorsiflexion (figure 5.22). This total flexion usually continues until the baby is upright. However, as the baby develops more abdominal, hip, and knee control, knee extension begins to occur with the hip flexion (figure 5.23). This is more predictable at six months and will be discussed further in that chapter.

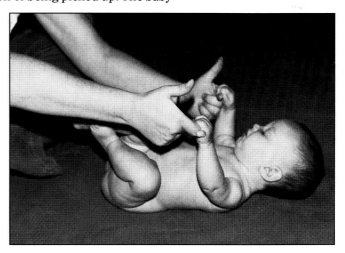

*Figure 5.22. The 5-month-old continues to use visual fixing to reinforce head stability and still cannot independently lift the head in supine. However, the baby can flex the head and lift it when actively grasping the examiner's fingers.*

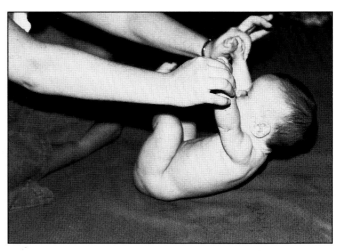

*Figure 5.23. As the baby develops more abdominal, hip, and knee control, knee extension begins to occur with hip flexion.*

# Sitting

Once the sitting posture is achieved (figure 5.24), the baby demonstrates increasing balance between the flexors and extensors. Erect sitting at five months is possible only when the baby's hands are held (figure 5.24) or the trunk is supported. When holding the examiner's hands, the baby can maintain trunk (spinal) extension with the chin tucked, the arms flexed forward, and the scapulae abducted. (Compare figures 5.24 and 4.25.)

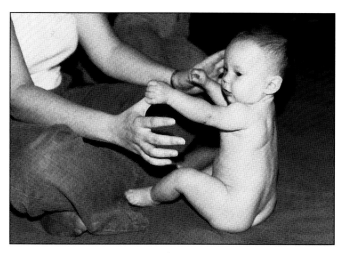

**Figure 5.24.** *Erect sitting at five months is possible only when the baby's hands are held or the trunk is supported. There is increasing balance between the flexors and extensors.*

## Head

During hand-held erect sitting, the 5-month-old has good head control. The baby can flex the head while maintaining cervical extension and can rotate the head without affecting the balance. Cervical mobility has increased, resulting in less weight shifting during rotation. The baby can even right the head laterally when tipped to the side during hand holding.

## Trunk

Although balance between the flexors and extensors is increasing, trunk extensor muscles are still the stronger group. This is demonstrated by the continued use of a forward-leaning posture. Forward leaning eliminates the need for abdominal action and uses the extensor muscles. The biomechanical theory that the body deviates toward the direction of muscle weakness, eliminating the need for action by that muscle group (Brunnstrom 1979), is useful in analyzing trunk muscle and motor development, activation, and balance.

Although the trunk is erect and the baby is maintaining weight on the ischial tuberosities, the spine is not fully extended (figure 5.24). Symmetrical extensor muscle activity is seen in the cervical and thoracic spinal muscles. The lumbar spine is noticeably kyphotic due to lack of extensor muscle activity. The pelvis is perpendicular.

The 5-month-old has only minimal rotational and lateral spinal mobility when sitting. The trunk muscles still contract with bilateral symmetry to provide stability with minimal mobility. This minimal mobility, along with the increased adducted position of the lower extremities, may result in the baby's falling laterally or sideward. This was not true at four months.

## Upper Extremities

When the baby holds on with hands, the flexor muscle activation is reinforced and balances the extensor muscle activation. When the hand grip is released, the baby will adduct the scapulae for stability and fall backward.

## Lower Extremities

When the pelvis is perpendicular to the supporting surface (figure 5.24), the legs are maintained in hip flexion, slight abduction, and external rotation, with knee flexion and ankle dorsiflexion. The pelvic-femur position causes elongation of the hamstrings at their origin and thus increases knee flexion. Ankle dorsiflexion is unchanged.

# Propped Sitting

When placed in sitting, the 5-month-old can briefly sit unsupported by propping forward on the extended upper extremities (figure 5.25). The upper extremities are thus yoked to the postural system.

The 5-month-old continues to lean forward in order to use the cervical and thoracic extensors to right the body. Hip flexion mobility and lack of resistance from the hip extensors also contribute to the forward leaning. Hip extensor muscles are becoming more active in stabilizing the pelvis and in contributing to the increasingly erect posture.

### Head

The 5-month-old holds the head erect and steady during upper extremity-propped sitting. The baby can also actively extend, rotate, and flex the head without becoming unbalanced. This enables the baby to be active in visual reaching and searching up, down, and sideward. In previous months, head and ocular muscles were intimately involved with stability rather than function.

### Trunk

The trunk muscles (spinal extensors) are very active during upper extremity propped sitting, making scapular adduction unnecessary for reinforcement. The cervical and thoracic erector spinae muscles contract bilaterally and symmetrically to right the head and trunk and prevent forward collapse. The anterior trunk muscles (abdominals) are not active during this phase of sitting. This is compensated for by the forward leaning of the trunk.

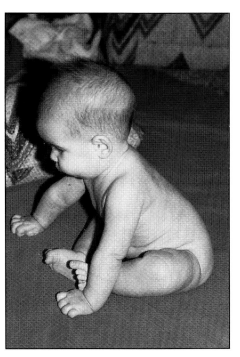

*Figure 5.25.* When placed in sitting, the 5-month-old can briefly sit unsupported by propping forward on the extended upper extremities. The upper extremities are yoked to the postural system.

The capital, cervical, and thoracic spinal extensor muscles are active in sitting (figure 5.28). The lumbar spine is still flexed. The pelvis is neutral, being neither anteriorly nor posteriorly tilted. Weight is borne on the ischial tuberosities. The forward position of the trunk occurs because of hip flexion, not trunk flexion.

#### Indications of Possible Disturbances in Motor Development

At five months, it is normal for the baby to assume forward trunk flexion during sitting. However, as the baby becomes older, a more erect position is normal. Constant maintenance of forward trunk flexion after six or seven months would indicate a problem in the normal development of abdominal, erector spinae, and hip muscle control. On the other hand, a baby's inability to sit in a forward leaning position at five months may indicate abnormal tone in the hip extensors.

### Upper Extremities

At five months of age, the baby has sufficient shoulder girdle and elbow muscle control to reinforce the postural system and provide upper extremity stability when leaning forward in sitting. When the upper extremities are used as part of the postural system, the baby can use freer head and eye movements. According to Barnes, Crutchfield, and Heriza (1978), upper extremity propping is actually a positive supporting reaction which has shown developmental progression in prone. Thus extended-arm propping in sitting occurs at the same time as extended-arm weight bearing in prone.

Upper extremity propping requires components of movement similar to prone extended-arm weight bearing. There is bilateral activation of the same four muscle components: serratus anterior, shoulder cuff muscles, pectoralis major, and triceps brachii. The triceps may not be active if the elbows are locked in extension. The wrists are extended, but the fingers are loosely flexed. Although the upper extremity components for propping and prone extended-arm weight bearing may be similar, the postural requirements are very different.

Although the upper extremities are being used for postural stability, the baby is beginning to experiment with freeing one hand to reach for toys while in this position. In order to free one hand, the baby must preadjust the posture to assure that the trunk and hip extensors will stabilize the upright posture. This is feedforward.

### Lower Extremities

The lower extremities provide positional stability for independent sitting, due to their increased range of mobility into hip abduction and external rotation (figure 5.25). The position of the lower extremities, therefore, provides a wide base of support and stabilizes the pelvis from marked displacement.

As in previous months, the baby leans forward during sitting because of the hip flexion mobility and lack of resistance from hip extensors. However, hip flexion is not as marked as it was in previous months because of the developing hip extensor muscle activation. As the hip extensors become more active, they contract to bring the pelvis into a perpendicular position and stabilize it there.

The development of hip extensor activity is an important step in the development of erect, independent sitting and sitting balance. Touwen (1976) noted that hip control is directly related to sitting balance. The hip muscles and femoral positions influence the position, mobility, and control of the pelvis. The pelvic positions subsequently influence the superincumbent spinal curves.

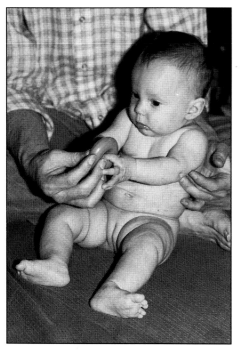

*Figure 5.26. With support, the baby can reach forward with both upper extremities by actively flexing and adducting the shoulders while extending elbows, wrists, and fingers.*

# Supported Sitting

In supported sitting, the baby's upper extremities are more functional in interacting with the environment. When the trunk is supported, the baby can reach forward with both upper extremities by actively flexing and adducting the shoulders while extending the elbows, wrists, and fingers (figure 5.26).

A primitive palmar grasp is still used (figure 5.27). Once the toy is grasped, the 5-month-old cannot yet manipulate it or transfer it, but the baby can flex the elbow, rotate the forearm, and bring the toy to the mouth for mouth manipulation (figure 5.27). At four months, the baby brought the mouth to the toy, and the arm without the toy mirrored the action of the one holding the toy (figure 4.28). At five months, each arm can function independently (figure 5.27).

# Standing

At five months of age, the baby has increased head and trunk control during standing, and the lower extremities take almost full weight (figure 5.28). The 5-month-old can maintain the erect posture when held by the hands or trunk. The baby uses this increased proximal control to move the head and upper extremities purposefully.

Although the lower extremities are fairly static in extension, the 5-month-old is beginning to alternate between knee extension and collapse (figures 5.28, 5.30). The baby is beginning to use sagittal plane movements to move the body over the lower extremities, which provides new proprioceptive and kinesthetic feedback.

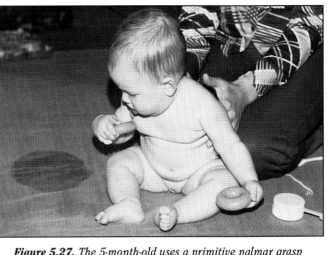

*Figure 5.27.* The 5-month-old uses a primitive palmar grasp and, having grasped a toy, cannot yet manipulate it or transfer it. However, because each arm now functions independently, the baby can flex the elbow, rotate the forearm, and bring the toy to the mouth.

### Head

Head control in trunk-supported standing is nearly fully developed. The 5-month-old can extend, flex, and rotate the head, using all the muscles that have become active.

As in other positions, head movements affect the whole body. Head extension increases back extension. Head flexion (capital flexion) elongates the capital extensors and enhances elongation of the neck (figure 5.28). Head rotational mobility has increased and affects the trunk and lower extremities in standing, causing rotation in the adjacent vertebrae.

### Trunk

Active extension is increasing throughout the trunk. Extensor muscles are becoming active in the lumbar area and hips, leading to an increase in the lumbar lordosis (figure 5.28). There is no abdominal activity yet in standing.

Although head rotation facilitates adjacent spinal rotation, spinal rotation mobility is still very limited. It does, however, cause a lateral weight shift to the face-side leg.

### Upper Extremities

When the 5-month-old is supported at the trunk, scapular adduction is no longer needed to reinforce spinal stability; therefore, the arms can hang loosely at the sides or in slight abduction without shoulder elevation (figure 5.29).

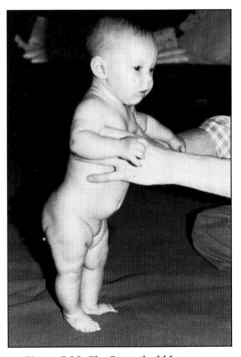

*Figure 5.28.* The 5-month-old has increased head and trunk control during standing, and the lower extremities take almost full weight. Trunk extensor muscles are becoming active in the lumbar area and hips, leading to an increase in lumbar lordosis. Knee and back extension are primarily responsible for maintaining the upright posture.

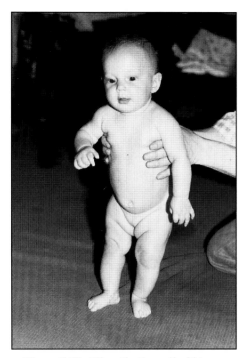

*Figure 5.29. When the 5-month-old is supported at the trunk, scapular adduction is no longer needed to reinforce spinal stability; therefore, the arms can hang loosely at the sides or in slight abduction without shoulder elevation. Hip extensors do not appear to be very active, so the baby leans forward when less support is given. The feet are pronated.*

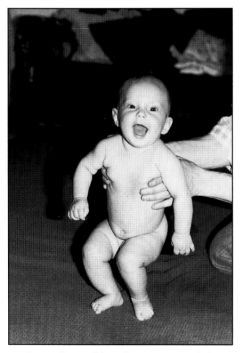

*Figure 5.30. Although contraction of the knee extensors (quadriceps) is apparently strong, the 5-month-old is beginning to flex the knees by releasing the extensor activity and collapsing into flexion.*

When the baby's hands are held during standing, elbow flexion, rather than scapular adduction, is used to maintain the position. Scapular adduction may occur if the baby tries to move while the hands are held. Scapular elevation (shoulder elevation) usually does not occur, suggesting active contraction of the lower trapezius for scapular depression.

## Lower Extremities

At five months, the baby bears almost full weight on extended legs. The legs are now in line with the body in the frontal planes (figure 5.29). The hips are adducted and slightly externally rotated, the knees are extended, and the feet are flat and slightly pronated and everted.

In the sagittal plane (figure 5.28), it is obvious that the hips are not yet in line with the shoulders. Hip extension is not yet complete. As range into hip extension increases, the iliopsoas muscle elongates. Lack of full elongation of the iliopsoas and active lumbar extensor muscles are responsible for the increasing lumbar lordosis. Knee and back extension are primarily responsible for maintaining the upright posture (figure 5.28). Hip extensors do not appear to be very active, so the baby leans forward when less support is given (figure 5.29).

Although contraction of the knee extensors (quadriceps) is apparently strong, the 5-month-old is beginning to flex the knees by thus releasing the extensor activity and collapsing into flexion (figure 5.30). Until now, the baby has experienced only flexion of the lower extremities on the body. This is the first movement of the body on the lower extremities.

From the flexed position, the baby can re-extend the knees by contracting the quadriceps. The feet remain in contact with the floor. The baby is experimenting with the new ability to alternate between contraction and release of specific muscles without disturbing the muscles in the rest of the body.

The up-and-down movement provides vestibular, proprioceptive, and kinesthetic stimulation, all of which will continue to enhance motor development. The alternating contract-release activity of the quadriceps may be a precursor of active lower extremity bouncing observed in later months.

# The Sixth Month

During the sixth month, the baby further develops voluntary asymmetrical, dissociated, and reciprocal movements, and coordinates and integrates previously developed movement components. The baby also uses newly developed synergistic muscle control in prone and supine, which seems to replace positional stability. These advances in neuromuscular maturation and control enable the baby to be more functional at six months than in previous months.

The baby is more active in prone and supine and utilizes less positional stability. Antigravity extensor control continues to improve and is more obvious in the hips and lower extremities. Increased antigravity flexor control enables the baby to flex the head and lift it in supine without first grasping the examiner's fingers. This increased balance of the extensor and flexor control enables the baby to further develop frontal plane lateral control as well as dissociated movements of the extremities.

Because of the increased trunk control, head control is fully developed by the sixth month, enabling the baby to easily extend the head in prone, flex in supine, and laterally flex in side lying. These movements, or righting reactions, continue to be enhanced by the vestibular and optical systems. Increased cervical spine mobility leads to decreased and more subtle biomechanical effects on the rest of the spine and trunk during head movements.

The baby's symmetrical (anterior-posterior, sagittal plane) and asymmetrical (lateral, frontal plane) righting reactions are becoming stronger because of increased muscle control. By the sixth month, the baby is starting to combine the righting reactions when diagonal weight shifting occurs (transverse plane movement) and is beginning to respond with rotation. At six months, equilibrium reactions are possible in prone.

Prone is a functional, mobile position for the 6-month-old, who can push up onto extended arms, weight shift on extended arms, and reach in front and to the side for toys. The baby can also pivot in a circle. Once a toy has been grasped, the baby can crudely manipulate it, finger it, or bring it to the mouth. Because of the dynamic muscle stability of the scapula on the trunk and the humerus on the scapula, more refined and specific forearm and hand movements are beginning to develop. Hand movements are also developing because of the experimenting and practicing that the baby has been doing with the hands.

The baby's increased proximal and synergistic muscle control enables more specific and dissociated extremity movements to be developed. The lower extremities are becoming more active and more mobile. In prone, the baby can actively weight shift in the pelvis and actively move the legs into dissociated positions. Increased proximal (trunk and pelvic) synergistic muscle control and better hip muscle control enable the baby to begin to assume pushup and/or quadruped positions from prone. The lower extremities are still used for positional stability in sitting and standing.

Antigravity flexor control is more mature and enables the baby to independently flex and lift the head, reach with the arms, flex and lift the hips and bring the feet to the mouth, and play with the feet in space over the chest. The 6-month-old, therefore, has equal ability to flex in supine and extend in prone. The flexion activities continue to elongate the extensor muscles, enabling equal mobility for flexion and extension activities. Increasing flexor control enables the 6-month-old to roll from supine to prone, activate equilibrium reactions in prone, and initiate equilibrium reactions in supine. The improved balance of flexors and extensors enables active and prolonged lateral flexion of the head and trunk in side lying.

Increased control for lateral flexion allows the 6-month-old to shift weight in the trunk and pelvis and assume dissociated lower extremity positions. This enables the baby to roll toward side lying and maintain the position there. Side lying is a more functional position for upper extremity use. The baby is also beginning to use the lateral and dissociated movements to lift into quadruped from prone. These dissociated lower extremity movements mobilize the lumbar and thoracic spine. Mobility throughout the spine, pelvis, and hip joints is necessary to achieve reciprocal extremity movements during locomotion. Counterrotation in the spine is also needed for reciprocal movements of the extremities.

The 6-month-old can pull to sitting when holding the examiner's hand. The baby has sufficient antigravity and synergistic flexor control to flex and lift the head, arms, and legs independently. In the process of coming to sit, the baby integrates extension components while maintaining the flexion component. The baby gradually extends the knees while the hips remain flexed, then subtly extends the hips, which helps to tip the body forward to sitting.

The 6-month-old can now sit independently without external support and without propping on forward extended arms. The baby can assume a nearly erect posture because hip extensor muscles help to stabilize the pelvis perpendicular to the floor and thus provide a stable base for trunk extension. The 6-month-old continues to lean slightly forward from the hips, still using bilateral symmetrical trunk extensors for stability and thus moving mainly in the sagittal plane. Lack of balance between trunk flexors and extensors in sitting makes active trunk lateral flexion in sitting difficult. Therefore if weight is shifted laterally during sitting, the baby falls sideways.

The 6-month-old continues to use lower extremity positional stability to maintain the sitting posture. This stabilizes the pelvis and trunk, enabling the baby to free the arms from the postural system and thus begin to reach with the arms and grasp and hold toys while sitting.

When placed in standing and supported by the trunk or the hands, the 6-month-old takes full weight on the legs. Although standing is essentially a static posture, the baby is beginning to bounce by flexing and extending the knees, thus moving on the sagittal plane. The baby is also beginning to reach for toys when the trunk is supported.

# Indications of Possible Disturbances in Motor Development

When evaluating for disturbances in motor development, it is imperative to consider the baby's normal abilities as well as problem areas. Analysis of the normal components required in each movement will give a more accurate picture of the problem.

By the sixth month, the baby should be integrating muscle control and movement patterns and producing a great variety of movements. Failure to do so would indicate a problem in motor development.

Functional muscle integration begins with antigravity lateral flexion of the head and trunk. Lateral flexion occurs by integrated and coordinated action of unilateral flexors and extensors. Inability to laterally flex actively in prone and side lying would indicate that flexor and extensor muscle control have not developed equally. Subtle problems in motor development in prone and/or supine would have been present in previous months.

At six months, the baby's inability to laterally flex the head and trunk actively while in prone and side lying indicates that flexor and/or extensor muscle control is not normal. This has many implications and may cause serious movement problems, because subsequent development requiring integration of these muscle groups cannot be normal.

The consequences of inability to laterally flex in prone and side lying include (1) inability to right the body laterally, (2) inability to weight shift on upper extremities and/or lower extremities, (3) inability to actively assume dissociated extremity positioning and movements, (4) inadequate development of trunk-spinal mobility, and (5) inability to develop and/or elicit equilibrium reactions.

The 6-month-old may manifest other signs of problems in motor development. Inability to roll from supine to prone, or rolling by using neck hyperextension and rotation, indicates poor development of antigravity flexor muscles.

Inability to sit independently also indicates problems in motor development, either too little or too much hip extensor muscle activation. Too little hip extensor activation causes the baby to lean very far forward, with no pelvic and, therefore, no trunk stability. The baby with exaggerated hip extensor muscle activity or tight hip extensors will have difficulty sitting because the hip extensors will pull the pelvis into a posterior tilt behind neutral. This will cause the baby to fall backward.

# Supine

In supine, the 6-month-old has antigravity flexor control which enables independent flexing and lifting of the head. The baby can pull to sitting with the arms while flexing, lifting, and maintaining the legs extended above the body. The baby can reach the hands toward the lifted feet and play in mid-positions of flexion (figure 6.1). The extremities can be flexed at the distal joints while the proximal joints are flexed (figure 6.1).

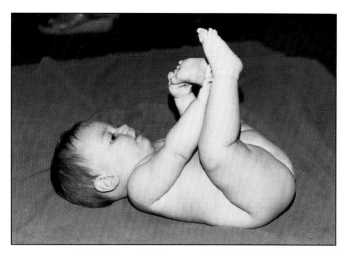

**Figure 6.1.** *The 6-month-old can reach the hands toward the lifted feet and play in mid-positions of flexion. The baby can extend the extremities at the distal joints while flexing at the proximal joints. There is minimal spinal flexion, even though the abdominal muscles are active.*

These flexed positions enable the baby to bring the upper and lower extremities together, enriching body exploration, tactile stimulation, visual awareness of the body, and antagonistic muscle elongation. Note: this antigravity flexion is accomplished with minimal spinal flexion (figure 6.1).

In addition, the 6-month-old can assume a variety of positions in supine, thus expressing the emerging muscle control and voluntary use of the muscles. The baby can roll from supine to prone and initiate equilibrium reactions in supine.

Symmetry and flexion are strong at six months, but they do not dominate the baby's repertoire of movements. The baby continues to play with dissociated and asymmetrical extremity positions as well as rotation and lateral flexion. Dissociated lower extremity play is often used to initiate rolling.

## *Head*

When the baby is playing in flexion, the capital and cervical flexor muscles contract while the capital and cervical extensors are elongated. The elongation of these muscles and all of the spinal extensor muscles becomes exaggerated as the buttocks are lifted higher in hand-to-foot and hand-to-mouth play (figure 6.1).

By the sixth month, the baby may actively and independently tuck the chin and lift the head against gravity without first grasping with the hands to reinforce head flexion, as at five months. Head lifting demonstrates antigravity control of the capital and cervical flexor muscles, and synergistic stability of the thorax by the abdominal muscles (Kendall, Kendall, and Wadsworth 1971). When the abdominal contraction is sufficient, shoulder elevation does not occur with head lifting. Flexion against gravity is a vital component of antigravity head control.

The increased capital and cervical muscle control and increased cervical spine mobility lead to improved head control and dissociated movements of the head from the trunk. Subsequently, the neck righting reaction will no longer be active, but optical righting, labyrinthine righting, body righting reaction on the head, and body righting reaction on the body will continue to be active.

## *Trunk*

During flexion, there is minimal spinal flexion, even though the abdominal muscles (rectus abdominis, external and internal obliques) are active (figure 6.1). The rectus abdominis lifts the pubis and brings it closer to the sternum (Kendall, Kendall, and Wadsworth 1971), simultaneously causing elongation of the lumbar extensor muscles. The oblique abdominals also contract and contribute to pubic lifting in addition to providing thoracic and pelvic stability. Stability of the thorax and pelvis enables upper extremity adduction and lower extremity flexion.

The oblique abdominal muscles must become increasingly active to control the side-to-side swaying of the lower extremities, which occurs when the legs are lifted over the trunk. When the legs sway to the side, the obliques bring them back to midline and help to maintain them there. Activation and development of the oblique abdominal muscles is important for the development of isolated rotation of the pelvis to each side, upper and lower extremity dynamic stability and reciprocal movements, the development of equilibrium reactions, shaping of the rib cage, and respiration.

## Upper Extremities

Upper extremity movements of the 6-month-old are similar to those used by the 5-month-old during flexion. However, the 6-month-old seems to be stronger and have more voluntary control of the upper extremity musculature. This may be due to improved abdominal muscle control, which provides synergistic stability to the thorax during humeral movements.

Shoulder girdle muscles can move and stabilize the humerus through a greater range of flexion in supine. (Compare figures 6.1 and 5.1.) Increased dynamic humeral stability can provide the basis for increased isolated elbow movements. With the humerus stabilized by the shoulder muscles, the triceps brachii can extend the elbow more effectively during shoulder flexion (figures 6.1, 6.2). As control of shoulder adduction with elbow extension increases, the baby can reach into and across midline.

Reaching is still accomplished with forearm pronation and wrist and finger extension (figure 6.2). Forearm supination mobility is increasing. However, active isolated forearm supination mobility and ability are still limited. Forearm supination may be accomplished through shoulder external rotation, as occurs when the baby reaches for and holds onto the foot.

*Note:* Just as dynamic scapular stability enables further refined development and isolated movement of the humerus, dynamic humeral stability enables further refined development and isolated movement of the elbow and forearm. This refine-

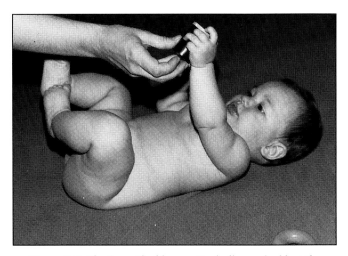

ment will occur within the next six months of the baby's life. (The serratus anterior is especially important in dynamic scapular stability for reaching; the cuff muscles, deltoid, and pectoralis major are especially important in dynamic humeral stability for reaching.)

## Lower Extremities

At six months, flexion of the lower extremities in supine occurs with the baby's hips more adducted and less externally rotated than at five months. (Compare figures 6.1 and 5.1.) Although marked hip flexion mobility is still possible, the baby can adjust the range more easily and can play between flexion and extension. The baby's ability to bring the hips closer to 90° of flexion requires balanced contraction of the hip flexors and extensors.

*Figure 6.2. The 6-month-old can actively flex and adduct the shoulder with slight external rotation, actively controlling and stopping the movement anywhere in its range.*

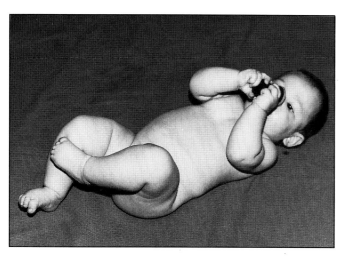

**Figure 6.3.** *The 6-month-old still lacks grading and isolated control of the wrist and finger musculature, usually holding an object tightly once it has been grasped. The baby can dissociate the lower extremities in supine, placing one foot on the opposite knee.*

Range in hip flexion is frequently reduced when the knee is actively extended above the body. Active knee extension may elongate the hamstring muscles at the knee and subsequently cause movement (extension) at the hip. Active knee extension also seems to cause ankle plantar flexion, which may be due to a stretch on the gastrocnemius.

When the baby plays in the hands-to-feet position (figure 6.1), integration of muscle action on the two sides of the body and movement into and through midline are enhanced. This enhances the development of diagonal muscle action (transverse plane movement) in the trunk and causes asymmetrical weight shifting in the pelvis.

The 6-month-old can dissociate the lower extremities in supine. Dissociation occurs when the baby places one foot on the opposite knee (figure 6.3). This position provides tactile stimulation to the foot and opposite leg and is part of body exploration.

## Indications of Possible Disturbances in Motor Development

As discussed at five months, a baby's inability to achieve and practice flexion activities in supine (bringing the feet to the mouth and, concurrently, the hands to the feet) suggests a problem in motor development. Failure to practice flexion activities could be due to tight head, back, and/or hip extensor muscles, or to insufficient control/strength of the abdominals and hip flexor muscles. If the baby cannot reach hands to feet, it may also be due to poor shoulder girdle control, including tight scapular adductors and poorly developed humeral flexors (pectoralis major, clavicular portion).

In addition to bringing the feet to the mouth, it is important for the 6-month-old to sustain the extended legs over the body (figure 6.1). Inability to sustain this mid-position for hand-to-foot play would indicate that the baby is not developing a balancing interplay of the hip flexor and extensor muscles. This will inhibit normal development of co-contraction of the muscles around the joint and will eventually lead to problems in hip control and stability.

By the sixth month, it is important for the baby to play with two hands on one foot. Failure to do so indicates poor development of midline awareness and poor ability to cross midline. It also indicates poor integration of muscle action on the two sides of the body.

Hand-to-foot play is also important from a sensory (tactile and visual) perspective. Failure to explore the feet with hands and eyes may result in poor development of body awareness and body scheme. Lack of tactile desensitization by hand-to-foot play may lead to problems in weight bearing during early stages of standing (Quinton 1976, 1977, 1978).

# Reaching in Supine

Shoulder girdle muscle control is quite good by six months, providing stability to the humerus. The baby can actively flex and adduct the shoulder with slight external rotation. The baby can also actively control and stop the movement anywhere in its range (figure 6.2), enabling reaching to be directed more precisely (von Hofsten 1990). The baby can now reach toward an object with one or both hands (Fagard 1990). As use of unilateral reaching increases, dissociation of the two extremities becomes more apparent. A palmar grasp or a radial palmar grasp is used (Erhardt 1984); manipulation is limited (figure 6.3).

The increased proximal muscle control of the humerus enables dynamic humeral stability and provides the basis for increased elbow and forearm control. The humerus is dynamically stable in most supine positions, allowing increasing refinement of forearm movements. The 6-month-old can control elbow extension and flexion through its antigravity range, regardless of the position of the humerus. Other forearm movements (active supination and pronation) are still limited. The 6-month-old uses primarily pronation and neutral rotation in supine reaching.

When reaching in supine, the 6-month-old extends the elbow and neutrally rotates the forearm (figure 6.2). Any increase in forearm supination with elbow extension that is observed may be attributed to increased shoulder external rotation.

The wrists are extended during reaching. The fingers are loosely extended and abducted; the thumb is beginning to be extended and abducted. The shape that the baby's hand assumes during the reaching is related to visual feedback and to the baby's prior experiences. The baby may use marked finger extension with abduction when reaching for unfamiliar objects, then use tactile and visual information to grasp the object. If the baby is familiar with the object and has had prior experience in grasping it, visual information may be used to preshape the hand to accommodate the object. At six months of age, preparatory adjustment of the hand occurs throughout the reaching phase (von Hofsten 1990).

The lower extremities may or may not flex during the reaching phase. Babies with low muscle tone often use lower extremity flexion to reinforce the abdominal contraction, which subsequently reinforces pectoral contraction (figure 6.2). Foot-on-foot contact also reinforces the stability.

## Grasp

At six months of age, closure of the hand around an object is visually and tactually controlled (Corbetta and Mounoud 1990). The baby may touch and feel the object before grasping it or may rely solely on visual information to begin to close the hand around the object. The baby can use a palmar or a radial palmar grasp, depending on the shape of the object (Erhardt 1984). The 6-month-old still lacks grading and isolated control of the wrist and finger musculature. Therefore, the baby usually holds an object tightly once the hand has grasped it (figure 6.3).

## Manipulation

The 6-month-old still lacks in-hand manipulation skill. The baby can grasp an object with one hand and explore it tactually with the other hand. However, most objects are still manipulated (explored) primarily by the mouth and tongue (figure 6.3).

The baby can often grasp a toy (such as a rattle) with one hand and bring it to the mouth for exploration. By using the face and the mouth as a point of stability, the baby may transfer the toy to the other hand (Nash 1991).

### Indications of Possible Disturbances in Motor Development

Reaching in supine is approaching an adult-like pattern (von Hofsten 1990). Therefore, infants who cannot reach and grasp in supine are demonstrating a delay in motor development. This may be due to delayed development of specific shoulder-arm muscles and/or delayed development of the synergistic postural muscles.

Problems in these areas would have been subtly present in the previous months, but by the sixth month, when each of the components should be integrated, their previous inadequate development becomes a major functional problem, such as poor or no reaching in supine.

By six months of age, the baby wants to interact with the environment. If unable to control the arm in space, the baby may compensate by adducting the arm to the side to stabilize it. This static stability of the humerus enables the baby to use the forearm and hand. However, static stability of the shoulder and humerus requires additional compensatory movements in the elbow, forearm, wrist, and hand. Elbow extension, forearm supination, wrist extension, and thumb and finger movements will be poorly developed because of the compensatory movements that must be adopted for the hands to interact with the environment and toys.

# Equilibrium in Supine

The 6-month-old is beginning to develop and utilize equilibrium reactions (tilting reactions) in supine (Barnes, Crutchfield, and Heriza 1978). Expression of equilibrium reactions requires antigravity control of the flexor muscles. By the sixth month, the baby can flex the head, shoulders, and hips against gravity. Therefore, most of the muscle activation needed to recover disturbed balance in supine is present.

Traditionally, equilibrium reactions—especially tilting reactions—have been considered to be a feedback response in that they are elicited when the center of gravity is disturbed and the vestibular system is stimulated (Weisz 1938; Martin 1965). They are usually tested on a tilting board (Barnes, Crutchfield, and Heriza 1978).

Equilibrium reactions also include feedforward motor control (Nashner 1985; Horack and Nashner 1986). When feedforward control is used, the baby can adjust the posture prior to the weight shift, which suggests that the baby can anticipate the weight shift and the disturbances that it will cause.

For this text, a tilting board was not used to evaluate the emerging equilibrium reactions. Equilibrium reactions are described as they emerge during the baby's normal playing activities, not as seen during a test on an equilibrium board.

The feedback response is demonstrated in how well the baby adjusts the posture once the weight is shifted. For example, in supine when flexed legs initially sway to the side, the baby may fall to the side and then readjust to assume supine flexion. The feedback experiences help the baby learn the consequence of the weight shift, which eventually leads to feedforward postural adjustments. The feedforward response is seen in how well the baby makes compensatory postural adjustments in anticipation of the leg sway and thus prevents falling to the side.

# Rolling

The 6-month-old can roll from supine to prone. Components of this milestone have been achieved and practiced in previous months, and the baby can now combine the various components and complete the entire movement.

## *Initiation of Rolling*

Rolling from supine to prone is initiated by flexion, rotation, and a lateral weight shift. These components occur most frequently in the head and the lower extremities (figure 6.4). This causes the baby to roll to side lying, as described for the fourth and fifth months.

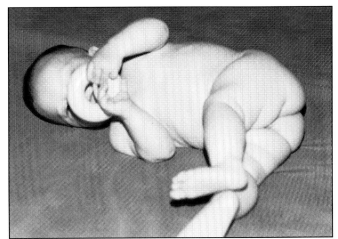

The head rotates and subtly flexes. The top arm comes across the body, utilizing shoulder flexion and adduction with scapular abduction. The bottom arm remains at the baby's side, often with the elbow flexed.

The lower extremities move with bilateral, symmetrical hip flexion with knee extension. This lower extremity movement was also observed at five months of age (figure 5.6).

The flexion movements of the head, upper extremities, and lower extremities help to facilitate trunk flexion and abdominal contraction. Activation of the oblique abdominals is of primary importance in the transitional phase.

*Figure 6.4.* Rolling from supine to prone is initiated by flexion, rotation, and a lateral weight shift, which occur most frequently in the head and the lower extremities.

## *Transition in Rolling*

The baby uses side lying to make a transition from symmetrical flexion to extension, which is needed to complete the movement to prone. The transition in side lying is made through active lateral flexion, which combines flexor and extensor muscles (figure 6.5).

The head laterally flexes against gravity as a result of stimulation from several sources: (1) **optical righting reaction** (visual feedback is used to orient the eyes with the horizon); (2) **labyrinthine righting reaction** (stimulation to the labyrinthine system causes the head to be brought into the proper position against gravity, resulting in lateral head righting); and (3) **body righting reaction on the head** (asymmetrical tactile stimulation to the body causes the head to right itself, thus also stimulating the lateral head-righting response) (O'Connell and Gardner 1972; Barnes, Crutchfield, and Heriza 1978).

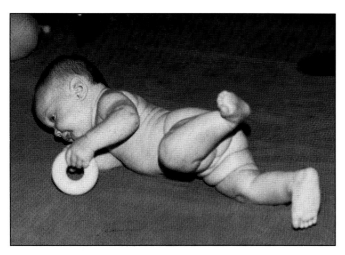

*Figure 6.5.* The transition from side lying to prone is made through active lateral flexion. The bottom arm is adducted biomechanically, and the top arm actively adducts as the baby reaches across the body. The top leg abducts, and the bottom leg extends at the hip and usually at the knee as the entire lower side elongates.

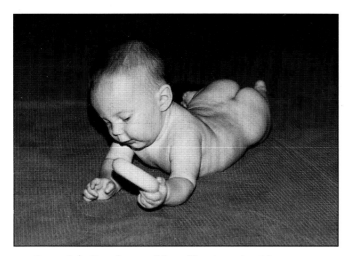

*Figure 6.6.* Completion of the rolling is made with extension. Both upper extremities flex forward into forearm weight bearing.

Lateral flexion of the head against gravity requires synergistic action of the oblique abdominals to stabilize the thorax (Kendall, Kendall, and Wadsworth 1971). Lateral flexion of the head facilitates a lateral response in the spine. Subsequently, the trunk also laterally flexes against gravity. The hip abductor muscles are also needed to stabilize the pelvis to the thigh, to provide a fulcrum for trunk lifting (Kendall, Kendall, and Wadsworth 1971).

In side lying, both arms adduct. The bottom arm is adducted biomechanically, and the top arm is adducted actively as the baby reaches across the body. As the head and trunk laterally flex, the weight-bearing humerus abducts and may assist with trunk raising. As the trunk is raised sideways, weight is taken off the bottom arm, freeing it to abduct further and move out from under the body to assume a forearm weight-bearing position (figures 6.5, 6.6).

In side lying, the lower extremities change from a symmetrical to an asymmetrical dissociated position (figures 6.4, 6.5). The bottom leg extends at the hip and usually at the knee as the entire lower side elongates. The top leg abducts (figure 6.5). In order for the femur to abduct, the pelvis must be stabilized with synergistic contraction of the trunk muscles (Kendall, Kendall, and Wadsworth 1971).

## *Completion of Rolling*

Completion of the rolling movement is accomplished with extension and occurs from the laterally flexed position. From this position, the baby rotates and extends the head. The trunk follows the head movements.

The head position changes from lateral flexion to rotation and extension (figures 6.5, 6.6), while the trunk position changes from lateral flexion to symmetrical extension. Trunk elongation on the previously laterally flexed side is enhanced by forward flexion of the arm on the same side (which elongates the latissimus dorsi) and activation of the back extensors (Kapandji 1974).

Both upper extremities flex forward at the shoulders and adduct into a weight-bearing position (figure 6.6). The bottom upper extremity moves from adduction by the side to forward flexion and adduction. The top upper extremity moves from adduction across the body to forward flexion with adduction, thus assisting trunk extension.

The bottom lower extremity continues to extend and abduct. The top lower extremity goes through a transition from hip and knee flexion (figure 6.5) to hip abduction and extension with knee extension (figure 6.6).

### *Indications of Possible Disturbances in Motor Development*

The 6-month-old baby can roll from supine to prone by initiating the movement with flexion, transitioning through lateral flexion, and completing the movement with extension. Any deviation from this sequence may suggest that the baby is having difficulty in motor development. The transition in side lying is an important kinesiological component of the activity.

A baby who extends the head and trunk to roll may do so because of a lack of antigravity flexion and lateral flexion control. Rolling with extension interferes with further development of flexion and lateral flexion. Rolling with extension also provides abnormal feedback to the vestibular, visual, and proprioceptive systems.

Movements of the lower extremities often provide information about the status of the developmental process. Lower extremity dissociation during side lying and rolling is an important developmental milestone by the fifth and sixth months. Therefore, lack of lower extremity dissociation usually suggests a problem in motor development.

Maintenance of the lower extremities in symmetrical flexion blocks the baby from completing the roll to prone. Use of symmetrical lower extremity extension during the initiation phase of rolling eliminates the need to flex laterally in side lying. Symmetrical lower extremity extension also makes it difficult for the baby to remain in side lying, and the baby does not experience the sensory and kinesiological components developed in side lying.

If the baby has been using the ATNR functionally because of inadequate development of other movement patterns, head turning may stimulate the asymmetrical arm response. The face-side extremity assumes a position of retraction with humeral extension and abduction and elbow extension. It is difficult to roll over this arm position. The skull-side arm assumes a position of retraction with scapular adduction, humeral extension and abduction, and elbow flexion. This shoulder/arm posture restricts the baby from rolling when the head rotates. This response, whether subtle or marked, indicates a lack of development of antigravity bilateral symmetrical flexor muscle control in the neck, trunk, and shoulders. The baby cannot roll with the shoulder girdles retracted. Babies who use this pattern cannot practice rolling to the side or to prone, and they will subsequently miss the experience of side lying.

# Prone

In prone, the 6-month-old is more functional and more mobile than at five months. The baby has strong antigravity extensor control. The Landau reaction is mature; therefore, head extension reinforces back and hip extension. These extensor muscles are strong now even without reinforcement from the Landau reaction, enabling them to remain active while the head rotates, laterally flexes, and flexes.

Shoulder girdle control has continued to improve, and the arms are capable of various weight-bearing positions and various movements while weight bearing. The 6-month-old can bear weight and shift weight on extended arms and reach forward. The baby can also push backward with both arms or sideward with one arm. The baby is beginning to pivot, pulling the upper trunk laterally by strongly adducting the weight-bearing arm.

Spinal and hip extensors are becoming balanced by abdominal activation in prone. This enables a reduction in the lumbar lordosis during extended-arm weight bearing. Dynamic synergistic contraction of the hip and trunk muscles enables the baby to begin to assume a hands-and-knees position and to utilize equilibrium reactions in prone.

Balance of flexors and extensors is demonstrated as lateral righting of the head and trunk. The 6-month-old spends much of the time in prone with the weight shifted laterally and the head and trunk laterally righted. This is preparation for creeping, crawling, and climbing.

## Indications of Possible Disturbances in Motor Development

Babies at six months enjoy the prone position because they are becoming very functional in this position, pushing up onto extended arms, weight shifting and reaching for toys, and grasping and holding toys of various sizes. Difficulty with any of these activities may indicate a problem in motor development.

Poor tolerance to the prone position and poor control in this position would have been evident in earlier months. Such intolerance could be due to poor head lifting, tightness in the scapular-thoracic muscles, tightness in the scapulo-humeral muscles, tightness in the hip flexors, or lack of hip extensor activity for stability.

Elongation of the hip flexors and activation of the hip extensors are critical components needed for the baby to attain forearm and extended-arm weight bearing. If the hips remain flexed, the baby's weight is shifted forward and prevents elevation of the upper trunk. If the hip extensors (especially gluteus maximus) do not contract sufficiently to stabilize the pelvis, head and upper trunk lifting cannot occur. The hip extensors are needed to provide an anchor to the skeletal system for prone extension.

If there is tightness around the scapulae muscles and/or the muscles between the scapula and humerus, the baby will not be able to flex the arms forward past 90° for forearm or extended-arm weight bearing. Poor shoulder flexion in prone subsequently leads to increased tightness of the muscles between the scapula and humerus and poor scapulo-humeral dissociation (Quinton 1976, 1977, 1978). As the cycle continues, all reaching patterns will be affected, and the baby will have to develop compensatory reaching patterns.

Failure to achieve shoulder flexion in prone also leads to problems in trunk extension. Normal shoulder flexion activates the lower trapezius and elongates the latissimus dorsi. The lower trapezius helps with active thoracic extension (Kendall, Kendall, and Wadsworth 1971), and elongation of the latissimus biomechanically assists with thoracic-lumbar extension (Kapandji 1970a). Babies who do not practice active shoulder flexion in prone often have difficulty with achieving thoracic extension, and they have difficulty achieving continuous extension between the thoracic and lumbar spines. These babies usually use excessive lumbar extension to compensate for the poor thoracic extension.

Inability to accomplish extended-arm weight bearing will also have an effect on the hands. Without weight bearing and weight shifting on the hands, the intrinsic muscles of the hand are not elongated, and these muscles—especially the thumb muscles—may become tight. Inability to weight shift on weight-bearing hands may contribute to poor development of the palmar arches and poor development of the dissociated movements in the hand, such as quieting of the ulnar side when the radial digits function (Nash 1991).

# Extended-Arm Weight Bearing

The 6-month-old uses the shoulder girdle and upper extremity control to push up onto extended arms and open hands (figure 6.7). Shoulder girdle, upper extremity, back and hip muscle control, and spinal and hip mobility have all increased, enabling the baby to come up higher than at five months. The arms are also more adducted, bringing them in line with the body.

## Head

At six months, head control in prone is fully developed. The stable shoulder girdle provides the fulcrum from which the head moves. Head movements are dissociated from the shoulders and the trunk, and the baby can extend, flex, laterally flex, and rotate the head in prone with only subtle effects on the trunk.

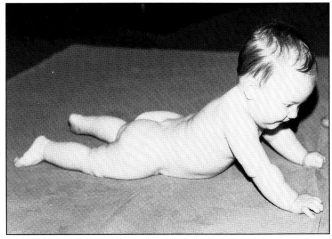

*Figure 6.7.* The 6-month-old uses shoulder girdle and upper extremity control to push up onto extended arms and open hands. Weight is borne on the heel of the hand.

Head and neck (capital and cervical) extension and hyperextension are possible at will, in or out of midline. When on extended arms or on forearms, the 6-month-old can extend the neck (cervical extension) and flex the head or tuck the chin (capital flexion) (figure 6.7). This results in elongation of the neck. Shoulder girdle depression and neck elongation suggest activity in the lower trapezius. Head and neck flexion during extended-arm weight bearing enhances downward visual gazing.

## Trunk

Spinal extensor muscle activity has increased. Range in spinal and hip extension has also increased, enabling the baby to push up higher on the arms. The hip extensors now actively stabilize the pelvis and provide the fulcrum and stability for forward elevation.

The anterior pelvic tilt is reduced by increased hip adduction and extension and by synergistic abdominal muscle activation. The abdominals provide anterior stability to the pelvis and contract in synergy with the gluteus maximus during extended-arm weight bearing.

### Upper Extremities

The same muscles are active in extended-arm weight bearing at six months as were active at five months. However, these muscles are now stronger and work more efficiently with each other to produce more functional results.

The triceps brachii contract to extend the elbows. The wrists extend biomechanically. Finger extension mobility has increased, and the 6-month-old can maintain an open hand (finger extension, abduction) when the wrist is extended. Weight is borne on the heel of the hand (figure 6.7), and the baby can make raking movements with the fingers (Erhardt 1984).

Weight is maintained on both arms when the baby pushes up onto extended arms. Head rotation during extended-arm weight bearing causes weight to be shifted to the same side to which the face turns (figure 6.9). This face-side weight shift causes weight to be shifted to the ulnar side of the face-side hand, freeing up the radial digits. The weight on the skull-side hand is shifted to the radial side, elongating the thenar muscles.

### Lower Extremities

Active extension occurs in the hips, knees, and ankles when the baby pushes up onto extended arms (figure 6.7). Active hip extension (gluteus maximus) and abdominal muscle contraction work together to neutralize and stabilize the pelvic position.

As activity levels increase, the baby practices weight-shifting activities; subsequently the lower extremities no longer maintain a posture of bilateral symmetry. Thus, dissociation of the lower extremities rather than symmetry is much more common at six months.

Ankle dorsiflexion and plantar flexion still occur in synchrony with the hip and knee. Ankle dorsiflexion accompanies active hip or knee flexion, and ankle plantar flexion accompanies active hip or knee extension.

## Pivot-Prone Extension

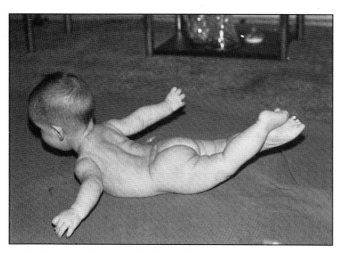

**Figure 6.8.** *The 6-month-old continues to use the pivot-prone position.*

The 6-month-old baby continues to use the pivot-prone position (figures 6.8, 6.10). At six months, pivot-prone extension is a full manifestation of the mature Landau reaction. Head extension continues to contribute to back extension through the labyrinthine system (Cupps, Plescia, and Houser 1976) and now also contributes to hip extension. According to EMG studies by Cupps, Plescia, and Houser (1976), hip extension is not a consistent component of the Landau reaction.

At the fourth and fifth months, the baby could alternate between pivot-prone extension and forearm weight bearing. At six months, the baby alternates between pivot-prone and extended-arm weight bearing (figures 6.8 to 6.11), using the increased shoulder girdle and upper extremity control.

Pivot-prone extension may be the baby's most automatic position of prone postural stability. The 6-month-old, like the 5-month-old, seems to use pivot-prone as a reinforcing position prior to movements which use marked effort (figures 6.8 to 6.11). This position may also elongate the anterior shoulder muscles in preparation for efficient contraction. According to Brunnstrom (1979), elongation of a muscle almost always occurs when a sudden burst of tension in the muscle is needed.

# Pivoting in Prone

Pivoting in prone usually occurs by the sixth or seventh month of age. It uses the new ability to weight shift on extended arms and enables the baby to reach out and move without rolling. This activity should not be confused with the pivot-prone position.

Until now, reaching in prone has been accomplished solely by forward shoulder flexion (sagittal plane movement), with the toy in or close to midline. This is the baby's first prone experience in reaching for a toy with shoulder abduction/adduction (frontal plane movements). Movement of the body over the arm is another new upper extremity weight-bearing experience.

Visual interest usually influences the baby to rotate and laterally flex the head (figure 6.12). Head and cervical spine lateral flexion stimulates spinal lateral flexion. Back extension, upper trunk elevation, and shoulder stability are maintained during each phase of prone pivoting.

## Upper Extremities

The upper extremities utilize many new movement combinations during prone pivoting. For the first time in prone, the two upper extremities perform dissociated frontal plane actions (figure 6.13).

Head and trunk lateral flexion causes the weight to shift to the arm on the face side (figure 6.12), resulting in increased shoulder adduction. The face-side weight-bearing arm can then assist the movement by adducting and pulling the body over the arm. The skull-side arm may assist the movement by abducting and pushing the trunk away from the arm. The elbows remains semi-extended. The wrists extend.

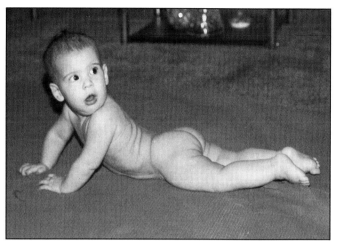

*Figure 6.9.* At six months, the baby alternates between pivot-prone and extended-arm weight bearing.

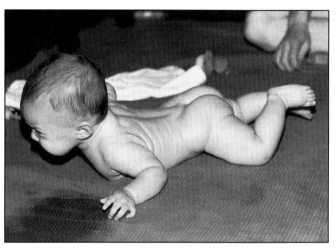

*Figure 6.10.* The 6-month-old, like the 5-month-old, seems to use pivot-prone as a reinforcing position prior to movements which use marked effort.

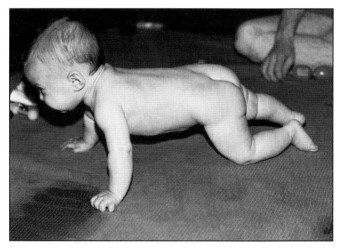

*Figure 6.11.* Pushups often occur when the baby moves out of the pivot-prone posture and places the hands near the shoulders. Strong elbow extension causes the baby to lift into a pushup position.

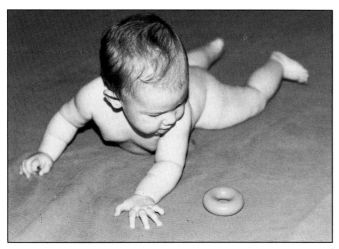

*Figure 6.12. Visual interest usually influences the baby to rotate and laterally flex the head. Head and trunk lateral flexion causes the weight to shift to the arm on the face side, resulting in increased shoulder adduction. The face-side weight-bearing arm can then assist the movement by adducting and pulling the body over the arm. The skull-side arm may assist the movement by abducting and pushing the trunk away from the arm. The elbows remains semiextended; the wrists extend.*

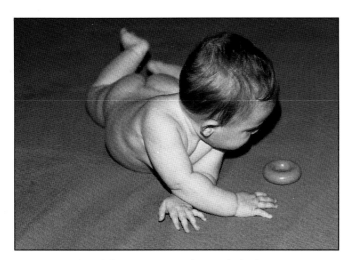

*Figure 6.13. If the wrist stays in line with the forearm, weight will be shifted to the ulnar side of the hand, freeing the radial digits, and the shoulder will externally rotate.*

If the wrist stays in line with the forearm, weight will be shifted to the ulnar side of the hand, freeing the radial digits, and the shoulder will externally rotate (figure 6.13). If the wrist goes into ulnar deviation, lateral weight shifting in the upper extremity may be positionally blocked (figure 6.12). If the weight is not shifted to the ulnar side of the hand, the radial digits are not freed, and the shoulder does not externally rotate but remains internally rotated. Ulnar deviation of the wrist is usually used when the baby has difficulty controlling the weight shift. This is often seen in low-toned babies of normal ability. However, this is also seen in abnormal motor development.

The skull-side arm assumes a position of humeral abduction, extension, and internal rotation as the body moves away. The elbow is extended and the forearm pronates, shifting weight to the radial side of the extended wrist and hand. This further elongates the thenar muscles of the hand.

The skull-side upper extremity may also push the baby into pivoting (frontal plane movement). This is a new pushing experience for the baby. Until the sixth month, upper extremity pushing was limited to pushing up into extended-arm weight bearing and pushing backwards with bilateral shoulder flexion (sagittal plane movements). Using this new pushing, the baby actually moves the body away from the weight-bearing arm.

As the trunk moves away from the skull-side upper extremity, the anterior shoulder muscles become slightly elongated. From the elongated position, the baby adducts and reaches the skull-side arm across the body, and it becomes the weight-bearing arm (figure 6.13). As weight is shifted to the skull-side arm, the face-side arm is free to reach with humeral abduction and internal rotation, elbow extension, and wrist and finger extension. This is the baby's first experience of reaching with shoulder abduction and of reaching away from the midline (frontal plane movement).

### Lower Extremities

The lower extremities are less active during pivoting. They seem to respond to the movement rather than initiating it. When the baby initiates the movement with head and trunk lateral flexion, the leg on the face side responds with flexion, abduction, and external rotation at the hip, and flexion at the knee and ankle. The other leg becomes extended, adducted, and neutrally rotated at the hip in response to elongation of the entire side (figure 6.13). Knee flexion and ankle dorsiflexion may be maintained.

# Forearm Weight Bearing

Although the 6-month-old can assume an extended-arm weight-bearing position, the baby more frequently uses forearm weight bearing (figures 6.14, 6.15). The hands are more functional in this position.

The same shoulder girdle muscles are active in forearm weight bearing as were active at five months. Because the lower trapezius seems to be increasingly more effective in maintaining scapular depression, the neck roll described at four and five months of age is not seen at six months (figure 6.14).

Humeral stability in forearm weight bearing is maintained by activation of the shoulder girdle muscles and by the biomechanical effect of weight bearing. Consequently, the elbow and forearm have increased freedom for independent movement (figures 6.14, 6.15). Through weight bearing, the humerus is mechanically stabilized and the baby can flex and extend the elbow to reach for a toy and bring it to the mouth (figures 6.14, 6.15). Active forearm supination is also seen when the humerus is mechanically stabilized.

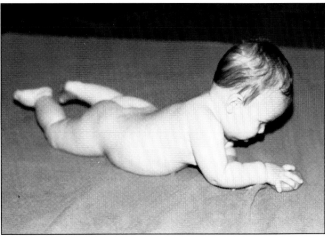

**Figure 6.14.** *Although the 6-month-old can assume an extended-arm weight-bearing position, the baby more frequently uses forearm weight bearing.*

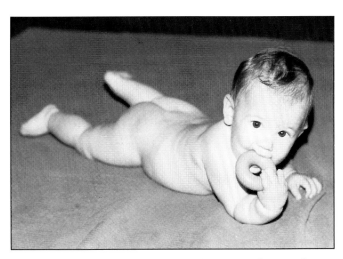

**Figure 6.15.** *The 6-month-old's hands are more functional in forearm weight bearing. The humerus is mechanically stabilized, the elbow and forearm have increased freedom for independent movement, and the baby can flex and extend the elbow to reach for a toy and bring it to the mouth.*

# Weight Shifting and Reaching in Prone

The 6-month-old has sufficient trunk, shoulder girdle, and upper extremity muscular control in prone to weight shift on forearms and extended arms. Upper extremity weight shifting can be initiated by head rotation that causes the weight to be shifted to the face side (figure 6.12), and/or shoulder girdle weight shifting that causes the weight to be shifted away from the face side (figure 6.18). The latter is a more mature weight shift in that it utilizes feedforward control and the righting reactions to free the face-side hand for reaching.

In the first weight shift, the baby turns the head toward a toy and traps the arm, which prevents reaching. In the second weight shift, the baby adjusts the posture away from the face-side arm prior to or in synchrony with head turning. Subsequently the face-side arm is free to reach. This suggests that the baby can anticipate the consequences of head rotation (for example, weight shift to the face-side arm) and thus make postural adjustments prior to the weight shift. Postural adjustments that are made prior to or in synchrony with movements are a result of feedforward information (Kelso 1982). This ability to make automatic postural adjustments for weight shifting prior to movement enables the baby to reach in many different directions.

## Upper Extremities

Increased proximal trunk and shoulder girdle control provides dynamic humeral stability, which enables further development of forearm, wrist, and finger movement components. The 6-month-old is beginning to use an increasing variety of distal movement components when reaching in prone.

### Reaching

The 6-month-old can reach for toys that are close to the body (figure 6.14) and away from the body (figure 6.16). Each of these movements uses slightly different proximal and distal movement components which are influenced by the position, size, and shape of the toy (Corbetta and Mounoud 1990). The 6-month-old can use visual information to adjust the hand during the reaching approach (von Hofsten 1990). Prior experience with the toy may also contribute to the preadjustments. Hand adjustments that are made synchronously with the reach occur as a result of feedforward information.

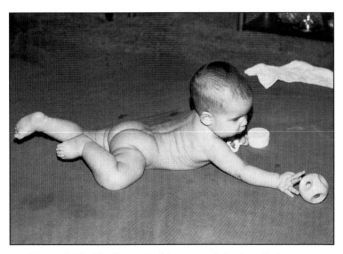

*Figure 6.16.* The 6-month-old can reach for toys that are away from the body using shoulder flexion with abduction, elbow extension, and wrist and finger extension.

The 6-month-old can functionally reach with elbow extension (figure 6.16) or with elbow flexion (figures 6.14, 6.17), whichever is appropriate for the position of the toy. Forearm pronation is usually used when the baby reaches in prone, whether the elbow is extended or flexed.

The wrist position varies according to the position of the toy and the approach of the arm to the toy. Wrist extension is the most common component (figure 6.16), but wrist flexion is used if the baby's arm or forearm comes down over the toy (figure 6.14).

Finger components of reaching are fairly consistent, whether the elbow is extended or flexed. The fingers approach the toy with MP and some degree of IP extension and abduction. The baby's hand is prepared to grasp the toy, regardless of its size or shape (figure 6.17). After experiencing and practicing grasping toys of different sizes and shapes, the baby will be able to preshape the fingers for each specific grasping pattern and combine this with the reaching components. Active wrist and finger extension is more pronounced when the baby approaches a toy with the arm resting on the surface (figure 6.16).

The position of the thumb varies, but it is almost always abducted away from the palm to some degree (figure 6.17). This prevents the thumb from interfering with finger grasping (Vogtle and Albert 1985).

## Grasp

Although the grasping pattern is influenced by the toy's size and shape, the 6-month-old usually uses a radial-palmar grasp (Erhardt 1984). The grasp is accomplished by active finger flexion (especially the radial fingers) and slight wrist extension. Wrist extension provides a tenodesis effect which strengthens the finger flexion. The 6-month-old can maintain sufficient power in the finger flexors to hold a toy even when the wrist is flexed (figures 6.14, 6.15).

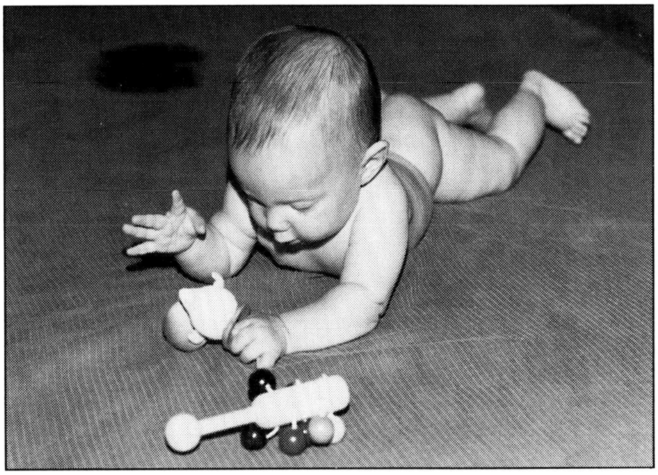

## Manipulation

The 6-month-old still has trouble manipulating toys in prone. Once the toy has been grasped with the radial digits, the baby can actively supinate the forearm to inspect the toy visually (figure 6.6), bring it to the mouth (figure 6.15), or finger it with the

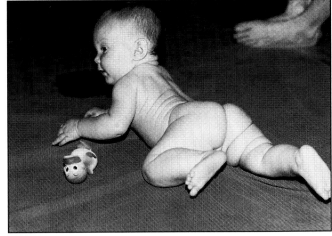

*Figure 6.17. The 6-month-old can reach functionally with elbow flexion. The baby's hand is prepared to grasp the toy, regardless of the toy's size or shape. The thumb is almost always abducted to some degree away from the palm, which prevents it from interfering with finger grasping.*

other hand. The wrist and fingers work in synchrony with the forearm, rather than in isolation. Elliott and Connolly (1984) describe this type of manipulation in which the hand is moved as a whole through movement of the arm as "extrinsic hand movement."

## *Head and Trunk*

The head and trunk respond to the shoulder weight shifting with a lateral body righting reaction which includes elongation on the weight-bearing side (figure 6.18). This response is stimulated by the asymmetrical tactile input which facilitates the body righting reaction on the head and by the labyrinthine and optical righting reactions which have been discussed previously.

The head moves with slight lateral flexion and rotation toward the reaching arm, which allows the baby to watch the reaching hand. Head rotation facilitates cervical spine rotation which, in turn, affects the thoracic spine, trunk, and pelvis. As the head and spine laterally flex and rotate away from the weight-bearing side, the trunk actively laterally flexes.

The trunk elongates on the weight-bearing side. The greater the weight shift, the greater the elongation. At the same time, the unweighted side of the trunk laterally flexes (figure 6.18).

Elongation on the weight-bearing side is important for controlled lateral flexion on the contralateral side of the trunk and for lower extremity dissociation. Elongation occurs in the muscles between the scapula and humerus, the ribs, the ribs

*Figure 6.18. The head and trunk respond to the shoulder weight shifting with a lateral body righting reaction which includes elongation on the weight-bearing side. At the same time, the unweighted side of the trunk laterally flexes. Dissociation of the lower extremities is common, and the baby may appear to be trying to creep forward.*

and pelvis, and the pelvis and femur. Tightness in any of these areas will affect the quality of lateral flexion and dissociation on the opposite side. This is an important principle used in treatment.

Lower trunk and pelvic weight shifting and lateral flexion are prerequisites to the development of dissociated and independent lower extremity movement components. These movements are precursors to functional movements in prone (such as creeping and crawling) and upright functional movements (such as walking and climbing).

## Lower Extremities

As the baby becomes more active with weight shifting, the lower extremities no longer maintain a posture of bilateral symmetry. Dissociation of the lower extremities is much more common (figure 6.18). By six months of age, there is increased mobility and increased muscle control around the lumbar spine, pelvis, hips, and knees, which enables the baby to respond to lateral weight shifting with dissociated lower extremity movements. The lower extremity on the weight-bearing side extends, adducts, and internally rotates to neutral (figure 6.18). The opposite lower extremity flexes, abducts, and externally rotates. These dissociated reactions occur as a part of the lateral body righting reaction.

When the trunk laterally flexes or laterally rights itself, the lumbar spine laterally flexes and rotates slightly. Biomechanically, this causes the pelvis to flex laterally and rotate backward on the unweighted side. These frontal and transverse plane movements (lateral flexion and rotation) of the pelvis and spine continue into the hip joint. The result is hip flexion (sagittal plane), abduction (frontal plane), and external rotation (transverse plane) of the unweighted leg, and hip extension (sagittal plane), adduction (frontal plane), and internal rotation (transverse plane) of the weight-bearing leg.

As the weight-bearing hip becomes more extended, adducted, and internally rotated, knee extension and ankle plantar flexion increase. Femoral adduction elongates the abductor muscles, helping to stabilize the pelvis on that side. Hip internal rotation increases the weight shift to that side. Each of these movements is subtle but very important for proper weight shifting.

The biomechanical importance of the subtle femoral rotation in weight shifting cannot be overemphasized. However, it must be noted that internal and external femoral rotation have different effects when the baby's position in space changes. In prone, external rotation of the right femur causes the weight to shift to the left, and internal rotation of the left femur causes the weight to shift to the left side. In supine and sitting, the opposite is true; external rotation of the right femur causes weight shift to the right, and internal rotation of the left femur causes weight shift to the right. These principles can be used in treatment.

During dissociated lower extremity movements, the baby may appear to be trying to creep forward (figure 6.18). Although these are precursor movements to creeping, the 6-month-old does not yet have sufficient motor control to actually creep on the belly.

The 6-month-old can also play with isolated knee flexion/extension movements (figure 6.19). To actively flex and extend the knee perpendicular to the floor, the hip must internally rotate to neutral; it cannot remain externally rotated. Active flexion and extension of the knee requires antigravity control of the hamstring muscles and mobility of the quadriceps muscles, especially the rectus femoris. The hip muscles must stabilize the hip in neutral rotation.

Ankle dorsiflexion and plantar flexion are still affected by movement at the hip and knee. Dorsiflexion accompanies active hip or knee flexion, and plantar flexion accompanies active hip or knee extension (figure 6.18).

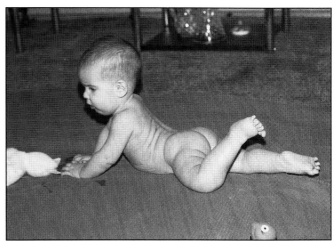

*Figure 6.19. The 6-month-old can play with isolated knee flexion/extension movements in prone.*

## Indications of Possible Disturbances in Motor Development

A 6-month-old who has difficulty assuming or maintaining lower extremity dissociation may be having problems in motor development. These problems could be caused by poor mobility in the spine, pelvis, hip, and/or knee, or by inadequate muscle control. Inability to actively weight shift and reciprocally dissociate the lower extremities will lead to serious problems in further development of pelvic and trunk control and the development of reciprocal creeping, crawling, climbing, and walking skills.

A common deterrent to lower trunk weight shifting is the prolonged maintenance of hip external rotation and ankle dorsiflexion with eversion. Marked hip abduction may or may not accompany the external rotation. When this lower extremity position is maintained in prone, the baby positionally blocks lateral weight shifting to the side. Consequently, the baby becomes discouraged from trying such movements and compensates with more symmetrical movements. Another compensation is excessive movement of the rib cage over the pelvis with lateral flexion on the weight-bearing side.

Another long-term effect of this fixing position is the lack of elongation of the hip abductor muscles. Subsequently the muscles will not become fully efficient in stabilizing the pelvis on the femur. This leads to many problems in pelvic-femoral movement and stability in crawling, walking, and standing on one leg.

Bilateral internal rotation of the femurs also signals problems in motor development. Internal rotation is usually accompanied by hip extension and adduction. As was mentioned previously, inability to actively externally rotate each femur independently will interfere with the development of active pelvic and lower extremity weight shifting. If the baby cannot actively externally rotate each femur reciprocally, the baby will not be able to initiate isolated hip flexion with abduction and will not develop dissociated lower extremity movements in prone.

Babies who continually assume an asymmetrical lower extremity position in prone, with inability to switch to the other side, may be experiencing a problem with movement control. Asymmetrical lower extremity positioning will cause asymmetrical weight bearing and weight shifting, which will eventually lead to asymmetrical development of subsequent movements.

# Pushups

By the sixth month, the baby has a strong desire to move forward but cannot yet pull forward. Efforts to move forward usually result in pushing backward on strongly extended arms, which reinforces total body extension (figure 6.20), or pushing backwards into a pushup position (figure 6.11). Moving the body forward over the arms for creeping requires many combinations of movements which most 6-month-olds have not yet developed. These will be seen in the seventh and eighth months.

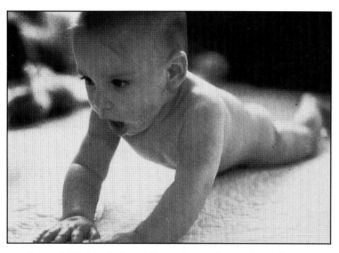

*Figure 6.20.* The baby's efforts to move forward usually result in pushing backward on strongly extended arms, which reinforces total body extension. As the baby pushes backward, shoulder flexion and elbow extension are increased. Contraction of flexor muscles (for example, abdominals) balances the extensor muscles.
(photo by Joan Mohr)

## Pushing Backward

As the baby pushes backward, shoulder flexion and elbow extension are increased (figure 6.20). The serratus anterior and lower trapezius are used to abduct and upwardly rotate the scapulae. Marked shoulder flexion elongates the pectoralis major and minor muscles and the latissimus dorsi, as well as all of the muscles between the scapula and humerus. This muscle elongation may facilitate more refined dissociated movements between the scapula and humerus.

Strong upper extremity action facilitates the oblique abdominals to contract synergistically to stabilize the thorax. As the abdominals contract, they counterbalance the strong back extensor activity, reduce the anterior pelvic tilt, and lift the abdomen from the surface (figure 6.20). The back extensors and abdominals thus co-contract to stabilize the trunk.

The lower extremities stabilize the trunk during the pushing. During this stability, the lower extremities maintain a position of external rotation. This rotation is due in part to the continued tightness of the soft tissue around the hips. External rotation of the hips during extension also suggests contraction of the gluteus maximus (Brunnstrom 1979).

Pushing backward in prone is primarily an extensor activity; however, it uses flexor muscle components. In figure 6.20, the extensor activity is obvious: widely opened eyes and mouth, and extended arms, back, and legs. The flexor activity is less apparent but still critical: shoulder flexion with adduction, lifting of the abdomen, and flattening of the lumbar spine.

## Pushing Up

The pushup phase appears between the sixth and seventh months of age, just prior to the baby's ability to move forward. It may be a precursor to the assumption of quadruped.

Pushups often occur when the baby moves out of the pivot-prone posture and places the hands near the shoulders. Strong elbow extension causes the baby to lift into a pushup position (figures 6.10, 6.11). The humeri are strongly adducted by contraction of the clavicular portion of the pectoralis majors, which synergistically activates the abdominals.

The wrist is biomechanically hyperextended as the humerus becomes perpendicular to the shoulder. The marked stretch on the finger flexors may actually cause an increase in finger flexion (figure 6.11).

As the baby pushes up, the legs stiffen, suggesting co-contraction of the muscles around the hips and knees. The gluteus maximus seems to contract with the hip flexors and knee extensors (such as the quadriceps) (figure 6.11). This stiffness interferes with the baby's moving in this position.

# Assumption of Quadruped

The 6-month-old's dissociated lower extremity movements are often precursors to assumption of quadruped (figures 6.21, 6.22). However, additional control is needed in the muscles of the trunk, pelvis, and hips for the baby to lift the hips to quadruped from the dissociated position. Most, but not all, 6-month-olds have this muscle power.

Good shoulder girdle and upper extremity control are critical for assumption of quadruped from the lateral position. The weight-bearing arm assists in lifting the trunk. The unweighted arm assists through its forward-reaching action. The upper extremities must work with each other and with the trunk and both lower extremities.

As the baby reaches forward with the unweighted arm, the latissimus dorsi and the laterally flexed side of the trunk are elongated. The reaching arm helps to pull the trunk forward and helps to lift the pelvis by stretching the latissimus dorsi. This action may facilitate lumbar hyperextension, which must be counterbalanced simultaneously by abdominal and hip adductor contraction for the baby to rise to quadruped.

Diagonal trunk muscle activity seems to occur during the lifting (figures 6.21, 6.22). The left upper extremity works with the right lower extremity, and the right upper extremity works with the left lower extremity. The development of diagonal muscle activation in the trunk is the precursor of more subtle trunk postural reactions and reciprocal and contralateral extremity movements.

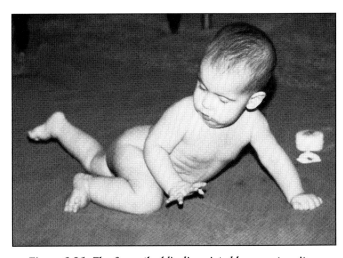

*Figure 6.21.* The 6-month-old's dissociated lower extremity movements often are precursors to assumption of quadruped.

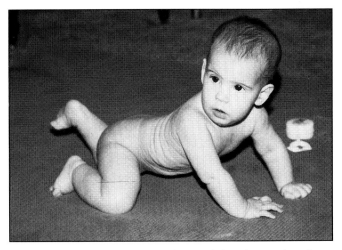

*Figure 6.22.* Additional control is needed in the muscles of the shoulder, trunk, pelvis, and hips for the baby to lift the hips to quadruped from the dissociated position. Diagonal trunk muscle activity seems to occur during the lifting.

Both lower extremities work to elevate the pelvis to quadruped. The leg muscles must coordinate contraction with the upper extremity and trunk muscles. The flexed leg moves toward adduction, extension, and internal rotation to neutral. Grading of this movement must be provided by eccentric action of the hip abductors, flexors, and external rotators so that the movement is not overshot.

The original weight-bearing leg also goes through a transition of muscle use. This leg helps to push the pelvis laterally and up by actively abducting, externally rotating, and extending against the floor. The gluteus maximus and gluteus medius seem to assist with the elevation.

Although 6-month-olds can assume quadruped, the baby cannot move in this position. The hip flexors are frequently used to stabilize the hip joints and assure pelvic-femoral stability. This usually results in a lordosis and an anterior pelvic tilt. Fixing or co-contraction is often used to provide stability when the baby assumes a new position or posture. Through experimentation with various synergistic muscle combinations, the baby will develop more dynamic muscle control in quadruped, which will ultimately enable movement in the position.

# Rolling from Prone to Supine

The 6-month-old can roll from prone to supine. However, most babies rarely practice this because they are more functional in prone. The baby is more willing to practice rolling from supine to prone, and although this motion requires more complex motor control, the baby is more proficient at it. Rolling from prone to supine continues to resemble a primitive act of falling (figures 6.23, 6.24).

Rolling from prone continues to be primarily an extension activity. Rolling occurs when the baby shifts the weight laterally and backwards and is unable to stabilize the weight on the shoulder or to counterbalance the weight shift with the trunk and lower extremity muscles (figures 6.23, 6.24). When the baby has sufficient anterior trunk and lower extremity flexor muscle control to counterbalance the backward weight shift, an equilibrium reaction occurs, and the baby recovers the original position.

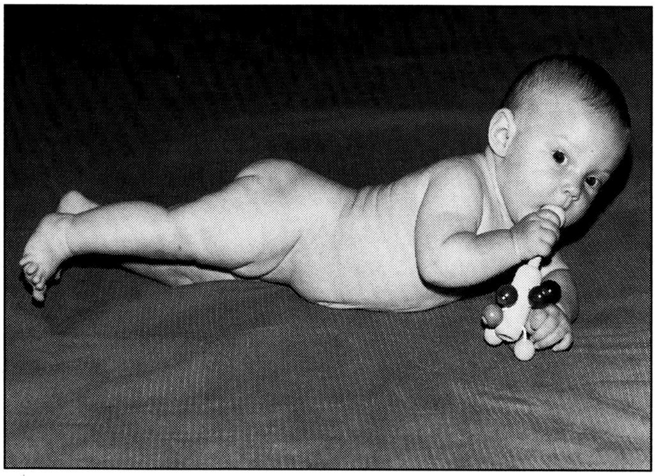

Extension is the primary initiating component for rolling from prone. It occurs in the head, the trunk, and possibly the hip (figure 6.23). These extension components, however, are becoming more balanced by antagonistic flexion components. Therefore, rolling (falling) from prone to supine is not as traumatic for the 6-month-old as it was for the 5-month-old.

*Figure 6.23. Rolling from prone continues to be primarily an extension activity. Rolling occurs when the baby shifts the weight laterally and backwards and is unable to stabilize the weight on the shoulder or to counterbalance the weight shift with the trunk and lower extremity muscles.*

## Head and Trunk

Head control is fully developed at six months. Therefore, head extension is easily and automatically balanced by flexion and lateral flexion, and head control is not lost when rolling.

Although trunk extensors are becoming more balanced by trunk flexors (abdominals), this balancing interaction does not occur as automatically as it does in the head and neck muscles, especially if trunk extension is reinforced by hip extension (figure 6.23). If the trunk and lower extremity flexors balance the extensors, an equilibrium reaction—rather than a falling reaction—usually occurs and the baby recovers the original position.

### Upper Extremities

Although at times the baby may not be able to maintain the lateral weight shift on the shoulder, the 6-month-old does have good shoulder girdle control. Humeral flexion and adduction work strongly to keep the arms forward and to counterbalance

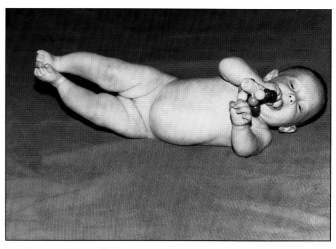

*Figure 6.24.* Rolling from prone to supine continues to resemble a primitive act of falling.

the extensor components of scapular adduction and shoulder girdle retraction during the roll. This counterbalance is maintained from the initiation to the completion of the fall. (Compare the upper extremity positions in figures 6.23 and 6.24 with 5.20 and 5.21. Of course, the fact that the 6-month-old is holding a toy may increase the flexor control.)

### Lower Extremities

Action in the lower extremities often determines whether the baby will roll to supine or will recover balance and stay in prone. Extension in the legs reinforces the total extension and usually results in the baby falling backward (figures 6.23, 6.24). Flexion in the unweighted lower extremity usually occurs when there is more abdominal activity. Therefore the baby usually does not fall backward.

# Equilibrium Reactions in Prone

By the sixth month, the baby usually has sufficient control to manage weight shifts in prone. Equilibrium reactions are used in a feedback role to recover balance when the center of gravity is disturbed. When weight is displaced laterally and backward in prone, the baby can respond with counterbalancing flexor muscle activity, restore equilibrium, and bring the body forward to its original position.

Less obvious equilibrium reactions are demonstrated in a feedforward mode. In these cases, the baby uses prior experiences with weight shifting to preadjust posture in anticipation of a weight shift, such as during reaching.

# Side Lying

By the sixth month, the baby has mastered antigravity extension in prone and antigravity flexion in supine and is now ready to combine them with antigravity lateral flexion in side lying. The baby has been practicing such precursory activities

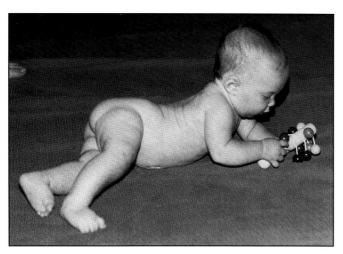

**Figure 6.25.** *Side lying includes elongation on the weight-bearing side and lateral flexion on the unweighted side. The unweighted lower extremity can easily flex, abduct, and externally rotate in conjunction with lateral flexion of the pelvis. The unweighted arm is free to grasp the toy.*

as lateral flexion during the transitional phase of rolling, and lateral flexion (righting) in response to lateral weight shifting in prone. This control now allows the baby to roll voluntarily to the side and maintain a laterally flexed posture (figure 6.25).

Side lying includes elongation on the weight-bearing side and lateral flexion on the unweighted side (figure 6.25). Elongation includes the muscles between the scapula and humerus, between the ribs, between the thorax and pelvis, and between the pelvis and femur.

As antigravity lateral flexion is practiced in side lying, the baby strengthens the muscles and the ability to recruit lateral righting reactions automatically in this and all other positions in space. Lateral righting in side lying is enhanced by feedback from the vestibular, optical, and somatosensory systems.

To activate lateral flexion in side lying, the required muscles and joints must be able to respond appropriately. The ability to respond should have been developed by previous motor activities. If there is a breakdown in any of these precursors, the 6-month-old will have difficulty achieving and maintaining lateral flexion in side lying. Therefore, failure to achieve lateral flexion in side lying indicates a disturbance in motor development.

In addition to assuming side lying, the 6-month-old can move while in side lying, demonstrating dynamic control—rather than fixing control—of muscles. Assumption, maintenance, and movement in side lying each requires progressively more control in the muscles of the head, neck, trunk, pelvis, and upper and lower extremities.

### Head and Trunk

Head control in prone is fully developed by the sixth month. Therefore, the head can adjust smoothly to other movements in the body.

Trunk control is not as well developed. The extensor muscles are still stronger and more easily recruited than the flexors, especially the abdominal muscles. Therefore the baby often uses the extensors in the side-lying position, accentuating the lumbar lordosis (figures 6.25, 6.26).

### Upper Extremities

Ability to weight shift and maintain weight on one upper extremity is a prerequisite for side lying. The baby has been practicing this since the fifth month and now has good dynamic shoulder girdle stability (figure 6.25).

While side lying, the baby's unweighted arm is free to move, reach, grasp, and play with toys. The ability to use one arm freely is an incentive for the baby to continue to practice side lying. Subsequently this posture becomes part of the reaching-grasping pattern.

## Pelvis and Lower Extremities

At six months, the baby has increased pelvic and lower extremity mobility and control. Therefore, when the baby is in side lying, the unweighted lower extremity can easily flex, abduct, and externally rotate in conjunction with lateral flexion of the pelvis (figure 6.25).

Active hip abduction and extension occur through contraction of the gluteal muscles. The gluteus medius and minimus abduct the hip and the maximus extends it (Brunnstrom 1979; Daniels, Williams, and Worthingham 1964; Kendall, Kendall, and Wadsworth 1971). Each of these muscles originates on the pelvis. Therefore, the pelvis must be fixed (or stabilized) for these muscles to work efficiently. Pelvic stability is achieved through oblique abdominal activation and positional stability. Both are needed in the initial phase of the movement. Gradually, positional stability is replaced by synergistic muscle control.

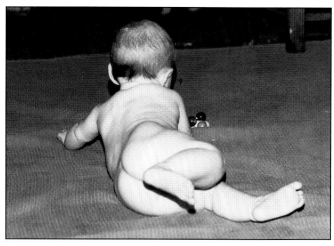

*Figure 6.26.* The baby often uses the extensors in the side-lying position, accentuating the lumbar lordosis. The baby may play with lower trunk movement while the upper trunk is stable, a movement initiated through lower extremity abduction and alternating hip flexion and extension.

While in side lying, the baby may kick and play with lower trunk movement while the upper trunk is stable. This kicking is initiated through lower extremity abduction and alternating hip flexion and extension (figure 6.26).

During kicking, pre-positioning the bottom lower extremity into hip flexion provides mechanical stability and counterbalances the backward rotation of the pelvis and trunk. The hip flexors can be used to help stabilize the pelvis and control the extension so that when the baby kicks backward, falling backward will not result (figure 6.26). If the bottom leg remains extended in side lying (figure 6.23), the baby may become unbalanced and fall backward when kicking the top leg.

Pre-positioning demonstrates feedforward postural adjustments. It indicates that the baby is aware of the consequences of weight shifting (such as falling backward). Feedforward postural adjustments become more subtle as trunk control improves.

## Indications of Possible Disturbances in Motor Development

At six months, babies who have difficulty achieving and maintaining side lying with lateral righting are demonstrating problems in motor development. The components for this activity should have been developing in previous months for integration at six months. Failure to achieve the components should have been noted in earlier months. A 6-month-old who has not integrated this postural control may be experiencing delayed or abnormal motor development.

The source of the disturbance should be analyzed for problems in muscle control, muscle and joint mobility, and integration of the sensory feedback. Possible problem areas could include poor upper extremity weight bearing, inability to weight shift on the upper extremities, poor lower trunk/pelvic stability, inability to weight shift in the lower extremities, inability to dissociate the lower extremities, and lack of awareness that a weight shift has occurred.

A problem in one or more of these areas will cause compensatory problems in the other areas. If the baby cannot weight shift to side lying from prone, the hands will not be able to be used skillfully. This may lead to problems in fine motor and play development.

If the baby cannot weight shift in the pelvis and dissociate the lower extremities, compensatory patterns for locomotion (such as bunny hopping and other abnormal gait patterns) may develop. In addition, the baby will have difficulty in coming to stand and with climbing activities.

# Pulled to Sit

At six months of age, the baby has sufficient muscle control to pull to sitting when someone holds the baby's hands. Increased antigravity flexor muscle control is evident throughout the body. As the baby pulls to sitting, integration of flexion and extension components becomes evident.

### Initiation

The baby actively participates in being pulled to sit by initiating flexion and reaching to the examiner (figure 6.27). The baby reaches with both arms, using shoulder flexion, adduction, and elbow extension. The 6-month-old can reach accurately to grasp and hold the examiner's fingers. Active finger flexion (grasp) automatically facilitates the biceps to contract (Brunnstrom 1979) and thus provides the initiation of upper extremity pulling. The lower extremities assume a position of flexion (bilateral flexion of the hips, knees, and ankles). The baby presets the body for the action. (This is another example of using feedforward action to prepare the posture for the anticipated disturbance.)

In addition, the baby tucks the chin and lifts the head from the surface. The capital flexor muscles are now strong enough to maintain the tucking of the chin. The abdominals contract with the capital flexors and the shoulder muscles to stabilize the thorax and pelvis, providing a stable base on which the head and arms can flex.

### Transition

Muscle strength plus feedback from the vestibular and visual systems enables the 6-month-old to lift independently from supine while holding the examiner's fingers. Midway in the action, the baby switches from total flexion and superimposes extension in the lower extremities (figure 6.28). It is important to note that, although the abdominal muscles contract strongly, the trunk does not flex but remains extended (figure 6.28).

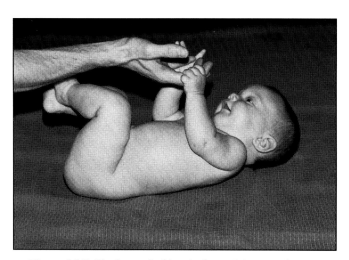

*Figure 6.27. The 6-month-old actively participates in being pulled to sit, initiating flexion and reaching to the examiner. The baby can direct the reach to grasp and hold the examiner's fingers.*

The lower extremities are most active during the transition phase as they move from total flexion toward hip, knee, and ankle extension (figures 6.27, 6.28). Although the hips remain flexed, they are starting to extend in conjunction with knee extension.

Active knee extension, by contraction of the quadriceps muscles, elongates the hamstring muscles. The stretch of the hamstrings at the knee may contribute biomechanically to hip extension.

### Completion

Completion of the forward movement to sitting is accomplished as the arms pull the trunk forward and the lower extremities extend. Lower extremity extension tips the pelvis and trunk forward because of the maintained contraction of the iliopsoas muscle.

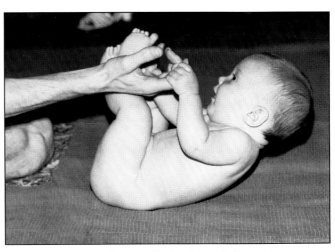

**Figure 6.28.** *Muscle strength plus feedback from the vestibular and visual systems enable the 6-month-old to lift independently from supine while holding the examiner's fingers. Midway in the action, the baby switches from total flexion and superimposes extension in the lower extremities.*

The baby's lower extremities assume a position of bilateral hip flexion, abduction, and external rotation, with knee flexion and ankle dorsiflexion. The lower extremity posture assures some stability in sitting.

# Sitting

The 6-month-old has sufficient trunk and hip control to sit erect without support (figure 6.29). The baby uses a ring position of the lower extremities for stability. The upper extremities are freed from the postural system and can be used for reaching, manipulation, or forward protective extension.

### Head and Trunk

While sitting, the 6-month-old has control of the head and trunk movements on the sagittal plane (extension and flexion). On the transverse and frontal planes, the baby has head control but not trunk control (figures 6.30, 6.31).

When the baby rotates the head while sitting, weight is shifted to the same side to which the head turns (figure 6.30). This frequently causes the baby to fall to the side, because trunk-hip control is not advanced enough to balance the weight shift.

If the weight shifts laterally on the frontal plane, the baby can respond by righting the head with lateral flexion (figure 6.31). The baby does not have the trunk-hip control to balance the weight shift and frequently falls with this direction of weight shift.

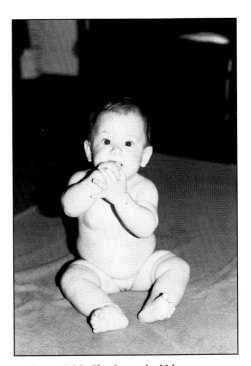

**Figure 6.29.** *The 6-month-old has sufficient trunk and hip control to sit erect without support. Ring sitting, with the hips symmetrically flexed, abducted, and externally rotated and the knees flexed, provides marked positional stability to the pelvis.*

## Upper Extremities

The 6-month-old has sufficient trunk control and lower extremity positional stability to free the upper extremities from the postural system and use them for reaching. The baby is most efficient when reaching for toys in front of the body because of some control of sagittal plane movements of the trunk. The baby can grasp the toy, flex the elbow, and bring the toy to the mouth. When attempting to reach for toys to the side, the baby often falls because of the inability to control frontal plane, lateral movements of the trunk.

The 6-month-old can prop forward on the arms but cannot yet prop sideways on one arm, which is a frontal plane movement. The baby has practiced components similar to forward propping (upper extremity weight bearing in prone, pushing backward in prone) and has sufficient shoulder girdle and trunk control to maintain the weight in the sagittal plane.

## Lower Extremities

The lower extremities play an important role in sitting. Hip muscle control and lower extremity positioning affect the stability of the pelvis and thus of the trunk. At six months, hip joint mobility has increased, enabling the thighs to rest on the supporting surface. Ring sitting, with the hips symmetrically flexed, abducted, and externally rotated and the knees flexed (figure 6.29), provides marked positional stability to the pelvis. Minimal muscle activation is needed.

This positional stability guards against lateral weight shifting of the pelvis and enables the baby to use bilateral symmetrical trunk muscles to move forward and back in a sagittal plane. Although the positioning of the lower extremities guards against frontal plane weight shifting in the pelvis (figure 6.31), it does not always guard against transverse plane weight shifting at the pelvis (figure 6.30). Transverse weight shifting is initiated by head and trunk rotation (figure 6.30). This weight shift must be controlled by strong hip external rotation, which may not be developed at six months. Therefore the baby will fall when rotating the head.

If the baby laterally shifts the weight in the trunk but does not shift the weight in the pelvis, the lower extremity pre-positioning of marked hip abduction and external rotation is usually sufficient to prevent lateral hiking of the pelvis and thus prevent the baby from falling sideward (figure 6.31). Active external rotation of the femurs is again used to stabilize the pelvis. If the lateral rotator muscles of the hip do not contract sufficiently to maintain the unweighted femur in external rotation and the femur internally rotates when the weight is shifted sideways (figure 6.32), the baby will fall.

Femoral rotation (active and passive) is very influential in weight shifting and weight bearing. In sitting, external rotation of the femur causes the weight to shift to the same side. Internal rotation of the

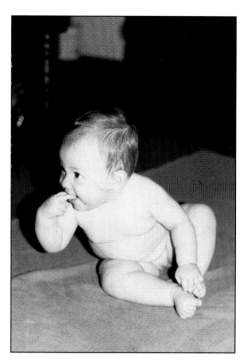

**Figure 6.30.** When the baby rotates the head on the transverse plane while sitting, weight is shifted to the same side to which the head turns, frequently causing a fall to the side.

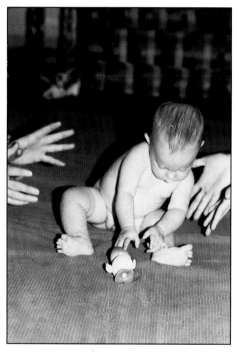

**Figure 6.31.** If the baby's weight shifts laterally on the frontal plane, the baby can respond by righting the head with lateral flexion. The 6-month-old does not have the trunk-hip control to balance the weight shift, but the positioning of the lower extremities guards against frontal plane weight shifting in the pelvis.

femur causes the weight to shift to the opposite side (figure 6.32). Bilateral symmetrical external rotation of the hips stabilizes the pelvis in neutral and blocks weight shifting (figures 6.29, 6.31).

Changes in the weight-shifting patterns in sitting are similar to those seen in prone and supine. Early weight shifting in prone and supine was initiated by head movements. As increased head and trunk control developed, weight shifting was initiated in the shoulders and pelvis, and head movements had minimal effect on the weight shift. Similarly, in sitting, head movements initiate weight shifting in the trunk. As the baby develops more trunk and hip control, head movements will have minimal effect on the weight shift, and weight shift will be initiated in the pelvis and hips.

# Protective Extension Forward

The 6-month-old consistently demonstrates forward protective extension responses in the upper extremities when the weight is displaced forward. According to Barnes, Crutchfield, and Heriza (1978), forward protective extension reactions, also called parachute reactions, appear at six to seven months and remain throughout life.

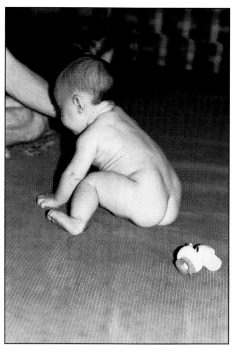

*Figure 6.32.* If the lateral rotator muscles of the hip do not contract sufficiently to maintain the unweighted femur in external rotation, and the femur internally rotates when the weight is shifted sideways, the baby will fall.

### *Indications of Possible Disturbances in Motor Development*

Babies at six months who have difficulty maintaining a sitting posture independently (with or without upper extremity propping) are demonstrating possible disturbances in motor development. Inability to maintain an independent sitting posture could be due to a number of problems that would have been subtly demonstrated in previous months: poor head and trunk control, poor upper extremity weight bearing, limited mobility in the hip joints, and poor development of hip musculature.

Subtle problems in hip musculature development become obvious in sitting. Normal development of the hip extensor muscles is needed to stabilize the pelvis posteriorly. If the hip extensors do not develop, the baby will always lean forward in sitting, relying on upper extremity propping for stability. If there is accompanying difficulty in maintaining weight on the upper extremities, the baby will not be able to sit independently.

If the baby has excessive extensor muscle activity, the hip extensors will posteriorly tilt the pelvis behind the perpendicular position. The weight is then thrown backward, and because there is not appropriate abdominal muscle activity to counterbalance the extensor pull, the baby falls backwards and cannot sit independently. Babies with excessive extensor muscle activity and poor flexor activity and mobility also tend to have difficulty maintaining supported sitting.

# Standing

Standing is still a static posture for the 6-month-old. Although there is increasing head, trunk, and hip muscle control, the baby cannot move out of the standing position. The baby is limited to sagittal plane movements of bouncing by flexing

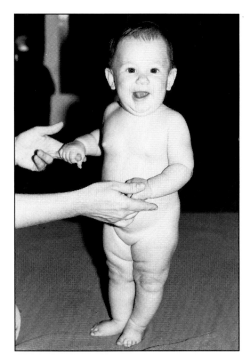

**Figure 6.33.** *The 6-month-old will take full weight on the legs and can be supported in standing by being held by the hands. Slight scapulae adduction reinforces trunk extension.*

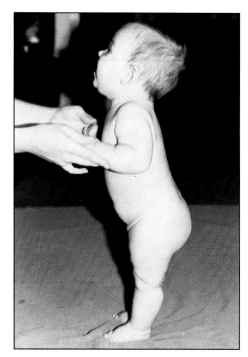

**Figure 6.34.** *The 6-month-old leans the trunk forward in standing, using back extensors for stability. The baby lacks the mobility and muscle strength to extend the hips fully in standing.*

and extending the knees. The 6-month-old can be supported in standing by being held at the trunk or the hands (figure 6.33). With either type of support, the baby will take full weight on the legs.

## Head and Trunk

Head control in standing is fully developed. When supported, the 6-month-old has sufficient active trunk control to provide a stable basis for head rotation, extension, and flexion.

Trunk control has increased, but the baby continues to rely primarily on bilateral symmetrical extensor muscle activation to maintain the standing posture. Just as in sitting, the baby leans the trunk forward in standing, using back extensors for stability. The trunk also leans forward because the mobility and muscle strength to extend the hips in standing is incomplete (figure 6.34).

As spinal extensor and hip extensor activity continues to increase, the baby will develop a lumbar lordosis. This will enable the hips to come under and align with the shoulders.

## Upper Extremities

The baby's increased spinal-trunk control allows more freedom for the scapulae. Bilateral scapular adduction is now rarely needed to reinforce thoracic extension in trunk-supported standing.

When holding an adult's hands, the baby's humeri are usually in line with the shoulders. The humeri may be slightly abducted away from the body but are more adducted than they were in previous months. The baby is beginning to flex the shoulders actively. However, shoulder extension and scapular adduction are still the strongest, most easily activated movement components and, therefore, are elicited when effort is involved.

When the trunk is held, giving more stability to the thorax, the baby may actively flex the arms. The shoulders (and thorax) may be elevated with the humeral flexion. Lack of fixation of the thorax by the abdominals suggests that the baby has the appropriate shoulder girdle muscle control for reaching in this position but not the synergistic postural control needed to stabilize the rest of the body. Therefore, further development of the shoulder and upper extremity muscles in standing is dependent on development of synergistic postural muscle activity.

It is important to note that the baby's ability to use the arms in one position (such as sitting) does not imply that they can be used in other positions. Each position and each individual activity has different but specific synergistic postural requirements.

In standing, the baby uses the hands to hold on for stability. However, when the trunk is supported, the baby can grasp a toy and bring it to the mouth.

## *Lower Extremities*

The 6-month-old bears full weight on extended legs. However, the hip extensors are not yet sufficiently active to fully extend the hips (figure 6.34). The hips are more adducted than they were at five months. The tibia are externally rotated. The knees are extended and the feet are pronated (figure 6.33).

Although the quadriceps muscles are still the major source of lower extremity extension, the hip extensors (gluteus maximus) are beginning to become more active. Contraction of the hip extensors helps the baby to remain more upright when less support is given (figure 6.33).

The 6-month-old has more control of knee flexion and extension (that is, movement on the sagittal plane) in standing than at five months. The baby no longer collapses during this activity as at five months. In addition, instead of always locking the knees into extension, the baby is beginning to grade and eccentrically contract the quadriceps. The 6-month-old still relies heavily on the external trunk or hand support to maintain the posture. As the hip extensors become more active in standing, they will work in synergy with the abdominals and quadriceps to extend the hips (Kapandji 1970b).

The feet remain on the floor during the bouncing (that is, knee flexion and extension). The posture of the feet continues to be one of pronation (dorsiflexion, abduction, and eversion). The increased effort of the movement usually results in fixing with toe flexion.

# The Seventh Month

The variety of movements and positions 7-month-olds can achieve is remarkable, as are the differences among 7-month-old babies. At this age, most babies are very active against gravity—rolling, pivoting, assuming quadruped and bear-standing, trying to crawl, coming to sitting, and pulling to stand. Up to this point, most babies have been content to have things brought to them and in exploring their bodies. Therefore, differences in motor activities among babies were less obvious. Now, however, the baby has more incentive, desire, and capability to move into the environment to secure toys or people, to explore the environment, or just to experience body movements. Therefore, the noticeable differences in abilities of babies at this age are probably related to both motivation and motor proficiency.

Practice in horizontal positions has enabled the development of antigravity movements in all three planes (sagittal, frontal, and transverse). Now the baby will begin to repeat similar components in more vertical positions such as sitting, standing, and quadruped. However, because of the different orientation to gravity, the components that were learned in the horizontal positions will have to be relearned with different synergistic postural activity.

By the seventh month, the baby usually has learned to roll from supine to prone, rarely staying in supine for very long. Play in supine is limited to exploration of small, lightweight toys, hands-on-foot play, and hands-on-body exploration.

In prone, the 7-month-old baby can achieve extended-arm weight bearing, upper extremity weight shifting, reaching on forearms and extended arms, lateral righting reactions with pelvic weight shifting, and lower extremity dissociation. The use and coordination of these components depends on the baby's trunk and extremity control and motivation. Often these components are expressed by the baby in pivoting activities.

Increased trunk and pelvic-femoral control enables the baby to assume quadruped, rock in this position, and eventually crawl. However, some 7-month-olds, especially low-tone or large babies, pull themselves along the floor by creeping on the belly rather than assuming quadruped. These babies still practice lifting the tummy from the floor and pushing up onto either their knees or feet.

Because of increased motor control, the 7-month-old can begin actively to explore the spatial and sensory characteristics of the environment. The baby can begin to learn about heights, distance, and space (Fritts 1990).

Babies with good shoulder control and strong righting reactions will spend much time playing in the side-lying position. When shoulder control is not as developed, the baby will play in more symmetrical positions in prone, such as forearm weight bearing, or will play mostly in sitting. Only a few babies will retain supine play.

The 7-month-old is very involved in play activities. Increased visual and hand control enables the baby to inspect toys. The baby enjoys new discoveries and playing with toys that change, as well as with small objects and household items. Dropping toys has also become a favorite activity (Fritts 1990).

During the seventh month, the baby is learning how to sit from quadruped. This transition requires and generates marked mobility at the hip joints as the femurs move under the pelvis. Therefore dynamic trunk-pelvic stability is required.

The 7-month-old can sit independently with the back and pelvis straight. Because of increased trunk and hip control, unsupported sitting is becoming a more functional position in which the baby can hold and manipulate toys. However, the baby does not yet have full sitting balance (or equilibrium). When balance is disturbed forward, the baby can use forward protective extension. If balance is disturbed in other directions, the baby usually responds with bilateral scapular adduction, which may throw the body backward. The 7-month-old continues to maintain the lower extremities in a posture of flexion, abduction, and external rotation, which provides positional stability to the pelvis. However, the knees are becoming more extended, modifying the earlier ring-sitting position.

Some babies pull themselves to stand at seven months, accomplishing this by transitioning from quadruped to kneeling while leaning on furniture. Once the upper extremities are stable, the baby may maintain lower extremity symmetry or transition to half kneel, push down with the arms, extend the legs, and rise to standing.

Once in standing, the 7-month-old takes full weight on the lower and upper extremities. Using the upper extremities as part of the postural system, the baby can actively bounce by flexing and extending the knees while keeping the feet on the ground. Because of increased hip extensor control and mobility, the hips are now usually in line with the shoulders.

# Indications of Possible Disturbances in Motor Development

As mentioned earlier, babies under seven months of age are content to have things brought to them, and their explorations have been very limited. Therefore, differences in motor activities among babies were less obvious and seemed to have fewer consequences. However, by the seventh month, when the baby does have the drive to move, the previously subtle differences seem "suddenly" to have more significance. All babies learn to move, but as they move, they learn to compensate for deficiencies. They learn tricks to stabilize themselves if they do not have normal muscle stability in the needed postural muscles. They may also learn compensations if they lack normal mobility to move into or out of certain positions.

Compensations are not unusual, but they reflect lack of development of full control in some area. Some babies compensate with prolonged primitive movements until the motor control catches up to permit more advanced motor responses. Quality of movement may be compromised when compensatory movements are practiced and learned.

Prolonged and uncorrected compensations have consequences, the least of which is reduced or impaired motor coordination, and the consequences can be more serious. Most compensations can be corrected with early therapy to increase motor control and/or mobility where it is lacking. The seventh month therefore becomes important in identifying the previously more subtle motor problems because of the compensations they produce or require.

# Supine

By the seventh month, most babies have learned to roll from supine to prone. Therefore, 7-month-old babies rarely stay in supine very long. Play in supine is limited to exploration of small, lightweight toys, hands-on-foot play, and hands-on-body exploration.

Antigravity flexor control in supine is fully developed and is demonstrated by the baby's ability to lift the head independently in supine and sustain it briefly (figure 7.1). During head lifting, the neck is elongated, the chin is tucked, and the shoulders are depressed. Such controlled head flexion in supine requires additional synergistic action of the oblique abdominal muscles to lower and stabilize the rib cage, subsequently providing a point of stability on which the head can flex and lift. Shoulder depression may be due to action of the lower trapezius muscles.

The baby also has sufficient trunk antigravity flexor control in supine to lift and play with the feet. From the hands-to-feet position, the baby can drop the legs to the side and relift them without having to roll to the side. These lower trunk-leg movements require action of the oblique abdominals. Such trunk control enables the 7-month-old to use equilibrium reactions in supine. Note that during trunk antigravity flexor muscle activities, the spine does not flex (figure 7.1).

As mentioned, the 7-month-old usually quickly rolls out of supine. The baby can roll to the side or all the way to prone. In either case, the side-lying position is characterized by strong lateral neck and trunk flexion. Marked lateral flexion is an indication of the balance of the flexor and extensor muscles.

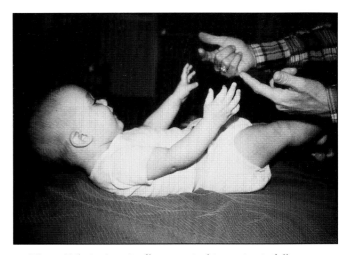

***Figure 7.1.*** *Antigravity flexor control in supine is fully developed and is demonstrated by the baby's ability to lift the head independently in supine and sustain it briefly.*

The side-lying position provides prolonged asymmetrical tactile input to the trunk, which may increase the stimulation of the body righting reaction on the head. This position also provides stimulation to the vestibular and visual systems for increased lateral head righting and lateral head control. With the increased lateral reaction, there is increased elongation of the underside.

### Indications of Possible Disturbances in Motor Development

By the seventh month, most babies are functional in prone and therefore prefer to be in prone rather than supine. If a 7-month-old baby prefers supine to prone, further observation of the baby's movements is suggested. Prone may be a difficult position. The baby may not be able to push up onto extended arms and/or may not be able to weight shift on the arms. If the baby cannot weight shift, the baby cannot reach, grasp, and manipulate toys. This is a basis for frustration which may cause the infant to prefer the supine position. The baby may need help to function in prone.

On the other hand, there may be cause for concern if a baby cannot function in supine. Low-tone babies may have difficulty flexing against gravity. They may not have the strength or control to flex their arms, head, or legs and engage in eye-hand-foot play. These problems would have been present at a much earlier age.

Babies with marked extensor tone also have difficulty in supine. They have tight extensor muscles and also lack antigravity flexor control. These problems would have been present at a much earlier age.

# Prone

Prone and quadruped are usually the preferred positions of 7-month-old babies. From these positions the baby is most independent and functional. In prone, the 7-month-old can weight bear, weight shift, and reach while on the forearms and extended arms. The baby can also weight shift in the lower trunk and pelvis and assume a position of lower extremity dissociation (figure 7.2). In addition, the baby can pivot in a circle (figures 7.3, 7.4).

In prone, the baby has sufficient trunk control and scapulo-humeral dissociation to reach in all directions for toys. Having grasped the toy, the baby often rolls to the side to play with the toy and bring it to the mouth (figure 7.2). The 7-month-old uses a radial-palmar grasp and an inferior scissors grasp with an adducted thumb and flexed fingers (Erhardt 1984).

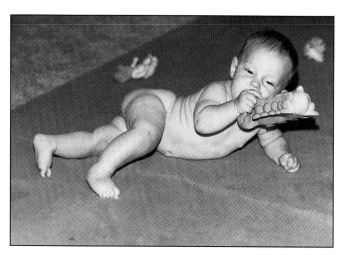

**Figure 7.2.** *In prone, the baby can weight shift in the lower trunk and pelvis and assume a position of lower extremity dissociation. Once a toy has been grasped, the 7-month-old often rolls to the side to play with the toy and bring it to the mouth.*

# Pivoting in Prone

During pivoting, both arms actively move on the frontal plane, alternating between abduction and adduction (figures 7.3, 7.4). Scapulo-humeral dissociation is needed for both pushing and reaching movements.

During the process, various weight-shifting experiences are facilitated in the hands. The arm to which the face turns is subtly, mechanically externally rotated, causing weight to be shifted to the ulnar side of the hand. This frees the radial digits for toy grasping. The skull-side arm becomes more internally rotated and the weight is shifted to the radial side of the hand, elongating the thenar muscles. These weight-shifting experiences provide varied and increased sensory stimulation to the arms, hands, and thumbs and may contribute to the development of the various palmar arches.

Pivoting is also an active means by which the baby can secure toys and explore the environment. Pivoting is not practiced by all babies. Babies who achieve quadruped early often do not pivot in prone.

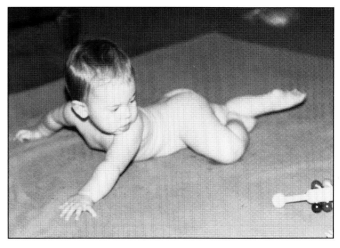

*Figure 7.3. The 7-month-old can pivot in a circle.*

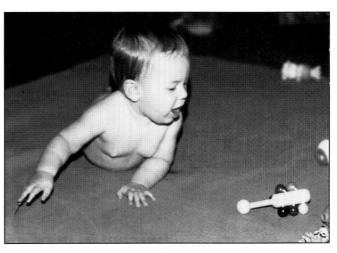

*Figure 7.4. During pivoting, both arms actively move on the frontal plane, alternating between abduction and adduction.*

# Weight Shifting in Prone

The 7-month-old spends much of the time in prone in a laterally shifted, asymmetrical posture (figures 7.2, 7.5). At six months, symmetrical postures were more common because they provided more stability. Postures which involve lateral weight shifting are important because they help to modify earlier, more primitive motor patterns. Laterally shifted postures provide varied sensory feedback through the vestibular, visual, and somatosensory systems, which may increase the activity of the body righting reactions and cause increased elongation on the weight-bearing side (figure 7.5). Much of the control for laterally shifted positions is provided by dynamic activity of the shoulder girdle and trunk muscles.

The 7-month-old with good shoulder girdle control frequently plays in the laterally shifted, asymmetrical position. The top arm is free for reaching, grasping, and manipulating toys. When trunk control is sufficient to prevent falling, the baby will also play with leg movements, abducting the top leg and swinging from flexion toward extension (figure 7.6). The 7-month-old does not yet have sufficient hip control to achieve full hip extension. At six months, hip movements in side lying caused the baby to fall backward (figures 6.23, 6.24).

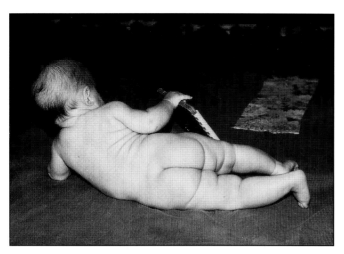

**Figure 7.5.** *The 7-month-old with good shoulder girdle control frequently plays in the laterally shifted, asymmetrical posture. The top arm is free for reaching, grasping, and manipulating toys.*

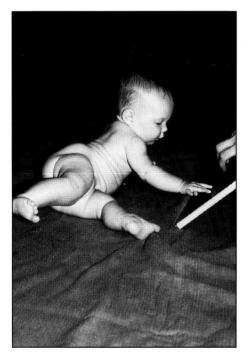

**Figure 7.6.** *The 7-month-old spends much of the time in prone in a laterally shifted, asymmetrical posture. When trunk control is sufficient to prevent falling, the baby will also play with leg*

Hip flexion and extension with the leg abducted require synergistic activity of the oblique abdominals to stabilize the trunk and pelvis. If the baby is lacking this synergistic stability from the oblique abdominals, as is often seen in abnormal motor development, hip abduction cannot be achieved.

### Indications of Possible Disturbances in Motor Development

Upper extremity weight bearing and weight shifting and lower extremity weight shifting with dissociation are critical features during the seventh month. If a baby cannot perform each of these movements, there is a problem in motor development. The baby who cannot weight bear and weight shift on the upper extremities will not be able to reach for or play with toys in prone or side lying. The baby who cannot weight shift and dissociate the lower extremities will have difficulty assuming quadruped, crawling, climbing, and walking.

# Assumption of Quadruped

During the seventh month, the baby is learning how to come to quadruped from prone. This is achieved by transitioning from prone to side lying, which includes lateral righting and lateral flexion of the unweighted side and elongation of the weight-bearing side (figure 7.7). This position enables upper and lower extremity dissociation. From the dissociated position, the baby transitions the weight over the flexed leg and pushes up to quadruped (figure 7.8).

The baby must extend and push up with the arm while abducting the extended hip and adducting the flexed hip. Hip abductors, flexors, and extensors must assist on the flexed leg to prevent overshooting.

Once in quadruped. the baby can rock forward, backward, and sideways. The rocking at first utilizes large movements with falling, then changes to smaller movements without falling. Rocking requires sufficient back stability to permit scapular freedom and mobility. Rocking provides vestibular, proprioceptive, and kinesthetic stimulation and strengthens the shoulder and hip muscles.

Most of the momentum and control for this rocking comes initially from the upper extremities. The lower extremities assume a stable position of flexion, abduction, and external rotation. Pelvic-femoral stability seems to be maintained by strong contraction of the hip flexors. In this initial fixing phase, the knees are flexed and the ankles are dorsiflexed, suggesting synergistic contraction of the hip, knee, and ankle flexors. Marked hip flexor action leads to anterior tilting of the pelvis and inhibition of the hip extensors.

As control of the trunk muscles in quadruped (especially the abdominals) develops, the baby will experiment with different muscle synergies to stabilize the pelvic-femoral joints. As the abdominals and hip extensors become more active, the baby will be able to rock forward through a greater range. The baby will also experiment with lateral and diagonal (contralateral) weight shifting (figure 7.10). As control increases in lateral and diagonal weight shifting, the baby will begin to crawl reciprocally.

Weight shifting on the hands while in quadruped also contributes to the development of the palmar arches of the hand (Nash 1991). According to Kapandji (1970a), the hand has three arches running in three different directions. The longitudinal arch runs from the wrist to the tips of the fingers, the transverse arch corresponds to the concavity of the wrist, and the oblique arch is formed by the thumb opposing the other fingers.

When first assuming quadruped, the baby rocks primarily in a forward/backward direction, due to fixing with the hip flexors. Forward and backward rocking in quadruped facilitates development of the longitudinal arches. As more trunk-hip control develops, the baby shifts weight laterally and diagonally. These directions of weight shift contribute to development of the transverse and oblique arches.

## Indications of Possible Disturbances in Motor Development

Babies who cannot assume quadruped by the seventh month may just be slow in gross motor activities. It is important to check if any other areas are slow to develop, or if in fact the baby is ahead in other areas, such as fine motor or speech. If other areas are not delayed, there is usually little cause for concern that the baby does not assume quadruped.

Inability to assume quadruped could be related to the baby's size. Heavy babies often stay on their bellies for a long time. Low-toned babies also frequently have difficulty assuming quadruped.

On the other hand, demonstration of delay in other areas could be cause for further evaluation. Problems that could contribute to the baby's inability to assume quadruped include poor upper extremity weight bearing, poor upper extremity weight shifting, poor lower extremity dissociation, poor ability to weight shift, and lack of interest.

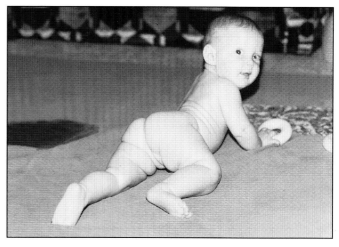

*Figure 7.7.* During the seventh month, the baby is learning how to move to quadruped from prone. This transition is initiated with lower extremity dissociation. Some babies begin to locomote by the primitive means of belly creeping.

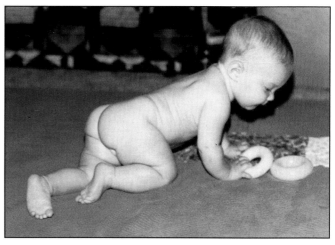

*Figure 7.8.* From the dissociated position, the baby transitions the weight over the flexed leg and pushes up to quadruped. When lower trunk-hip control is sufficient, crawling occurs.

The baby's posture in quadruped is significant regarding trunk control. When a baby first assumes quadruped, an anterior pelvic tilt is commonly seen. However, the anterior tilt is soon modified by increased control of the abdominals and hip extensors.

If the baby continues to fix with the hip flexors, the anterior tilt is not modified, and the baby is not using the abdominals and hip extensors. This leads to poor ability to rock forward, laterally, and diagonally. Subsequently, weight shifting over the hands is not practiced and development of the palmar arches may be affected.

Maintenance of the anterior tilt in quadruped also interferes with scapular and head control. Scapular winging and neck hyperextension usually occur as a result of anterior tilting of the pelvis in quadruped. Subsequently the baby will have difficulty crawling and may resort to bunny hopping.

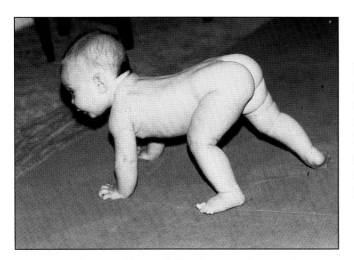

*Figure 7.9. From quadruped, the 7-month-old may push up into a "bear-standing" position. The position elongates the hamstring and gastrocnemius muscles.*

# Bear-Standing Position

From quadruped, the 7-month-old may push up into a "bear-standing" position (figure 7.9). This position requires stable shoulder girdle control and lower extremity mobility. The bear position elongates the hamstring and gastrocnemius muscles at their origins and insertions. This is a good position to work toward when treating infants with movement problems, especially those who have high tone.

# Creeping

Most babies assume quadruped by seven months and proceed to crawl on their hands and knees. However, some babies, usually large or low-tone babies, may locomote by creeping on their bellies. The obvious components necessary for belly creeping are upper extremity weight shifting, trunk righting reactions which can alternate between the right and left sides, pelvic weight shifting, and lower extremity dissociation (figure 7.7).

Creeping appears to be a movement progression developed in association with the body righting reaction (figure 7.7). Creeping has the background components of body righting: lateral weight shifting, trunk elongation and hip extension on the weight-bearing side, and trunk lateral flexion and hip flexion on the unweighted side. As the unweighted arm reaches forward, the flexed side is elongated, and it becomes the weight-bearing side. Consequently, the originally elongated side laterally flexes as a result of being unweighted, and the extremities assume their dissociated positions.

Creeping is a primitive means of moving. Some babies may start with creeping movements (figure 7.7) but advance to quadruped crawling when the lower trunk-hip control is sufficient (figure 7.8).

There is significant confusion regarding the use of the words *creeping* and *crawling*. The definitions used here have been taken from Brazelton (1969, 158): "Creeping is distinguished from crawling by the fact that the infant's abdomen is on the ground. A crawl results when a baby gets up on his elbows and bent knees."

# Crawling

For many 7-month-old babies, crawling on hands and knees is the primary means of locomotion. To crawl, the baby must be able to lift the trunk from the floor while weight bearing and weight shifting on extended arms and flexed hips.

Although these components may resemble those used in belly creeping, the synergistic postural stability needed in quadruped crawling is different from that needed for belly creeping. Upper and lower extremity weight bearing and weight shifting occur synchronously; therefore diagonal synergistic control of the trunk muscles is needed (figures 7.10, 7.11).

Reciprocal extremity movements, or simultaneous movement of contralateral upper and lower extremities (figure 7.10), utilize diagonal synergistic control of the trunk muscles and counterrotation of the spine. In order to perform this controlled movement, the baby must first be able to weight shift independently on the upper and lower extremities. These extremity movements prepare the spine for more controlled movements.

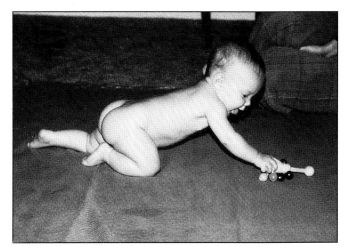

**Figure 7.10.** *Contralateral lifting of the extremities requires diagonal synergistic trunk control. To crawl, the baby must be able to maintain a lifted trunk while weight bearing and weight shifting on extended arms and flexed hips.*

When weight is shifted laterally from one weight-bearing extremity to another, there is concomitant rotation of the spine away from the weight-bearing extremity. This rotation is noticed when ipsilateral weight shift occurs in the upper and lower extremities (such as side lying) (figures 7.2, 7.7). However, this rotation is not noticed when contralateral weight shift, as in reciprocal crawling, occurs in the upper and lower extremities (figure 7.10). The rotation is not obvious because counterrotation occurs.

In counterrotation (figure 7.10), the upper spine rotates toward the unweighted upper extremity (here, the right). The lower spine rotates toward the unweighted lower extremity (the left). Neither direction of rotation is noticed because they balance out each other. According to Kapandji (1974), maximum rotation occurs in the disks immediately above and below the disk at T-7, T-8. Therefore, T-7, T-8 may be the pivotal point for counterrotation. Counterrotation is an important biomechanical

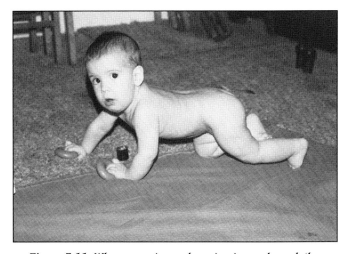

**Figure 7.11.** *When assuming and moving in quadruped, the baby frequently reaches for and carries toys in the hands.*

characteristic because it enables reciprocal extremity movements in creeping, crawling, and walking. This would suggest that thoracic spine mobility is important for reciprocal extremity movements.

When babies assume and move in quadruped, they frequently reach for and carry toys in their hands. The baby usually grasps the toy with a radial palmar grasp with adduction of the thumb (Erhardt 1984) (figures 7.10, 7.11). When crawling with a toy in the radial digits, weight is shifted to the ulnar side of the hand, which encourages forearm supination and/or shoulder external rotation. Toy transport is an important step in the baby's development of hand control (Nash 1991).

### *Indications of Possible Disturbances in Motor Development*

The most obvious problem in crawling would be demonstrated as bunny hopping. This mode of locomotion uses bilateral symmetrical movement of the lower and upper extremities. It is used by babies who have difficulty with lateral weight shifting, lower extremity dissociation, and diagonal trunk control. Babies who practice this method of crawling should be evaluated further, because this often is a precursor of problems in walking.

# Quadruped to Sitting

From quadruped, the 7-month-old baby may start to push back to sitting (figures 7.12, 7.13). This maneuver requires good upper extremity strength, good trunk control, and good hip control and mobility. Therefore, at seven months most babies transition from quadruped to prone, rather than to sitting.

The transition from quadruped to sitting is initiated with a lateral weight shift in which the unweighted lower extremity responds with flexion, abduction, external rotation, and knee flexion so that the foot is placed on the floor (figure 7.12). The head and trunk respond with lateral flexion. While weight bearing, the baby actively externally rotates the weight-bearing hip (figure 7.12, left hip).

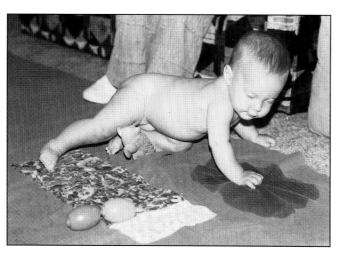

Active external rotation of this hip pulls the pelvis and trunk backwards to sitting (figure 7.13). The baby maintains the unweighted lower extremity in external rotation with the foot on the ground and thus controls the pelvic weight shift (figure 7.13). Active external rotation of the unweighted leg brings the baby up to sitting by weight shifting the pelvis and trunk.

As will be seen, the transition from quadruped to sitting (figures 7.12, 7.13) is the reverse of the transition from sitting to quadruped (figures 7.18, 7.19).

*Figure 7.12. From quadruped, the 7-month-old may start to push back to sitting.*

# Pulled to Sit

Because 7-month-olds dislike the supine position, it is usually difficult to get them into this position to pull them to sit. However, if babies do not deliberately roll out of the position, they can pull themselves up to sitting (figure 7.14). The baby independently flexes the head and actively pulls with the arms, and there may be slight scapular adduction and shoulder elevation to reinforce the upper trunk control. The abdominals contract, the hips flex, the knees begin to extend, and the ankles plantar flex. When the knees extend, the hamstrings are elongated. This may facilitate hip extension, which in turns brings the baby up to sitting.

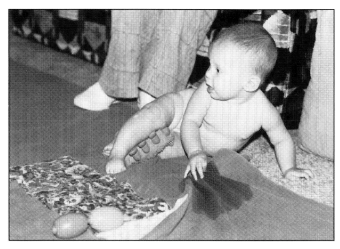

*Figure 7.13. Moving from quadruped to sitting requires good upper extremity strength, good trunk control, and good hip control and mobility.*

# Sitting

The 7-month-old finally has the trunk and hip control to sit independently and use the hands to reach out or to manipulate toys. Although pelvic-hip control has increased, the baby still uses lower extremity positional stability, especially when concentrating on fine motor tasks (figures 7.15, 7.16).

While sitting independently, the 7-month-old can reach out with one or both hands (figures 7.15, 7.16). When obtaining a toy is the primary objective, the baby establishes postural stability prior to reaching. Postural stability still includes lower extremity abduction, flexion, and external rotation. Prior establishment of postural stability is another example of the baby's increasing use of feedforward information to control and refine movements.

When the trunk is stable, the baby initiates the reach from the shoulder girdle (figure 7.16).

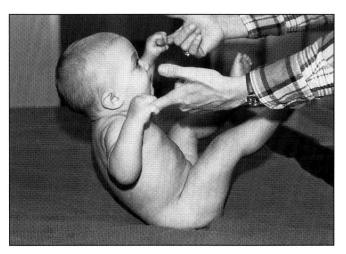

*Figure 7.14. The 7-month-old can pull up to sitting, independently flexing the head and actively pulling with the arms. The hips flex while the knees extend and the ankles plantar flex.*

The stable trunk provides the foundation from which the scapular muscles can contract. Dynamic scapular stability subsequently provides stability for humeral movements. Dynamic stability of the humerus enables variations in elbow-forearm movements. Therefore the baby can use forearm adjustments (elbow extension/flexion and forearm rotation) to orient the hand to different toys (figures 7.15, 7.16).

The baby grasps the toy with a radial palmar grasp, with thumb abduction/adduction (Erhardt 1984). Having grasped the toy, the baby can bang and shake it, visually inspect it by rotating the forearm, and transfer it from hand to hand (Fagard 1990; Corbetta and Mounoud 1990). The baby can also retain a toy in one hand and reach for another toy with the other hand. This demonstrates the increased dissociation between the two extremities. They are no longer dominated by mirrored reactions (Fagard 1990; Corbetta and Mounoud 1990).

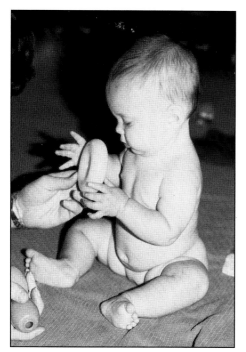

*Figure 7.15. The 7-month-old has the trunk and hip control to sit independently. The baby begins to use forearm supination during bilateral reaching. Postural stability is maintained by bilateral lower extremity abduction and external rotation.*

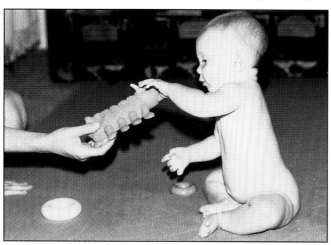

*Figure 7.16. When the trunk is stable, the baby initiates the reach from the shoulder girdle. The baby sits erect with beginning evidence of a lumbar curve.*

As increased pelvic-hip control develops, the baby begins to experiment with new lower extremity positions. This is usually done when the baby is not using the hands to inspect or manipulate toys (figure 7.17). The dominant lower extremity posture of hip flexion, abduction, external rotation, knee flexion, and ankle dorsiflexion with eversion is modified by increased hip adduction, knee extension, and ankle plantar flexion (figure 7.17). The narrower base in sitting is indicative of increased dynamic hip-pelvic-trunk postural control.

Increased spinal-trunk extension enables the 7-month-old to sit erect with some evidence of a lumbar curve (figure 7.16). The baby has full head control and can move the head in any direction. Head movements, however, have an effect on the trunk. Head rotation causes trunk rotation (figure 7.17). Initially the shoulder girdle and upper trunk rotate over a symmetrical stable pelvis, but as the baby develops more trunk and hip control, the entire trunk, including the pelvis, rotates over the femur (figure 7.17). Rotation of the trunk and pelvis over the femur is an important step in development, providing pelvic femoral mobility and helping to develop dynamic hip control.

Head and trunk rotation in sitting cause weight to be shifted to the same side to which the face turns (figure 7.17). The legs are used to prevent and/or control the weight shift (just as they were in early prone weight shifting). Initially, positioning of the legs in wide abduction and external rotation prevents movement of the center of gravity during head rotation in sitting. Next, the weight shift is controlled by active external rotation and abduction of the skull-side leg (figure 7.17). At this age, internal rotation of the skull-side leg, which is seen in later months, would allow the weight to shift too far to the face side and would result in the baby falling to the face side. Therefore, active hip external rotation and abduction are important early control mechanisms for postural stability in sitting. This postural stability must be established prior to the weight shift.

When the baby depends on lower extremity positional stability and symmetrical alignment, the trunk and reaching movements are limited to the sagittal plane (figures 7.15, 7.16). When pelvic-femoral control develops further, the baby will be able to reach while rotating (movement on the transverse plane) (figure 7.17). In sitting, lateral weight shift of the trunk (frontal plane movement) is the last to develop.

## Indications of Possible Disturbances in Motor Development

Inability to sit unsupported by the seventh month of age is an obvious developmental problem. In most situations the baby demonstrates problems in other areas of motor development as well.

Babies who do not have good pelvic-hip control continue to use the stable symmetrical lower extremity/pelvic posture. Exclusive use of this posture leads to the development of hypermobility of the thorax over the pelvis and prevents the development of pelvic-hip mobility. Maintenance of this posture also contributes to tightness of the hamstring muscles.

# Sitting to Quadruped

Once independent sitting is established, the 7-month-old initiates transitions from sitting to prone or quadruped. The baby makes this transition by moving the trunk and pelvis forward over the tibia (figures 7.18, 7.19). The leg is actively tucked under the trunk as the body reaches forward. As the weight shifts forward onto the hands, the nonweight-bearing leg stays in abduction and external rotation. Once the arms and trunk are stable, the unweighted leg moves toward adduction and neutral rotation, which brings it into line with the trunk. The weight-bearing leg actively moves toward hip internal rotation and extension.

The trunk remains symmetrical during these transitions and moves as a total unit on the sagittal plane over the hip joint (figure 7.18). Marked hip joint mobility, especially on the transverse plane (rotation), is needed. The weight-bearing hip remains markedly externally rotated during the transition and then actively internally rotates to neutral at the completion of the movement. The opposite leg is actively maintained in hip flexion, abduction, and external rotation with knee flexion. This position of the unweighted leg may stabilize the pelvis and trunk during the transition.

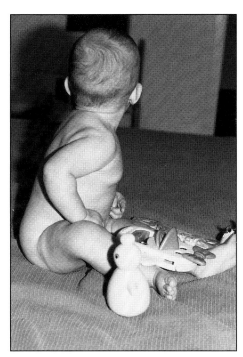

*Figure 7.17.* The 7-month-old has full head control and can move the head in any direction. Head rotation will cause trunk rotation.

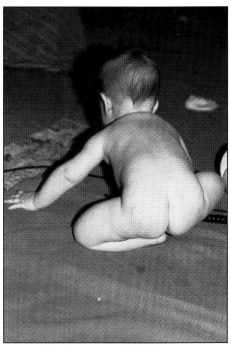

*Figure 7.18.* The baby makes the transition from sitting to quadruped by moving the trunk and pelvis forward over the tibia.

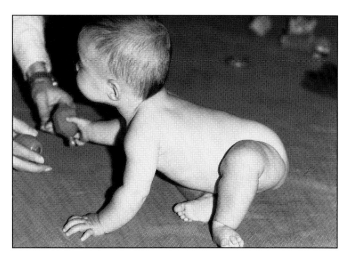

Figure 7.19. The 7-month-old actively tucks the leg under the trunk as the body reaches forward.

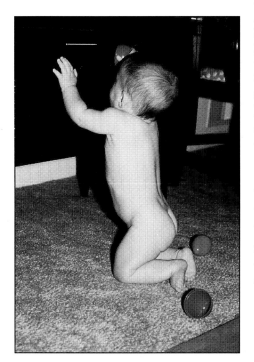

Figure 7.20. Rising to kneeling: the baby crawls to a support and stabilizes the lower trunk and center of gravity by tilting the pelvis anteriorly and fixing it there with the hip flexors. From this stable position, the baby can lift the hands to the furniture and assume a kneeling position.

Controlled upper extremity reaching and weight bearing, trunk stability, and marked hip joint mobility are needed for this transition to quadruped. Trunk symmetry with hip mobility is the distinguishing characteristic of the movement at seven months. Use of trunk rotation to transition to quadruped comes later. If shoulder, trunk, and hip control are not sufficient to allow movement to quadruped, the baby will transition to prone.

# Rising to Stand

By the seventh month, many babies are beginning to transition themselves to stand by pulling up on furniture or people. From the quadruped position, the baby crawls to furniture and stabilizes the lower trunk and center of gravity by tilting the pelvis anteriorly and fixing it there with the hip flexors. From this stable position, the baby can lift the hands to the furniture and assume a kneeling position (figure 7.20). The baby then pushes down with the hands, extends the legs, and lifts the body (figure 7.21). Some babies rise by symmetrically extending both lower extremities, others weight shift and assume a half-kneeling posture as they push down with their hands. Once standing, the baby maintains the weight on the upper extremities while adjusting the legs under the pelvis (figures 7.21, 7.22).

## Indications of Possible Disturbances in Motor Development

Upper extremity weight bearing is a critical component in the baby's rising to stand and in maintaining standing. Babies who have difficulty with upper extremity weight bearing and weight shifting cannot bring themselves to standing and cannot stand independently.

# Independent Standing

When the baby's legs are in a stable position, the arms are freed from their postural role and become more functional. The baby begins to try stabilizing with one hand as the other hand reaches, bangs, and pulls objects (figure 7.22). Good bilateral hand play is not yet possible because at least one arm is needed for stability.

When the baby reaches for a toy or looks at something while standing, the body follows the head movements. In early standing, head rotation facilitates upper body rotation but not lower trunk rotation. The lower trunk, pelvis, and lower extremities remain symmetrical and stable, assuring stability to the center of gravity (figure 7.22).

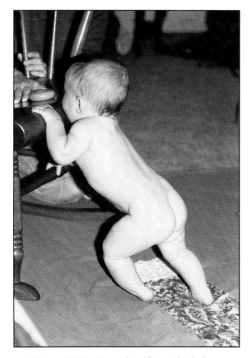

**Figure 7.21.** *From kneeling, the baby pushes down with the hands, extends the legs, and lifts the body. Once the baby is standing, the weight is maintained on the upper extremities as the baby adjusts the legs under the pelvis.*

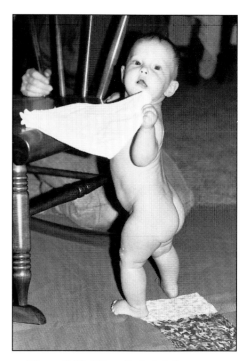

**Figure 7.22.** *When the baby's legs are in a stable position, the arms are freed from their postural role and become more functional. The baby begins to experiment, stabilizing with one hand as the other hand reaches, bangs, and pulls objects. The lower trunk, pelvis, and lower extremities remain symmetrical and stable, assuring stability to the center of gravity.*

Rotation of the upper trunk over the pelvis is also seen in sitting but soon changes so that rotation includes the pelvis rotating over the femur. If the change to trunk and pelvic rotation over the femur does not occur, the baby will develop abnormal mobility of the trunk over the pelvis, and normal pelvic-femoral development will not occur.

## Lower Extremity Weight Shifting: Cruising

Once babies can use the legs to stabilize themselves in standing, they begin to experiment with pelvic-lower extremity weight shifting. This experimentation usually includes sideward cruising along the furniture. Sideward cruising is movement on the frontal plane and requires hip abduction/adduction control. In addition, upper extremity stability and weight shifting are needed for this new, lower extremity, frontal plane movement (figure 7.23).

Sideward cruising along the furniture is initiated by lateral weight shifting in the pelvis. Active adduction brings the center of gravity over the nonmoving, weight-bearing leg (figure 7.23, left leg). The hip abductors must contact eccentrically and synergistically with the hip adductors to control the amount of weight shift. Once the weight is on this leg, the other leg is free to abduct. Hip abduction is usually accompanied by ankle/foot eversion.

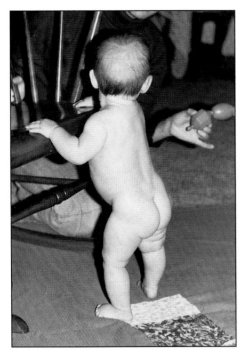

*Figure 7.23.* Once the baby can use the legs to stabilize the body in standing, the baby begins to experiment with pelvic-lower extremity weight shifting, which usually includes sideward cruising along the furniture.

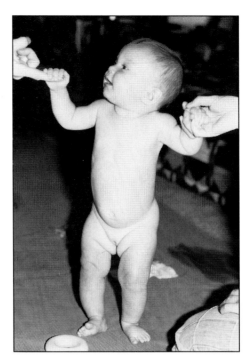

*Figure 7.24.* At seven months, the baby has sufficient trunk and hip control to take full weight on the legs when held by the hands.

As the nonweight-bearing leg abducts, the weight-bearing leg must also abduct to move the center of gravity. As the weight-bearing leg abducts, weight is shifted to the medial side of the foot and pronation increases. Once the nonweight-bearing leg is placed and begins to accept weight, it adducts to move the center of gravity, which permits the weight-bearing leg to unweight and adduct.

In early cruising, the feet may not participate in the weight-shifting activity but may remain pronated, with the weight shifted medially, throughout the activity. (At a later time, the weight-bearing foot inverts when weight is shifted onto it by hip adduction.) The baby who is unsteady during cruising may curl the toes to increase tone in the lower extremities and thus increase the stability. (Weight shifts in the foot will follow a pattern similar to that in the hand during extended-arm weight bearing.)

Although 7-month-olds can bring themselves to standing, they cannot yet lower themselves to the floor. This is accomplished by falling or "sitting down." Babies don't seem to mind the fall and thus are not deterred from standing up again. During the transition to the floor, the baby shifts the weight posteriorly, with a posture that resembles sitting down. The pelvis is well behind the shoulders and the feet, and the ankles are maintained at 90°.

## *Indications of Possible Disturbances in Motor Development*

Babies who have difficulty with weight shifting in prone will have difficulty with weight shifting in standing. If they try to reach with the arms and the legs do not adjust, they will fall. Cruising sidewards provides lower extremity practice in frontal plane control. Babies who do not cruise sidewards often have difficulty with forward walking.

# Supported Standing

When held in standing, the 7-month-old takes full weight on the legs. The baby can be held by the hands (figure 7.24) or around the chest (figure 7.25). The baby has sufficient trunk and hip control to manage this reduced support.

# Walking

By seven months of age, most babies attempt to walk when supported in standing (figure 7.25). Forward walking at this age is usually described by a steppage gait. The lower extremities are alternately flexed and extended while they are maintained in abduction and external rotation. Minimal step length is achieved with this posture, and the legs do very little to advance the body forward. The baby progresses forward primarily by leaning forward in the upper trunk and by depending on the supporting person to move forward (figure 7.25). Marked scapular adduction and a lordosis is often noticed in these early walking attempts.

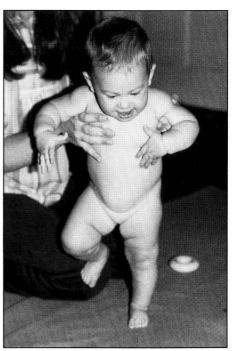

***Figure 7.25.*** *By seven months of age, most babies attempt to walk using a steppage gait when supported in standing. The baby progresses forward primarily by leaning forward in the upper trunk and by depending on the person who is supporting the chest to move the baby forward.*

# The Eighth Month

Babies at eight months are very busy and active in exploring the environment. They can transition through many positions and do not stay in any one position very long. They can crawl and move from sitting to quadruped and back. From quadruped, they can pull themselves to stand at furniture and cruise around the furniture. The desire to move and explore leads them more and more into the upright position. Therefore it is not unusual to find babies at this age climbing up onto low furniture or attempting to climb stairs. In the process of moving from quadruped to stand, the 8-month-old may now stop in the kneeling position and play.

Although there is a strong desire to move and explore independently, there is also increased interest in small objects. The baby uses the increasing finger and thumb dexterity to pick up small objects, manipulate them, explore them visually and tactually, and bring them to the mouth.

Sitting equilibrium reactions and sideward protective extension are present. Therefore the 8-month-old can achieve various independent sitting postures and changes in postures without difficulty. The 8-month-old can easily transition from sitting to prone or quadruped. The baby can freely rotate the trunk and pelvis because the trunk and hip control to support this movement has developed.

Most babies at this age enjoy and prefer standing activities. They also enjoy cruising around the furniture or walking with their hands held.

## Supine

Most 8-month-old babies do not like supine. When placed on their backs for diaper changes or dressing, they quickly try to roll over to get to a more functional independent position.

## Prone

Prone is a versatile position for 8-month-olds, but they are usually not content just to stay on the stomach and quietly play. When placed in prone, babies usually move quickly to quadruped to crawl or to sit.

# Sitting

Although 8-month-olds may use positional stability in sitting, they are no longer dependent upon it. The pelvic-femoral muscles and trunk muscles are sufficient to stabilize the posture. Subsequently, the baby experiments with and uses a variety of lower extremity positions when sitting. Variability is an important characteristic of normal development.

The ring-sitting posture is the most stable and usually is used when the baby is engaged in fine motor tasks (figure 8.1). Both lower extremities are flexed, abducted, and externally rotated at the hips, the knees are flexed, the ankles are dorsiflexed. When effort is involved, active extension or flexion of the toes often occurs, which indicates that the legs are actively involved in the postural control. Prolonged use of the ring-sitting position, with no variations of the lower extremity positions, may indicate that there is a problem in the development of pelvic-femoral muscle control.

As the pelvic-femoral muscles become more efficient in controlling the sitting posture, the baby narrows the base of support. The legs progress toward a long-sitting posture in which the hips are more adducted and less externally rotated and the knees are extended (figure 8.4).

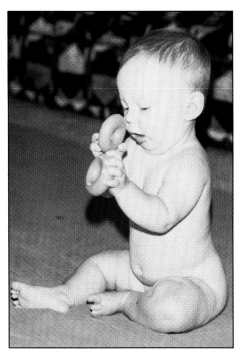

*Figure 8.1.* The ring-sitting posture is the most stable and usually is used when the baby is engaged in fine motor tasks.

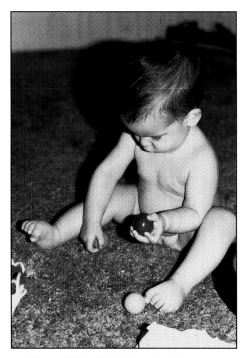

*Figure 8.2.* Initial attempts at long sitting often involve widely abducted legs with semi-knee extension. The 8-month-old is beginning to use active forearm supination, no longer needing to adduct the arm to the side to stabilize the humerus. The baby can grasp two objects simultaneously.

Initial attempts at long sitting often involve widely abducted legs with semi-knee extension (figure 8.2). When this posture is new, or when the fine motor activity is intense, the baby may try to compensate for the lack of positional stability at the hips by curling the toes. Toe curling increases lower extremity tone and stability. Strong, active external rotation of the hips is also frequently used to increase pelvic stability.

Another modification of the lower extremity posture is a combination of ring and long sitting (figure 8.3). One leg is flexed, abducted, and externally rotated at the hip, with knee flexion and ankle dorsiflexion. The other leg is more adducted and less externally rotated at the hip, and the knee is extended. The ankle may plantar flex. The asymmetry in the lower extremities causes a weight shift toward the leg that is flexed, abducted, and externally rotated. This weight shift becomes obvious when the baby tries to move (figure 8.5).

Long sitting with the knees straight and pelvis vertical requires mobility in the hamstrings (figure 8.4). When the quadriceps extend the knees, the hamstrings are stretched. As babies practice this posture, they gain pelvic-femoral-knee mobility.

If there is tightness in the hamstrings and the baby fully extends the knees, the pelvis will tilt posteriorly and the trunk will flex. This posture is not seen in normal development.

Because the baby no longer needs the legs for postural stability, the legs can be used to orient the body toward toys or people. Babies at eight months frequently use lower extremity movements to adjust the trunk orientation. The baby can realign the body so as to be facing the toy by actively abducting and externally rotating one hip while flexing the knee (figure 8.5). If the toy is out of reach, the baby can then lean the symmetrical trunk over the flexed leg to reach it (figure 8.5). Reorientation of the body allows the baby to move the trunk on the sagittal plane when reaching for the toy. At this age, this is a more stable method of reaching than moving the trunk on the other planes.

During the eighth month, the baby frequently practices trunk rotation (transverse plane movement) in sitting (figure 8.6). Head rotation causes the entire spine and pelvis to rotate over the femur. Rotation of the pelvis toward the face side is controlled by active external rotation of the skull-side hip (figure 8.6).

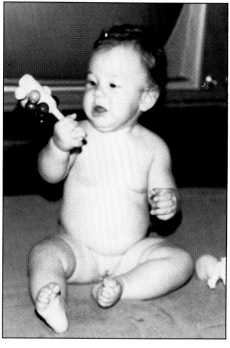

*Figure 8.3. Another modification of the lower extremity posture is a combination of ring and long sitting. One leg is flexed, abducted, and externally rotated at the hip, with knee flexion and ankle dorsiflexion. The other leg is more adducted and less externally rotated at the hip; the knee is extended. The 8-month-old practices supination/pronation movements with toys in the hand.*

## Indications of Possible Disturbances in Motor Development

By the eighth month, control in sitting is an indication of the baby's progress in motor development. Babies who cannot sit independently should be evaluated further. Inability to sit may be related to the baby's excessive use of head, trunk, and hip extension. Tightness in the hip extensor muscles (gluteus maximus and hamstrings) also makes it difficult for the baby to sit.

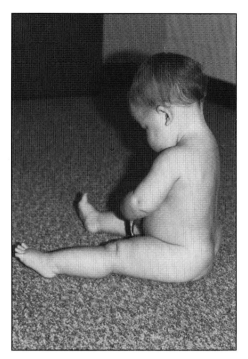

*Figure 8.4.* Long sitting with the knees straight and the pelvis vertical requires mobility in the hamstrings.

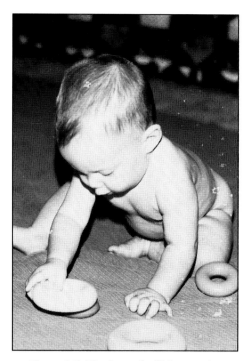

*Figure 8.5.* The 8-month-old frequently uses lower extremity movements to adjust the trunk orientation, realigning the body to face the toy by actively abducting and externally rotating one hip while flexing the knee. The baby maintains trunk symmetry while leaning over the tibia to reach the toy.

Inability to sit may be related to low tone, poor trunk extension, and poor pelvic-femoral stability, in which case the baby may lean far forward and prop on the arms to remain seated. Arm propping interferes with the development of upper extremity use.

More subtle problems may be present if the baby maintains the ring-sitting posture and cannot move out of it. This suggests that the baby has not developed sufficient trunk-pelvic-hip control to free the legs from the postural system. Maintenance of the symmetrical lower extremity posture limits the baby to trunk movements on the sagittal plane. If rotation is used, the upper trunk rotates over the stable pelvis, and abnormal mobility between the rib cage and pelvis develops. Diagonal trunk muscle control does not develop. Subsequently, the baby will have difficulty with reciprocal extremity movements.

## Side Sitting

As trunk and pelvic-femoral control continue to develop during the eighth month, the baby begins to allow the skull-side leg to internally rotate during trunk rotation (figure 8.7). Initially abduction control is maintained. Eventually the baby's leg will internally rotate and adduct, and the baby will side sit (figure 8.8).

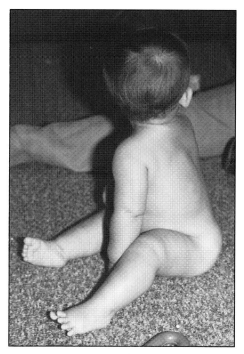

*Figure 8.6.* During the eighth month, the baby frequently practices trunk rotation (transverse plane movement) in sitting and uses active external rotation of the skull-side leg to control the pelvic weight shift.

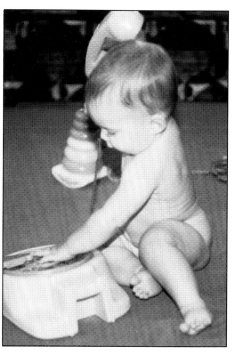

*Figure 8.7.* As trunk and pelvic-femoral control continue to develop during the eighth month, the baby begins to allow the skull-side leg to internally rotate during trunk rotation.

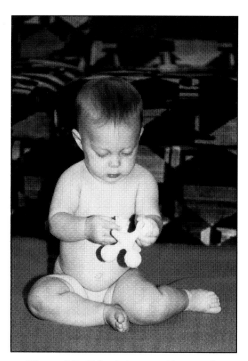

*Figure 8.8.* Side sitting provides a wide base of support, with one leg in the ring position and the other in the W position.

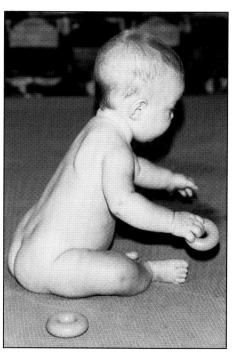

*Figure 8.9.* In the transition to quadruped, the baby tucks the leg under the body, then moves the pelvis and trunk forward as a unit over the lower leg.

**Side Sitting / 159**

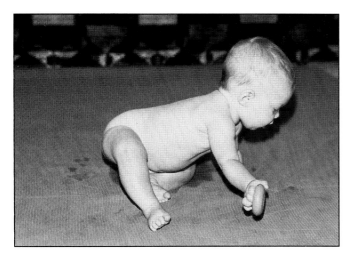

*Figure 8.10.* *The trunk remains symmetrically extended and movement occurs on the sagittal plane.*

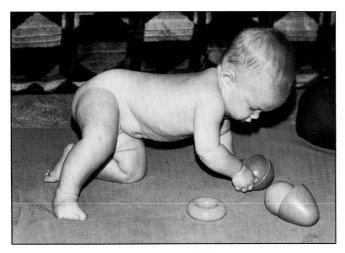

*Figure 8.11.* *Once the baby is shifted forward toward quadruped, the weight-bearing leg must internally rotate to align the leg with the trunk. The unweighted leg may remain flexed, abducted, and externally rotated with the foot on the floor.*

Side sitting is a transitional position for most babies, and they do not spend much time in this position. Most babies transition in and out of side sitting by actively alternating between hip internal and external rotation.

Early side sitting provides a wide base of support (figure 8.8). One leg is in the ring position and the other is in the W position. As the baby's control improves, side sitting will be maintained with a narrower base.

# Upper Extremity Use

Increased trunk and pelvic-femoral control in sitting enables the 8-month-old to reach in a variety of directions, with a variety of reaching patterns. The baby uses a radial-digital grasp, opposing the thumb and fingertips (figures 8.1 to 8.3) (Erhardt 1984). The baby also uses a scissors grasp with small objects, adducting the thumb to the side of the flexed index finger (Erhardt 1984). The baby can manipulate, transfer, and release the toy at will.

The 8-month-old seems to enjoy supination/ pronation movements and practices them with or without toys in the hands (figures 8.2, 8.3). Dynamic action of the scapula muscles provides humeral stability, which subsequently enables stability for forearm movements in a variety of positions in space. The baby no longer needs to adduct the arm to the side to stabilize the humerus for forearm movements (figure 8.2).

Babies at eight months like to use their increased finger dexterity, engaging a scissors grasp by adducting the thumb to the side of the flexed index finger to pick up small objects (Erhardt 1984). This skill is especially useful in self feeding. Manipulation skills have increased.

The 8-month-old can grasp two objects simultaneously (parallel activity) (figure 8.2) and bang them together (Corbetta and Mounoud 1990). According to Fagard (1990), banging two toys together indicates the baby's increasing ability to associate objects.

According to Corbetta and Mounoud (1990), the baby continues to use visual and tactile information related to the intrinsic properties of the object to refine hand control (opening, orientation, perception). Intrinsic properties of objects include size, shape, and texture.

# Sitting to Quadruped

The 8-month-old can move easily from sitting to quadruped, initiating this transition by tucking the leg and foot under the body (figures 8.5, 8.9). The other leg remains flexed, abducted, and externally rotated, providing stability to the pelvis (figures 8.5, 8.9, 8.10). Once the leg is tucked under the body, the baby moves the pelvis and trunk forward as a unit over the lower leg (tibia). The trunk remains symmetrically extended, and movement occurs on the sagittal plane (figures 8.5, 8.9, 8.10). Marked hip joint mobility is needed for this transition. Once the center of gravity is elevated and forward, the baby can bear weight on the arms and adjust the legs for crawling.

Once the baby is shifted forward toward quadruped, the weight-bearing leg must internally rotate to align the leg with the trunk (figure 8.11). The unweighted leg may remain flexed, abducted, and externally rotated with the foot on the floor (figure 8.11). Some babies crawl with this posture.

At the completion of the transition from sitting to quadruped, most babies adjust the abducted leg by adducting it to bring it into line with the pelvis and trunk (figure 8.12). Reciprocal crawling proceeds from this posture.

From quadruped, the baby can return to sitting by reversing the process described above. From quadruped, a lateral weight shift results in one leg abducting, flexing, and externally rotating so that the foot rests on the floor (similar to figure 8.11). The weight-bearing leg then actively externally rotates and the foot is tucked under the trunk. The action of the hip muscles pulls the pelvis and trunk backward to sitting (figure 8.13). Without active hip control, babies cannot bring themselves to sitting with this pattern.

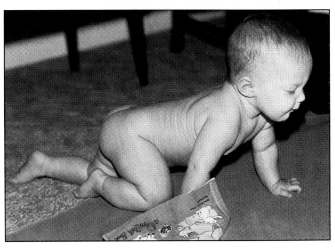

*Figure 8.12.* At the completion of the transition from sitting to quadruped, most babies adjust the abducted leg by adducting it to bring it into line with the pelvis and trunk. Reciprocal crawling proceeds from this posture.

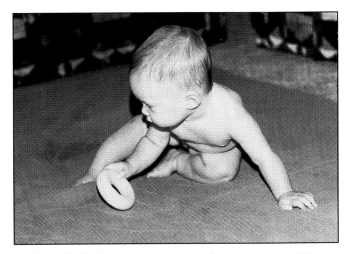

*Figure 8.13.* From quadruped, the baby can return to sitting: a lateral weight shift results in one leg abducting, flexing, and externally rotating so that the foot rests on the floor. The weight-bearing leg then actively externally rotates, and the foot is tucked under the trunk. The action of the hip muscles pulls the pelvis and trunk backward to sitting.

## Indications of Possible Disturbances in Motor Development

Babies who use ring sitting to stabilize their posture will have difficulty transitioning out of sitting. They lack the trunk control that is needed to free the legs from the postural system for their realignment. They also lack control of the pelvic-femoral muscles.

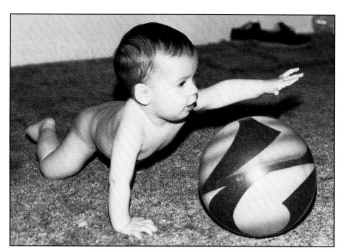

*Figure 8.14. When reciprocal extremity movements are used in crawling, opposite upper and lower extremities move simultaneously and counterrotation occurs in the trunk.*

# Crawling

Crawling is 8-month-olds' most efficient means of moving from place to place. They use reciprocal extremity movements in their crawling, which require diagonal and counterrotation control in the trunk (figure 8.14).

When reciprocal extremity movements are used in crawling, opposite upper and lower extremities move simultaneously (figure 8.14) and counterrotation occurs in the trunk. When the left arm is lifted, weight is shifted laterally to the right arm and subtle rotation of the upper trunk occurs toward the left. When the right leg is lifted, weight is shifted laterally to the left leg and subtle rotation of the lower trunk occurs toward the right. Therefore the upper trunk rotates to the left and the lower trunk rotates toward the right (opposite or counterrotation). Neither rotation is noticed because each is absorbed in the mid-thoracic region, T-7, T-8 (Kapandji 1974).

When the left upper and right lower extremities are lifted, the weight is redistributed to the right upper and the left lower extremities. Therefore there is an imaginary diagonal of control between the right upper and the left lower extremities. This diagonal of control involves the trunk, shoulder, and hip muscles. The synchronous action of these muscles seems to hold the body together. This diagonal control is quite significant in reciprocal crawling. Children who lack this diagonal control retain homolateral or ipsilateral crawling, which utilizes the more primitive lateral righting reactions in which all of the weight is just shifted laterally.

Crawling and its weight-shifting components provide varied input into the hand, which may contribute to the development of the palmar arches (Nash 1991). A lateral weight shift in the hand frees the radial digit for grasp. Therefore the 8-month-old often carries small toys in the hand when crawling. The baby is also beginning to push toys with one hand while crawling (Nash 1991).

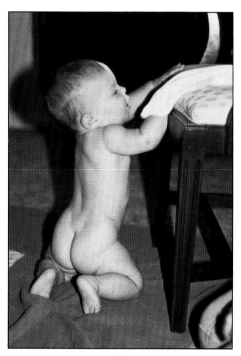

*Figure 8.15. In the process of pulling to stand from quadruped, the baby reaches up with the arms and places them securely on the furniture. In early attempts to pull to stand, the baby stabilizes the pelvis and hips with the hip flexors and synergistic knee and ankle flexors. This is noted by the strong anterior pelvic tilt and marked ankle dorsiflexion.*

# Rising to Stand

The desire to attain the upright is very strong in 8-month-olds, and they now have the motor ability to accomplish this desire. They will frequently pull themselves to stand on furniture and people, and they love to climb up onto furniture and stairs (figures 8.15 to 8.22). Good upper extremity control and strength are critical. Although the arms still do the majority of the work in this transition, the legs provide more assistance than they did at seven months.

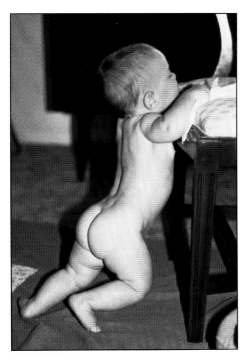

**Figure 8.16.** *Once the arms are stable, the baby pushes down with the arms to rise to stand. In initial attempts to stand, the baby may use symmetrical lower extremity extension to assist the process.*

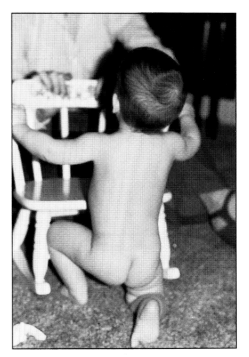

**Figure 8.17.** *The 8-month-old usually progresses to asymmetrical lower extremity postures in rising to stand. The baby's arms provide postural stability while pulling to stand, and the legs are free to adjust under the body during elevation. Elongation on the weight-bearing side (right) is incomplete because the weight-bearing hip remains slightly abducted and externally rotated.*

In the process of pulling to stand from quadruped, the baby reaches up with the arms and places them securely on the furniture (figure 8.15). This provides stability for trunk elevation. In early attempts to pull to stand, the baby stabilizes the pelvis and hips (and thus the center of gravity) with the hip flexors and synergistic knee and ankle flexors. This is noted by a strong anterior pelvic tilt and marked ankle dorsiflexion (figure 8.15).

Once the arms are stable, the baby pushes down with the arms to rise to stand. In initial attempts, the baby may use symmetrical lower extremity extension to assist the process (figure 8.16), but in a short period of time the baby changes to asymmetrical lower extremity postures (figure 8.17). Because the arms provide postural stability while the baby pulls to stand, the legs are free to adjust under the body during the elevation.

# Kneeling

Kneeling and half kneeling occur as natural steps in this transition to stand (figures 8.15, 8.17, 8.19). During early experiences in kneeling and half kneeling, the baby relies on the upper extremities for stability. The hip extensors are not yet active. Pelvic-femoral stability is maintained by the hip flexors and wide abduction of the legs. Activation of the hip flexors triggers synergistic action in the knee flexors and ankle dorsiflexors (figures 8.15, 8.17, 8.19). Therefore, marked ankle dorsiflexion usually suggests fixing at the pelvic-femoral joint with the hip flexors.

When the arms provide postural stability, the baby can experiment with letting go of the hip flexor fixing and practice hip extensor activity. Hip extension in kneeling and half kneeling is more difficult than hip extension in standing because of the knee flexion. Therefore early kneeling and half kneeling are accomplished with hip flexion rather than hip extension.

There are several reasons why it is difficult for the baby to extend the hips in kneeling. First, with a new posture, the baby relies on the hip flexors to stabilize the pelvis and hips in the vertical position. The 8-month-old needs time and practice to discover how to use the hip extensors and abdominals for this stability.

Second, it is difficult for the baby to extend the hips when the knees are flexed because of the elongation of the quadriceps, the rectus femoris. When the rectus femoris is tight and is stretched by knee flexion, it causes hip flexion. Therefore part of the process of achieving upright kneeling involves active elongation of the rectus femoris. (Initial elongation of the rectus femoris occurred at five months when the baby played with active knee flexion/extension while prone, figure 5.16).

Hip extension is achieved through contraction of the gluteus maximus, which works in synergy with the back muscles and lateral abdominal muscles (Kendall, Kendall, and Wadsworth 1971). As the gluteus maximus becomes more active and provides pelvic-femoral stability, hip flexor fixing is diminished and the hip flexors, including the rectus femoris, are actively elongated.

# Half Kneeling

For the 8-month-old to achieve half kneeling, the baby must be able to dissociate the lower extremities while in a weight-bearing position. The mobility and ability to dissociate the legs started at five months of age in prone, which is a nonweight-bearing position. Just as in prone, lower extremity dissociation for half kneeling is initiated by a lateral weight shift in the trunk and pelvis. The weight-bearing side elongates, and the weight-bearing hip extends (figures 8.17, 8.18). The trunk on the unweighted side responds with a lateral righting reaction (which includes subtle lateral flexion of the pelvis) and hip flexion, abduction, and external rotation (figure 8.17). This entire process is much more obvious in climbing activities (figures 8.18 to 8.21).

At eight months of age, elongation of the weight-bearing side is incomplete at the hip joint because the baby needs the stability of the wide base (figures 8.17, 8.18, 8.20). The weight-bearing hip remains slightly abducted and externally rotated. Therefore full weight shift is not achieved. To compensate, the baby may laterally flex the trunk on the weight-bearing side to unweight the leg that is to move forward.

Over time, as babies continue to practice this transition, they will achieve full elongation of the side. Such elongation requires increased control of the hip extensors (especially gluteus maximus), hip adductors, and rotators. In addition, eccentric control of the hip abductors is needed to prevent excessive weight shift.

After the lower extremities are positioned in half kneeling (figure 8.21), the 8-month-old uses the arms for stability and control to rise to standing. The baby continues to use this stability to adjust the legs under the trunk (8.22). When lower extremity stability has once again been achieved, the baby can free the arms from the postural system and use them for reaching and grasping (figure 8.23).

### *Indications of Possible Disturbances in Motor Development*

Kneeling and half kneeling are difficult tasks because they require trunk and hip postural control and upper extremity support. Babies who have difficulties in any of these areas will have difficulty transitioning to kneeling and half kneeling.

Babies who have sufficient upper extremity control but poor pelvic-femoral control may achieve kneeling by pulling up with their arms while fixing the lower trunk with the hip flexors. Although this is seen as part of the normal motor developmental sequence, it is abnormal when a baby cannot break out of the fixing. In this situation, the flexor tone gets stronger and the hip extensors do not take over.

Babies who use strong fixing patterns for stability in kneeling will not be able to weight shift and free one leg to move forward. Symmetry will be maintained and babies may pull themselves to stand by pushing down with the arms and symmetrically extending the legs. As was mentioned above, this pattern is often used in normal motor development (figures 8.15, 8.16). It becomes abnormal when a baby cannot vary the pattern and it becomes very stereotyped.

# Climbing

The 8-month-old's urge for the upright is not limited to pulling to stand. Fortunately, in most cases, the baby's urge to climb and explore is matched with the motor ability to accomplish these tasks. However, these maneuvers are accomplished without judgment and without the ability to climb back down. Furniture, stairs, and people are the usual obstacles the 8-month-old attempts to climb (figures 8.15 to 8.22). The choice is usually related to what toys or objects the baby is trying to secure. Therefore climbing may also be related to the baby's ability to scan the environment and perceive affordances.

Climbing demonstrates the baby's ability to problem solve how to manage the body on unfamiliar, uneven, and unsteady surfaces. The baby uses upper extremity stability and feedback information to regulate the progression. Climbing involves alternate weight shift from side to side, in both the upper and lower extremities. The entire process duplicates the sequences of kneeling, half kneeling, and standing (figures 8.17 to 8.23).

The components used by the 8-month-old to climb are a continuation of the components initiated by the 5- and 6-month-olds to achieve lateral weight shifting, lateral righting, and lower extremity dissociation. Those components include upper extremity and pelvic weight shifting, elongation of the weight-bearing side (including hip adduction and extension), lateral righting of the trunk and pelvis on the unweighted side, and flexion, abduction, and external rotation of the unweighted leg. (Compare figures 8.18, 6.18, and 5.18.)

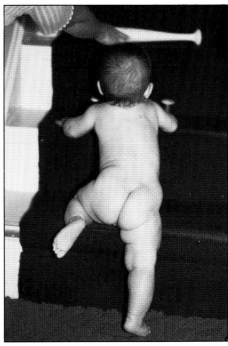

*Figure 8.18.* Climbing involves alternate weight shift from side to side in both the upper and lower extremities. When climbing is initiated from standing, the weight-bearing side (right) is elongated as the unweighted leg flexes, abducts, and externally rotates. This posture resembles that of the 5- and 6-month-olds (figures 5.19, 6.16).

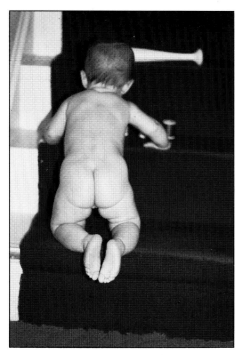

*Figure 8.19.* The 8-month-old's climbing is usually motivated by the desire to reach toys or objects that attract the baby's attention. During early kneeling, the baby uses a wide base of support with the arms and legs. Flexor muscle activity stabilizes the lower trunk and lower extremities.

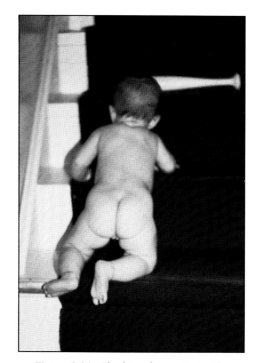

*Figure 8.20.* Climbing demonstrates the baby's ability to problem solve how to manage the body on unfamiliar, uneven, and unsteady surfaces. At eight months, elongation on the weight-bearing side (right) during the transition to half-kneeling (left) is incomplete because the baby needs the stability of the wide base. Dorsiflexion of the right ankle suggests fixing with the hip flexors.

# Standing

Once in standing, 8-month-olds are not content to stand. They now have the skills to shift the weight in the legs on all three planes. They can flex and extend the hips and knees, and rotate, abduct, and adduct the hips. They use each of these skills to secure toys, play with toys, and move through and explore the environment.

While standing, the baby abducts the legs to stabilize the posture (figures 8.22, 8.23). Lower extremity stability enables the baby to free the arms for reaching, grasping, and manipulation, as well as for cruising. However, the baby's upper extremities are frequently still needed to reinforce postural stability. Subsequently, fixing with shoulder girdle elevation may be seen. This becomes very obvious when the baby is cruising (figures 8.27 to 8.30).

Movement on the sagittal plane is used in rising to stand and in lowering to the floor to get a toy (figure 8.24). When lowering to the floor, the baby shifts the weight posteriorly, so that the hips are well behind the shoulders and feet. The trunk stays straight.

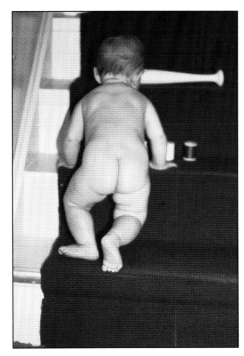 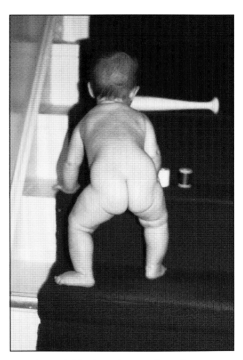

*Figure 8.21.* Once the forward foot (left) is stable, the baby shifts the weight to that side and unweights the back leg (right) to bring it forward. The baby uses upper extremity stability and feedback information to regulate the climb.

*Figure 8.22.* Once in standing, the baby abducts the legs and uses a wide base of support to stabilize the posture.

Lowering is initially controlled by eccentric contraction of the quadriceps but may end with the baby collapsing upon getting closer to the floor. The range of knee flexion that occurs before the baby collapses may be an indication of the baby's eccentric quadriceps control. Because the hips and center of gravity are shifted so far posteriorly, there is minimal movement of the tibia forward over the foot (dorsiflexion) (figure 8.24). The toes may curl, which indicates increased synergistic activity to augment stability.

Babies' initial attempts at rotation (transverse plane movement) in standing (figure 8.25) are consistent with their initial attempts at rotation in prone and sitting. Weight shift is initiated by head rotation. It is usually curiosity or interest in a toy which causes the baby to turn the head, with concurrent rotation of the trunk and pelvis over the femur. The shoulder girdle stays in line with the pelvis. Weight is shifted to the same side to which the face turns (figures 8.25, 8.27). Subsequently, the face-side leg assumes a position of hip external rotation, flexion, and subtle adduction, with weight on the lateral border of the dorsiflexed foot (the foot inverts). The skull-side leg begins subtly to internally rotate, extend, and abduct, with the weight on the medial side of a plantar-flexed foot (the foot everts) (figure 8.25). These lower extremity postures resemble and may be precursors to the mid-stance and terminal stance (pushoff) phases of gait.

At seven months of age, the trunk rotated over a symmetrical, stable pelvis. The shoulder and pelvic girdles did not stay aligned, and the pelvis did not rotate over the femur. No weight shift occurred in the legs or the feet (figure 7.22).

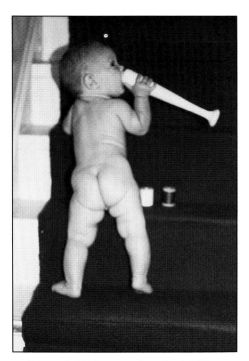

**Figure 8.23.** *Lower extremity stability enables the baby to free the arms for reaching, grasping, and manipulation.*

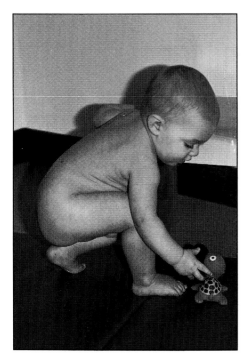

**Figure 8.24.** *Movement on the sagittal plane is used in lowering to the floor to get a toy. The baby shifts the weight posteriorly, so that the hips are well behind the shoulders and feet. The trunk remains straight. Lowering is controlled by eccentric contraction of the quadriceps. There is minimal movement of the tibia forward over the foot (dorsiflexion).*

For the pelvis to rotate over the femur, the hip muscles (the lateral rotators and the gluteus maximus) must dynamically stabilize the pelvis and the femur in the vertical position as well as rotate the pelvis over the femur. Rotation (transverse plane movement) at the hip joint is a critical component that facilitates full lower extremity dissociation. The extremities can move symmetrically on the other two planes (sagittal plane flexion and extension, and frontal plane abduction and adduction). The transverse plane components enable the integration of the sagittal and frontal plane movements.

Lower extremity weight shift on the frontal plane while standing is similar to upper extremity weight shift on the frontal plane while in prone. In standing, the lateral weight shift is initiated with the trunk and pelvic girdle (figure 8.26). This weight shift causes the side to elongate and the weight-bearing hip to adduct and extend with neutral rotation. Weight is shifted to the lateral border of the foot, causing the foot to invert. The other leg is unweighted and free to flex, abduct, and externally rotate.

Just as in prone, this lateral weight shift in standing seems to be used in a feedforward mode to free the face-side extremities (figures 8.26, 8.29). In prone, the weight shift occurred prior to movement of the reaching arm. The same is true in standing: weight shift occurs prior to movement of the reaching leg.

Hip control on the weight-bearing side must be sufficient to initiate the weight shift and stabilize the pelvis as the other leg is freed to move. The pelvic-femoral muscles must dynamically stabilize the pelvis and femur in the vertical position, rotate the pelvis over the femur, and maintain external rotation of the weight-bearing leg. If the hip muscles maintain the hip in extension and external rotation, the weight will be maintained on the lateral border of the foot. If hip muscle activity is insufficient to maintain the extension and external rotation, the leg will internally rotate and flex, and the weight will be transferred to the medial side of the foot. These lower extremity actions resemble and may be precursors to the midstance and swing phases of gait.

# Cruising

The 8-month-old baby is starting to combine the new pelvic-lower extremity movements to cruise around the furniture. During these new movements, the baby seems to reinforce postural stability by elevating the shoulders (figures 8.27 to 8.30). This fixing posture becomes most obvious when the baby tries to reach while standing or cruising (figure 8.30). The shoulder girdle will remain elevated until the baby has developed more trunk-pelvic-lower extremity control in standing and walking.

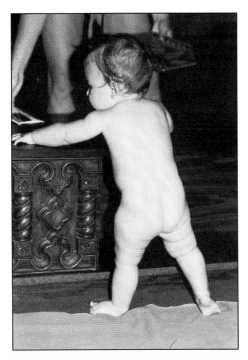

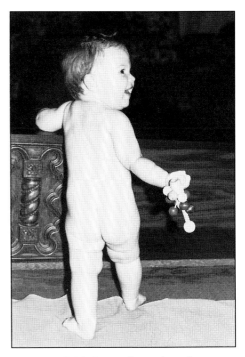

*Figure 8.25*. Weight shift in standing is initiated by rotation of the head. The shoulder girdle stays in line with the pelvis, and weight is shifted to the same side to which the face turns. The skull-side leg begins subtly to internally rotate, extend, and abduct with the weight on the medial side of a plantar-flexed foot.

*Figure 8.26*. In standing, a lateral weight shift is initiated with the trunk and pelvic girdle. This weight shift frees the face-side extremities to flex, abduct, and externally rotate.

When cruising along the furniture, the 8-month-old starts from a position of symmetry, facing the sofa. Interest in a toy causes the baby to rotate the head, trunk, and pelvis, a transverse plane movement (figure 8.27). Concurrently, the weight is shifted to the face-side leg which is slightly flexed, adducted, and externally rotated. Slight extension, internal rotation, and abduction occur on the skull-side leg. The shoulder and pelvic girdles stay aligned. Therefore the rotation occurs below the pelvis, at the hip joint.

The weight is then transferred laterally to the face-side leg and the baby adducts the back leg, both frontal plane movements (figure 8.28). Subsequently, weight is shifted back to the skull-side leg by the hip adductors, with synergistic control from the hip extensors and abductors.

Weight shift onto the skull-side leg includes rotation toward the unweighted side. This frees the face-side leg which subsequently moves on the sagittal plane with marked hip and knee flexion (figure 8.29). This is the swing phase of gait.

The body position of rotation and leaning enables the baby to advance along the sofa by extending the knee and placing the foot on the floor. Rotation at the hip joint produces lower extremity dissociation (figure 8.30). From this position, the cruising pattern is repeated.

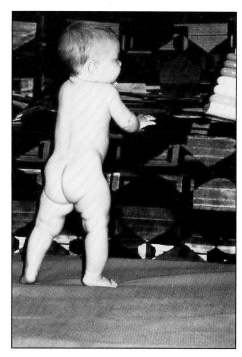

**Figure 8.27.** *Cruising is initiated when interest in a toy causes the baby to rotate the head, trunk, and pelvis toward the toy. Weight is shifted to the face-side leg, which is slightly flexed, adducted, and externally rotated. The position of the forward leg resembles the midstance position in gait. The position of the back leg resembles the terminal stance position.*

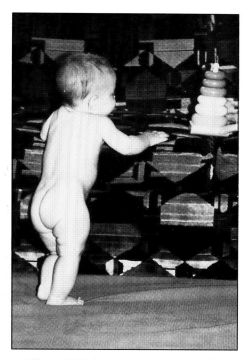

**Figure 8.28.** *As cruising continues, all of the baby's weight is transferred to the face-side leg, and the baby adducts the back leg. This is a frontal plane movement. Upper extremity weight bearing and weight shifting also occur.*

In figures 8.27 and 8.30, the positions of the lower extremities resemble the positions that will be assumed during the midstance and terminal stance phases of advanced gait. In figure 8.29, the positions of the lower extremities are more representative of the positions that will be assumed during the midstance and swing phases of advanced gait.

In figure 8.29, the baby's posture resembles the laterally righted postures that were first observed in prone at five and six months of age (figures 5.19, 6.18) and then repeated in half kneeling (figure 8.17) and climbing (figure 8.18).

Figure 8.30 demonstrates more advanced diagonal control of the trunk, similar to the crawling pattern (figure 8.14), which enables reciprocal extremity movement. The 8-month-old is in the transition phase toward increased trunk control.

# Walking

Babies at eight months can stand independently by holding onto someone's fingers, rather than others holding onto them (figure 8.31). However, this holding causes them to fix in the upper trunk with marked scapular adduction (figures 8.31, 8.32). The 8-month-old keeps the legs abducted and externally rotated, assuring a wide,

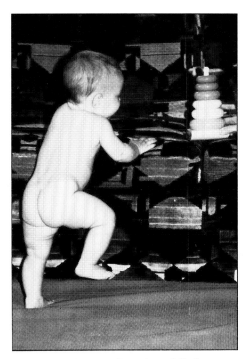

**Figure 8.29.** Weight is then shifted to the skull-side leg, freeing the face-side leg, which flexes for the swing phase.

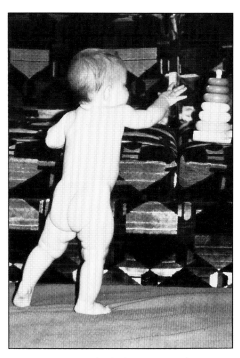

**Figure 8.30.** The body position of rotation and leaning enables the 8-month-old to advance along the sofa when the knee is extended and the foot is placed on the floor. The back leg extends and assumes a terminal stance posture.

stable base of support. The hips are more in line with the shoulders than in previous months, but this is accomplished by the marked trunk extension and lumbar lordosis rather than increased hip extension (figure 8.31).

The arms and shoulder girdles provide postural stability for walking, as demonstrated by the baby's continued dependence on upper extremity support from an adult. The arms and shoulder girdles can once again be described as being yoked to the postural system. By limiting the degrees of freedom in the upper trunk through scapular adduction, the baby seems to have increased control in the lower extremities.

Although this control is still limited, the baby's legs are more involved with the forward progression in walking at eight months than they were at seven months. However, the lower extremity control observed in cruising, especially transverse control, is not yet incorporated into forward walking.

The 8-month-old does not yet rotate the pelvis over the femur when walking forward. Lower extremity movements occur primarily on the sagittal and frontal planes. The steppage pattern of hip flexion, abduction, and external rotation is still used during swing (figure 8.32). The swing leg is hyperflexed as the hip, knee, and ankle move in synchronous flexion, which is followed by synchronous extension (Forssberg 1992). The stance leg remains abducted and externally rotated.

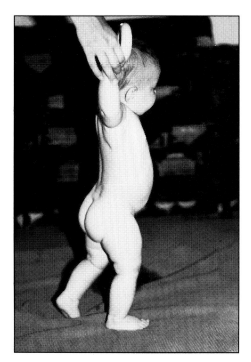

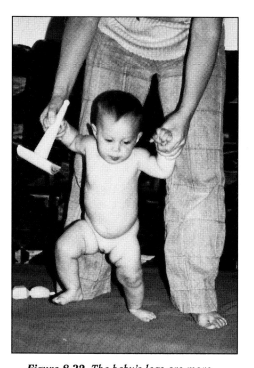

**Figure 8.31.** The 8-month-old can stand independently by holding onto someone's fingers. The scapulae are adducted. The hips are more in line with the shoulders because of marked trunk extension and lumbar lordosis rather than increased hip extension.

**Figure 8.32.** The baby's legs are more involved with the forward progression in walking at eight months than they were at seven months, but the steppage pattern of hip flexion, abduction, and external rotation is still used during swing. The lower extremities move primarily on the sagittal and frontal planes.

# The Ninth Month

**B**y the ninth month, the differences in skill levels among babies is ever increasing. Some babies are more active than other babies. Some babies concentrate more on fine motor than gross motor activities.

By this age, most babies are combining their gross motor and fine motor skills. It is an age of active sensory-spatial exploration (Fritts 1990). The baby detects many affordances in the environment (Gibson and Schmuckler 1989) and has the motor skills to explore these affordances. The 9-month-old is fascinated by new discoveries, toys that change, household objects, and small objects (Fritts 1990).

The 9-month-old is very versatile in sitting and can assume many sitting postures while engaging the hands in fine motor activities. The baby can also transition in and out of sitting while holding onto a toy.

Crawling is the 9-month-old's primary means of locomotion. Babies use this skill to secure toys that they notice across the room. Crawling skills are expanded to climbing skills. Through climbing, the baby experiments with the properties of furniture, discovering which ones are climb-on-able and which are not. Here, too, the baby is learning what the environment affords.

Standing and walking are primary drives for the baby. Much of the effort is put into coming to stand and cruising around furniture. The baby is also beginning to experiment more with lowering from standing.

## Sitting

Sitting is a functional position for the 9-month-old. Trunk control is well developed; therefore the legs can assume many varied positions. The baby can ring sit (figure 9.1), long sit (figure 9.2), side sit (figure 9.3), W sit (figure 9.10), and transition out of sitting (figure 9.4). Sitting is often a transitional state for babies as they continue to explore the environment actively.

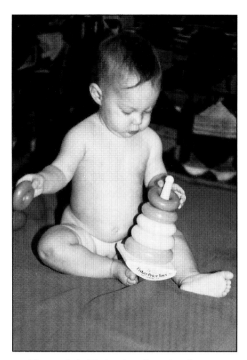

**Figure 9.1.** Sitting is a functional position for the 9-month-old. Ring sitting is one of the varied positions the baby can use. Increased trunk control frees the arms from the postural system and enables the baby to use a variety of shoulder and forearm movements.

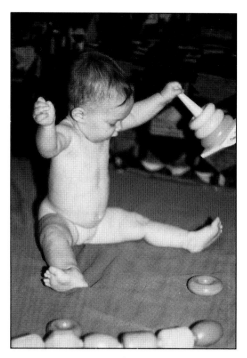

**Figure 9.2.** During long sitting, the baby's legs are abducted and externally rotated at the hips and extended at the knees. The pelvis is perpendicular or slightly anteriorly tilted. The baby can flex and abduct the shoulders without losing trunk control.

The increased trunk and pelvic control frees the arms from the postural system and enables the baby to use a variety of shoulder and forearm movements (figures 9.1 to 9.3). The baby can reach for objects out of reach while varying the reaching patterns and can flex the shoulders and reach overhead (Vogtle and Albert 1985).

The increased dissociation of the arms from the trunk enables the baby to begin to push objects and hold objects during transitions (Nash 1991). An inferior pincer grasp is emerging, with thumb adduction to the lateral border of the index finger (Erhardt 1984). Voluntary release is starting and the baby practices this by frequently dropping objects. A true hand-to-hand transfer is possible. The baby is beginning to make adjustments according to the weight of an object and is also beginning to hold two cubes (Corbetta and Mounoud 1990).

Long sitting is now achieved with increased knee extension. As the quadriceps extend the knees, the hamstring and gastrocnemius muscles are elongated. Elongation of the posterior knee muscles could cause hip extension or posterior pelvic tilting if the hamstrings are tight, or ankle plantar flexion if the gastrocnemius is tight. In 9-month-old babies, this is not a problem. The hamstrings and gastrocnemius muscles have been progressively elongated throughout the developmental process.

During long sitting, the baby's hips are abducted and externally rotated while the knees are extended (figure 9.2). The pelvis is perpendicular or slightly anteriorly tilted. The baby can move the pelvis and extended trunk forward from the hip joints

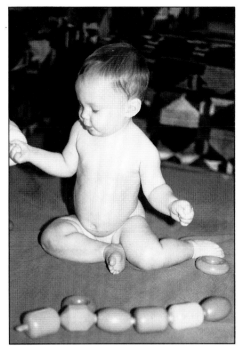

*Figure 9.3.* Side sitting is a new posture. It is assumed during trunk rotation when the skull-side leg is not needed to stabilize the pelvis. It provides a wide, stable base of support.

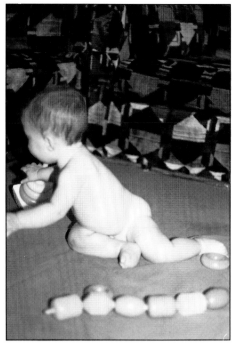

*Figure 9.4.* From side sitting, the 9-month-old can transition to quadruped by rotating the trunk and pelvis over the femur.

when reaching for toys (figure 9.5). Forward movement of the pelvis stretches the hamstrings and is subsequently followed by knee flexion (figure 9.5).

The 9-month-old is also beginning to play with active anterior (figure 9.6) and posterior (figure 9.7) pelvis tilting while sitting. Anterior pelvic tilting extends the trunk and stretches the hip extensors (hamstrings). Posterior pelvic tilting is a new activity which uses trunk flexion. Posterior pelvic tilting is usually seen when the baby looks down at a toy (figure 9.7). The baby is not limited to either position but practices alternation between anterior and posterior pelvic tilting.

From long sitting, the baby can rotate the trunk and pelvis over the face-side hip joint (figure 9.8). Active external rotation of the skull-side leg is still frequently used to control the pelvic weight shift.

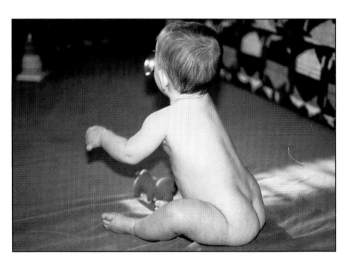

*Figure 9.5.* From long sitting, the baby can move the extended trunk and pelvis forward from the hip joints. This stretches the hamstrings and flexes the knees.

Movement of the face-side leg is also still used to reorient the body for reaching (figure 9.9). When the face-side leg flexes, abducts, and externally rotates from the long-sitting position, the trunk is simultaneously shifted to face the object. Pelvic-femoral mobility is needed for this maneuver.

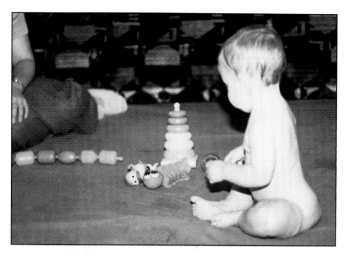

**Figure 9.6.** *The baby uses active anterior pelvic tilting during sitting, which extends the trunk and stretches the hamstrings.*

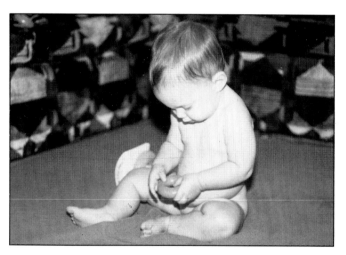

**Figure 9.7.** *Posterior pelvic tilting is a new activity which flexes the trunk. It usually occurs when the baby looks down at a toy.*

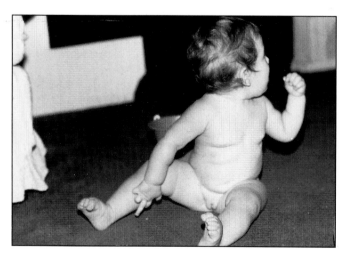

**Figure 9.8.** *From long sitting, the baby can rotate the trunk and pelvis over the face-side hip joint.*

Side sitting is beginning to emerge as another option. Side sitting (figure 9.3) usually occurs during the process of trunk rotation to obtain a toy or transition to quadruped (figure 9.4). As was mentioned earlier, trunk-pelvic rotation is usually controlled by active external rotation of the skull-side leg (figure 9.8). By nine months, however, because of increased trunk-pelvic control, the baby begins to experiment with reducing that external control. Therefore, if the baby feels stable during trunk-pelvic rotation, the baby will permit the skull-side leg to move from external rotation (figure 9.8) to internal rotation (figure 9.4). Internal rotation of the skull-side leg results in forward rotation of the pelvis and increased weight shift to the face side.

Initial experiences with side sitting utilize a wide base of support and thus stabilize the pelvis on the frontal plane. The face-side leg assumes a ring-sitting position (flexion, abduction, external rotation), while the skull-side leg assumes a W-sitting position (flexion, abduction, internal rotation). The baby can easily move out of the side-sitting posture by externally rotating the skull-side leg.

W sitting is another new sitting position that the 9-month-old may use (figure 9.10). W sitting is usually assumed from quadruped. It is used most frequently by babies with low tone, because it provides a wide, stable base of support for the trunk and thus the upper extremities.

Although W sitting is a normal position, it is not a good position for the lower extremities. This position exaggerates hip internal rotation and may thus enhance medial femoral torsion, which may later cause "knock-knees." W sitting also puts stress on the medial ligaments of the knees and may lead to knee instability.

When the baby rotates while in a W-sitting position, the upper trunk and rib cage rotate over the pelvis. Trunk rotation during W sitting does not include the pelvis rotating over the femur (figure 9.11). The pelvis is positionally stable; thus it cannot move. If the pattern is used over a period of time, or if it is used exclusively, it will lead to decreased control of the trunk and decreased control of the hips. Both W sitting and trunk rotation while W sitting should be discouraged.

Fortunately, the baby can easily move out of W sitting, transitioning to kneeling (figure 9.12). The baby uses the quadriceps to move between W sitting and kneeling. In order to sit down from kneeling, the baby must use grading and eccentric control of the quadriceps. These are new movements for the 9-month-old. The hip flexors, rather than the hip extensors, frequently work with the quadriceps during this transition. This is noted as anterior pelvic tilting and hip flexion.

The 9-month-old can easily transition from sitting to quadruped by continuing to use forward vaulting of the symmetrical trunk over the flexed leg (figure 9.13). This maneuver uses controlled upper extremity reaching to propel the body forward. The hip muscles, especially extensors and abductors, are used to stabilize the femur while the body is lifted. The weight-bearing femur stays abducted and may thus use the hip abductor muscles in a concentric contraction in conjunction with the hip extensors. The unweighted leg remains actively flexed, abducted, and externally rotated. This may stabilize the pelvis in a symmetrical position.

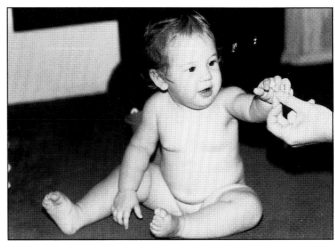

*Figure 9.9* *The baby uses active lower extremity flexion, abduction, and external rotation to reorient the body for reaching. The baby likes small objects.*

The 9-month-old can also transition to quadruped by rotating the trunk and pelvis over the femur (figure 9.4). This transition requires marked pelvic-femoral mobility. The baby must also have dissociated control of the legs to adjust them under the pelvis once weight is put on the arms.

## Indications of Possible Disturbances in Motor Development

Babies who cannot sit independently by nine months of age are demonstrating atypical motor development and should be evaluated further. Stereotypic sitting postures with no variety are also suggestive of a motor delay, as is the inability to move in and out of sitting.

Babies who can sit independently only when using a ring-sitting or W-sitting posture are demonstrating poor development of the pelvic-femoral muscles. They are using lower extremity positional or mechanical stability rather than dynamic muscle activity to stabilize the pelvis and thus the trunk.

Ring sitting and W sitting both contribute to tightness of the hip and knee muscles. Ring sitting contributes to tightness of the hip flexors, abductors, lateral rotators, and hamstrings. W sitting contributes to tightness of the hip flexors, adductors, medial rotators, and hamstrings. W sitting may also reinforce medial femoral torsion and stretching of the medial knee ligaments. This often results in a knock-knee position in standing.

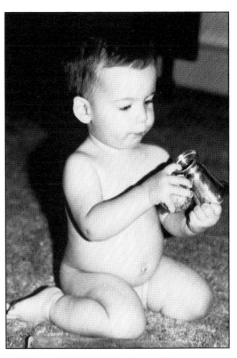

*Figure 9.10.* *W sitting is another new sitting position that the 9-month-old may use, usually assumed from quadruped. Although it is a normal position, W sitting is not a good position for the hips or knees. The baby can hold two objects and make adjustments for the weight of the objects.*

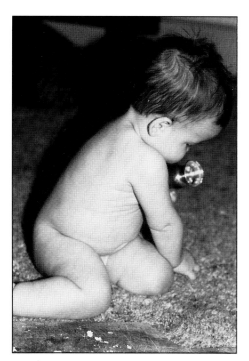

**Figure 9.11.** Trunk rotation during W sitting is accomplished primarily by rotation of the upper trunk and rib cage over the pelvis. It does not include the pelvis rotating over the femur. This may lead to excessive mobility between the ribs and pelvis, and it exaggerates hip internal rotation.

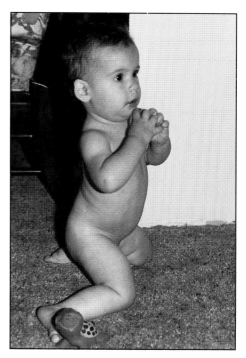

**Figure 9.12.** The 9-month-old can transition from W sitting to kneeling by contracting the quadriceps and hip flexors. Although the trunk is elevated, the hips are flexed.

Hamstring tightness can be a significant problem in babies with developmental delays and may be an early symptom of future problems. Tightness of these muscles inhibits long sitting. When the knee is straightened, the pelvis is posteriorly tilted, causing the baby to fall backward. The baby may compensate for this posterior tilt by flexing the trunk, causing a kyphosis, which leads to increased tightness in the rectus abdominis (Quinton 1976, 1977, 1978).

Hamstring tightness may also contribute to poor standing and walking. When the hamstrings are tight, it is difficult to flex the hip and extend the knee simultaneously. Hip flexion with knee extension is needed in the swing phase of gait.

Side sitting can also become a problem in infants with atypical motor development. Side sitting is a combination of ring sitting and W sitting. Both contribute to muscle tightness and abnormal use of positional stability, which block further development of the pelvic-femoral and knee muscles.

# Quadruped

By the ninth month, the baby has become quite proficient at crawling. Reciprocal extremity movements and trunk counterrotation continue to be used. Speed and control during crawling are quite refined. The baby can move at varied speeds and can quickly change directions. Crawling is the primary means of locomotion, and the 9-month-old uses this skill to explore the environment and to obtain and transport toys (figure 9.14).

From quadruped, the baby can easily come back to sitting by reversing the process used to assume quadruped (figures 9.14, 9.15). The weight must be shifted laterally (to the left in figures 9.14 and 9.15). With the weight on the left knee, the baby must actively externally rotate the left hip to tuck the foot under the trunk. The strong external rotation of the weight-bearing hip helps to pull the baby backward to sitting. The baby then extends the trunk on the stable pelvis and hips. The unweighted leg maintains a posture of flexion, abduction, and external rotation. This helps to stabilize the pelvis. Trunk control is quite stable; therefore the baby can retain toys in the hands during the process.

### Indications of Possible Disturbances in Motor Development

The baby who cannot assume quadruped and move is demonstrating an obvious problem in motor development. Crawling with a bunny-hop pattern is also indicative of a disturbance in motor development. Babies who use a bunny-hop pattern do so because they continue to fix with their hip flexors (Quinton 1976, 1977, 1978), which restricts hip extension. Fixing also restricts lower extremity dissociation and lateral weight shifting. Lateral weight shifting is needed to crawl with a reciprocal pattern.

# Kneeling

The 9-month-old may play in the kneeling position (figures 9.12, 9.16), using the quadriceps to extend the knees and elevate the trunk. The hip extensors

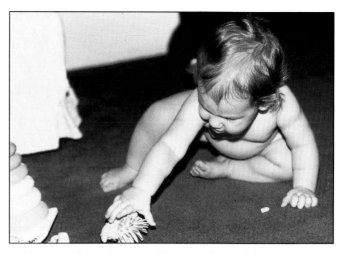

**Figure 9.13.** *The 9-month-old can easily transition from sitting to quadruped by continuing to use forward vaulting of the symmetrical trunk over the flexed leg. The unweighted leg remains flexed, abducted, and externally rotated.*

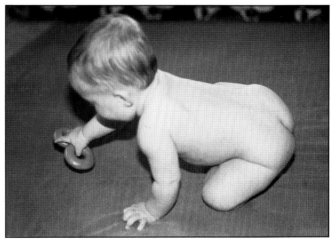

**Figure 9.14.** *The baby uses quadruped and crawling to obtain toys and explore the environment. From quadruped, the baby can come back to sitting by reversing the process used to assume quadruped. Weight is shifted laterally to the left, and the left leg is externally rotated, with the foot tucked under the trunk.*

may assist, but the hip flexors seem to be stronger. While kneeling, the baby maintains a posture of hip flexion, abduction, and external rotation. Strong contraction of the hip flexors is accompanied by synergistic ankle dorsiflexion and an anterior pelvic tilt (figure 9.16). When the baby is not fixing with the hip flexors, the ankles relax in plantar flexion.

The 9-month-old may also play in half kneeling (figure 9.17). To assume half kneeling, the baby must be able to control the trunk and hips while shifting weight laterally. As the weight shifts, there is concurrent elongation of the weight-bearing side and lateral righting and lateral flexion on the unweighted side. This enables

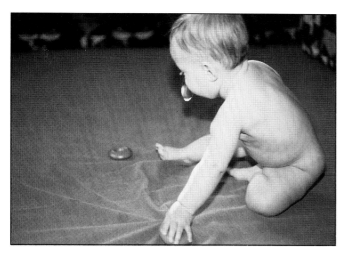

*Figure 9.15. The strong external rotation of the weight-bearing hip helps to pull the baby backward to sitting. The trunk remains symmetrically extended. The unweighted leg remains flexed, abducted, and externally rotated. The baby can hold the toys during the transition.*

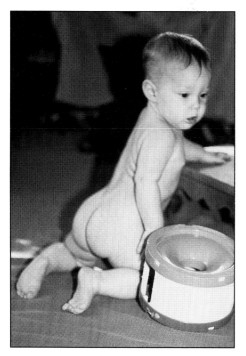

*Figure 9.16. The 9-month-old may play in the kneeling position, using the quadriceps to extend the knees and elevate the trunk. The hip extensors and hip flexors stabilize the pelvis. Anterior pelvic tilting and ankle dorsiflexion demonstrate a fixing pattern.*

the unweighted leg to come forward as part of a balance reaction. Because of the asymmetrical weight bearing, half kneeling is more difficult to maintain than kneeling. Therefore it represents more developed hip control.

# Climbing

Climbing is another skill that the baby uses to explore the environment. Increased pelvic-hip control enables the baby to stop and play in the various transitional phases, such as kneeling and half kneeling.

Stair climbing clearly isolates the movements used in climbing (figures 9.18 to 9.20). During stair climbing, each of the weight-shifting sequences is repeated over and over. The sequence is initiated with a lateral weight shift and elongation on the weight-bearing side, and lateral righting with hip flexion, abduction, and external rotation on the unweighted side (figure 9.18). This enables the baby to lift the leg up onto the step. This is followed by a lateral weight shift to the shortened side, with subsequent elongation of that side (figure 9.19). Subsequently, the opposite leg flexes as a part of the lateral righting reaction. The leg comes forward into a half-kneeling position (figure 9.19). This is followed by weight shift to the flexed leg, which facilitates extension of the knee and elongation of the side (figure 9.20). The baby can assume a standing posture or continue to flex the leg to the next step as in figure 9.18.

Although the 9-month-old has the motor ability to climb up stairs and furniture, the baby does not have the ability to come down. The 9-month-old also does not have the judgment to know that this is a dangerous position. Endeavors to descend usually include attempts to sit down by weight shifting the pelvis posteriorly (figure 9.21), which of course is unsafe and may cause the baby to fall.

Climbing into a small chair is a perceptual problem for the 9-month-old. The baby in figures 9.22 through 9.25 tries to use her known climbing schemes but ends up standing, rather than sitting, in the chair. The known scheme includes lateral weight shifting and lateral righting, kneeling, half kneeling, and standing (figures 9.18 to 9.20).

Sitting in the chair thus becomes a problem-solving event. The baby must experiment with her motor skills to figure out how she can sit, rather than stand, in the chair (figure 9.26). Early attempts to sit are usually unsuccessful. To sit in the chair, the baby must modify the previous kneeling sequence. Once the first leg is flexed onto the chair, the baby must rotate the pelvis and trunk over the leg. External rotation of the flexed hip is needed.

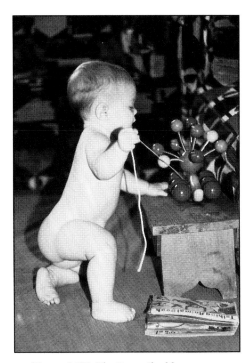

*Figure 9.17.* The 9-month-old may also play in half kneeling. To assume this position, the baby must be able to control the trunk and hips while shifting the weight laterally. Because of the asymmetrical weight bearing, half kneeling is more difficult to maintain than kneeling and represents more developed hip control.

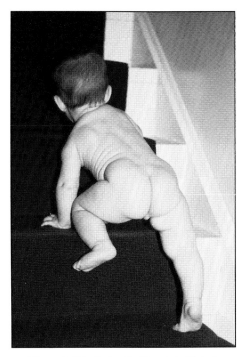

*Figure 9.18.* Stair climbing is initiated with a lateral weight shift and elongation on the weight-bearing side (right) and lateral righting with hip flexion, abduction, and external rotation on the unweighted side (left), which allows the baby to lift the leg onto the step.

## Indications of Possible Disturbances in Motor Development

Climbing is an important activity for the 9-month-old in that it provides the baby with the opportunity to explore the environment and practice new combinations of motor skills. It also reinforces the baby's motor problem-solving skills. Babies who cannot climb miss out on these experiences.

Inability to climb may be suggestive of a developmental delay. Babies who cannot weight bear and weight shift on the upper extremities or transition in and out of sitting and quadruped demonstrate motor delays. Therefore they will be poorly equipped to participate in climbing.

Babies who seem to have the motor components for climbing but reject the activity may be doing so for sensory-perceptual reasons. This is an age of active sensory-spatial exploration of movement (Fritts 1990). It is a time when the infant learns about heights, distances, and space. For some babies, this awareness produces fear. Some babies may need help to modify the fear and its basis.

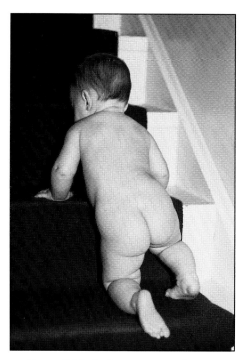 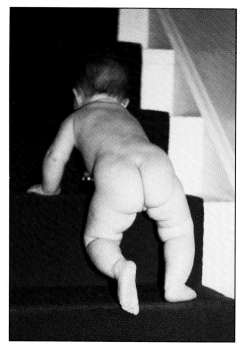

**Figure 9.19.** *As the process continues, weight is shifted laterally to the shortened side, with subsequent elongation of that side (left). The opposite leg (right) then flexes as a part of the lateral righting reaction, and the leg comes forward into a half-kneeling position.*

**Figure 9.20.** *The baby then shifts weight to the flexed leg (right), which facilitates extension of the knee and elongation of the side. The unweighted leg flexes to standing or continues the climbing process.*

Another possible reason that the baby may not engage in climbing activities is that the baby does not detect or perceive that these surfaces are affordable for climbing. Affordances for actions are learned through visual and tactile exploration (Gibson and Schmuckler 1989). Therefore babies who have limited mobility have limited exploratory experiences, which further limits their perception of what is possible.

# Standing

Standing and walking are primary drives for the baby. Much effort is put into coming to stand and cruising around furniture. The baby is also beginning to experiment more with lowering from standing. This is still done with a posterior weight shift into sitting.

The 9-month-old takes full weight on the legs in standing. However, a hand on the furniture still helps to stabilize the balance. The baby can anticipate the postural needs and assumes a wide base of support with the legs when engaging the hands with new or complicated toys (figure 9.27). If a toy falls, the baby can retrieve it from the floor. The 9-month-old still uses a marked posterior weight shift in the hips to lower to the floor (figure 9.28). The baby stabilizes the trunk, hips, and knees during the posterior weight shift. This usually facilitates a balance response of ankle dorsiflexion (figure 9.28).

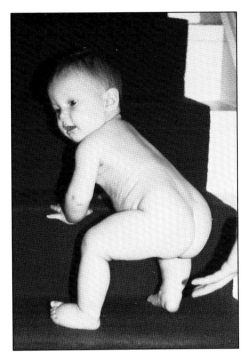

**Figure 9.21.** *Endeavors to descend usually include attempts to sit down by weight shifting the pelvis posteriorly, a dangerous maneuver that could result in a fall.*

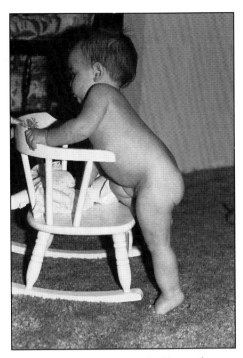

**Figure 9.22.** *The 9-month-old uses the skills that work for climbing stairs when attempting to climb into a chair. Weight is shifted laterally to the left, allowing the right leg to flex up onto the chair.*

Sitting down on the floor is not always planned. It also occurs when the baby loses balance while standing. Loss of balance often occurs when the baby becomes very involved with a toy. Toy manipulation may become more significant than balance control. Falling may occur if the baby uses two hands on the toy, giving up the balance hand. The fall does not seem to interfere with experimentation with the toy.

The 9-month-old continues to practice rotation in standing (figure 9.29). During rotation, the trunk and pelvis rotate over the face-side leg, causing external rotation of the leg and inversion of the foot. Inversion causes weight to shift to the lateral border of the foot. Concomitant with the rotation of the pelvis, the back leg subtly extends and internally rotates (figure 9.29). Hip internal rotation mobility may still be limited; therefore, to compensate for the movement, the back hip and knee flex as the pelvis rotates over the face-side leg. The rotation components become increasingly more evident during the ninth month and may contribute to the overall mobility of the hip joint.

# Cruising

The cruising pattern is becoming more refined, but upper extremity support is still critical. The baby now exhibits more frontal plane control of the legs while walking along the furniture. Hip abduction is accomplished with less hip flexion and more

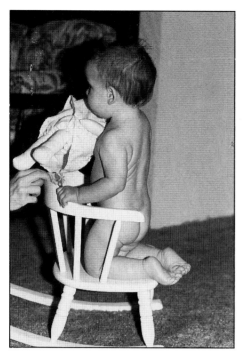

*Figure 9.23.* The known scheme for stair climbing puts the baby into a kneeling position in the chair.

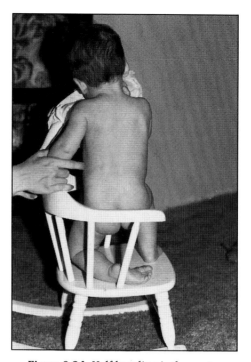

*Figure 9.24.* Half kneeling is the next step in the known scheme.

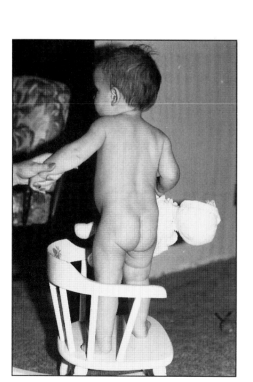

*Figure 9.25.* The final step in the known scheme of stair climbing puts the baby in a standing position in the chair, rather than sitting.

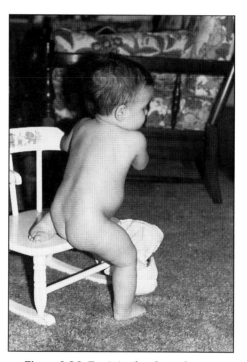

*Figure 9.26.* To sit in the chair, the baby must modify the previous kneeling sequence by rotating the pelvis and trunk over the flexed leg. Hip external rotation is needed.

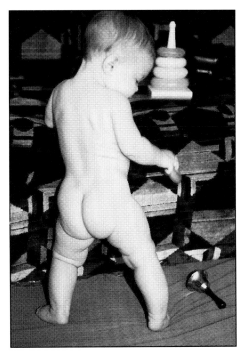

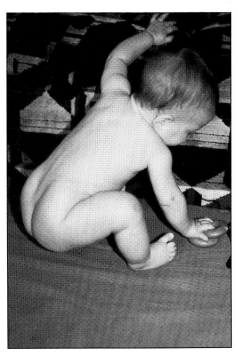

*Figure 9.27. The 9-month-old takes full weight on the legs in standing. However, the baby still uses a hand on the furniture for balance.*

*Figure 9.28. The 9-month-old still uses a marked posterior weight shift in the hips when reaching to retrieve a toy from the floor.*

knee extension. (Compare figures 9.30 and 8.29.) Observation of the pattern suggests that the tensor fascia lata is active in this movement. An anterior pelvic tilt still occurs during hip abduction, suggesting synergistic stability from the hip flexors.

From the position of hip abduction with flexion (figure 9.30), the baby brings the foot to the floor. Once the foot is on the floor, the baby shifts the weight laterally onto the leg using the hip adductor muscles (figure 9.31). The hip abductor muscles must contract synergistically to control the lateral weight shift. Once the weight is shifted, the other leg is unweighted and is free to adduct, thus continuing the cruising process.

Increased control by the hip adductors and abductors enables smoother lateral weight shifting as the baby alternates between abduction and adduction. This control also enables closer alignment of the leg with the trunk during single-limb weight bearing (figure 9.32). The change in the abduction/adduction pattern suggests increased control and mobility between the pelvis and femur. It may also suggest increased eccentric control of the hip abductors. Eccentric control is needed to control the lateral weight shift in standing.

In addition to hip control on the frontal plane, the baby is developing hip control on the transverse plane. This is demonstrated with the added component of rotation during the cruising process. Using the increased hip control, the 9-month-old can shift the weight laterally and then rotate toward the unweighted leg (figure 9.32). This posture resembles the midstance (left leg) and swing (right leg) phases of gait.

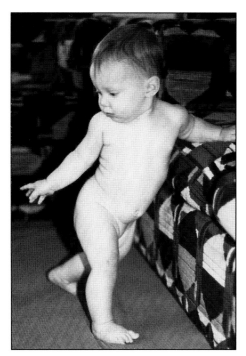

*Figure 9.29.* The 9-month-old continues to practice rotation. The trunk and pelvis rotate over the face-side leg, causing external rotation of the leg and inversion of the foot. Weight shifts to the lateral border of the foot, and the back leg subtly extends and internally rotates.

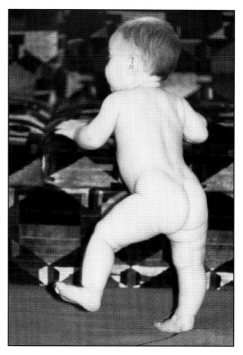

*Figure 9.30.* Upper extremity support during cruising is still important. Hip abduction is accomplished with less hip flexion and more knee extension.

This rotation is similar to that seen in forearm weight bearing where a lateral weight shift precedes reaching and thus frees the face-side hand to reach. It is also an example of a preplanned (feedforward) postural adjustment made prior to movement.

During this process, the pelvis rotates forward over the weight-bearing leg. The hip lateral rotator muscles, including the gluteus maximus, must contract simultaneously to keep the weight-bearing leg externally rotated and extended (Kendall, Kendall, and Wadsworth 1971). External rotation of the leg keeps the knee extended and the weight on the lateral border of the foot. If the hip lateral rotator muscles do not contract sufficiently, the hip internally rotates and flexes, the knee flexes, and the weight is shifted to the medial side of the foot, pronating the foot (figure 9.29).

This pattern of hip internal rotation, knee flexion, and foot pronation is seen early in the developmental process. However, if it is a pattern that is continued, it is suggestive of insufficient control of the hip extensor and lateral rotator muscles.

At the next step in the cruising process, the baby transfers weight onto the forward leg and rotates more toward the goal. Now the hip lateral rotators must stabilize the forward hip in external rotation. The increased rotation mobility at the hip joint permits the back unweighted leg to extend and internally rotate (figure 9.33).

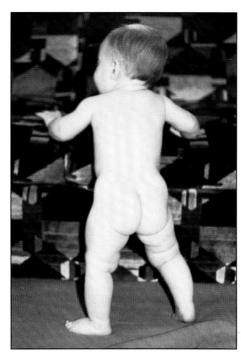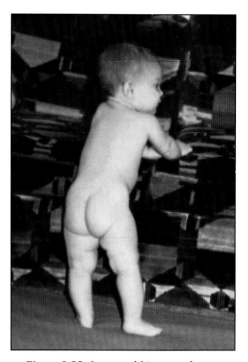

*Figure 9.31. Increased control by the hip adductors and abductors enables smoother lateral weight shifting. Once the knee extends, weight is shifted onto the abducted (left) leg by the hip adductor muscles. The hip abductors control the weight shift.*

*Figure 9.32. Increased hip control enables closer alignment of the leg with the trunk during single-limb weight bearing. This increased control on the frontal and transverse planes enables the baby to weight shift laterally and then rotate the body toward the unweighted leg. The left leg resembles the midstance phase of gait and the right leg resembles the swing phase.*

Increased hip extension, through action of the gluteus maximus, facilitates knee extension (Kendall, Kendall, and Wadsworth 1971) and ankle plantar flexion. On observation, the lower extremity position of the back side leg resembles the terminal stance (pushoff) phase of more mature gait and may thus be a precursor to it (figures 9.33, 9.34).

The standing rotation and cruising rotation patterns change quickly during the ninth month. Rotation changes the side-to-side cruising patterns to a forward walking pattern (figure 9.34). The components become more refined (figures 9.32 to 9.34). Rotation, or transverse plane movement, enables integration of the other two planes of movement. Therefore, as rotation of the pelvis over the femur becomes more controlled, there is more dissociation between the legs. As the legs become more dissociated, the sagittal plane (flexion/extension) and frontal plane (abduction/adduction) components become less conspicuous. The forward walking pattern utilizes lower extremity dissociation which is indicative of triplanar (sagittal, frontal, and transverse) control at the hip joint.

These patterns are just emerging during the ninth month and may not always be used. The cruising pattern with lower extremity abduction and upper extremity support is more common at this age.

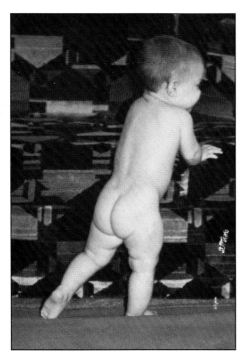

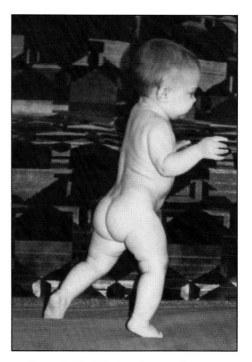

*Figure 9.33.* At the next step in the cruising process, the baby transfers weight onto the forward limb and rotates more toward the goal. Now the hip lateral rotators must stabilize the forward hip in external rotation. The increased rotation mobility at the hip joint permits the back unweighted leg to extend and internally rotate.

*Figure 9.34.* Rotation changes the side-to-side cruising patterns to a forward walking pattern. As rotation of the pelvis over the femur becomes more controlled, there is more dissociation between the legs.

### Indications of Possible Disturbances in Motor Development

A baby's standing and cruising pattern may demonstrate some atypical developmental components. These may include inability to stand because of too little or too much extensor tone. These are obvious signs of abnormal motor development.

More subtle problems are demonstrated in how the baby assumes and manages standing. A 9-month-old baby knows how to initiate and control weight shifting in the lower extremities while standing. When rotating and weight shifting to the face side, the baby can correct for the disturbances of balance, using feedback information. The baby can also preadjust posture in preparation for an anticipated disturbance of posture, using feedforward information.

Babies with subtle motor problems may not be able to use feedback information to make postural adjustments after their weight is shifted. Subsequently, the baby will fall as a result of head movements while standing.

Another problem is seen in the inability to use feedforward information to anticipate disturbances of the posture. This is observed as the baby's inability to laterally weight shift prior to rotation to unweight the face-side leg. This results in an inability to cruise along the furniture because the weight is always on the face-side leg.

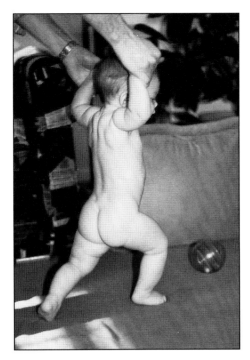

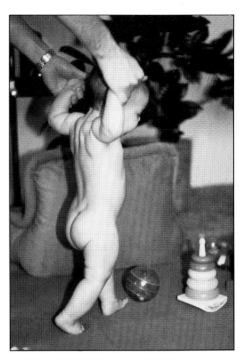

*Figure 9.35.* When supported for walking, the 9-month-old continues to fix the upper trunk with strong scapular adduction. Hip abduction and external rotation are maintained during both swing and stance phases of gait. The hip, knee, and ankle move synchronously, the right in flexion, the left in extension.

*Figure 9.36.* Scapular adduction facilitates spinal extension and an anterior pelvic tilt. The hips are under the shoulders (because of the lumbar extension and anterior pelvic tilt, not hip extension).

# Supported Walking

When supported for walking, the 9-month-old continues to fix the upper trunk and limit the degrees of freedom with strong scapular adduction (figures 9.35, 9.36). Scapular adduction facilitates spinal extension and an anterior pelvic tilt. The hips are under the shoulders because of the lumbar extension and anterior pelvic tilt, not because of hip extension. As a result of the anterior pelvic tilt, the hips remain flexed. Hip abduction with external rotation continues to provide a wide base of support.

The baby limits the degrees of freedom, or fixes, at the hips on the frontal and transverse planes. In other words, the baby maintains hip abduction and external rotation during both swing and stance phases of gait. The legs move primarily on the sagittal plane as the baby uses hip flexion and extension.

During swing, the baby moves the hip, knee, and ankle in synchrony with flexion, abduction, and external rotation. This is followed by synchronous extension, abduction, and external rotation (Forssberg 1992). Range into hip extension is still limited. Therefore the baby compensates with an anterior pelvic tilt (figures 9.35, 9.36). During stance, the baby utilizes hip abduction and external rotation to maintain a wide base of support for stability.

Hip external rotation limits the range of hip extension. Therefore the development of hip extension seems to be related to an increase in hip internal rotation. Although these changes are occurring as the baby cruises around the furniture (figures 9.32 to 9.34), they are not yet present in forward walking. In this more advanced skill, the baby still limits the degree of freedom around the hips. As the baby continues to practice supported walking, increased control of the hip muscles will develop. Subsequently, the need to fix with external rotation will decrease, and lower extremity dissociation will increase concurrent with an increase in pelvic-femoral rotation and hip extension.

# The Tenth Month

**B**abies at ten months are very busy, actively exploring the environment and practicing all of their motor skills. During this period they spend much time developing and playing with perceptual concepts, especially *in* and *out.* The 10-month-old usually likes all toys and enjoys inspecting them with the eyes and the hands. During this time, the baby is very interested in container play, putting things in and taking them out (spending most of the time taking things out). During the tenth month, the baby is also beginning to mimic gestures (Vogtle and Albert 1985; Fritts 1990; Nash 1991).

## Sitting

Static sitting is rare for 10-month-olds. When babies are quiet in sitting, they are usually eating or exploring a toy. They spend most of the time moving in and out of sitting, retrieving toys, and transporting toys to a new location.

By the tenth month, the baby can long sit with the legs in line with the body (figure 10.1). Long sitting is possible because of adequate length in the hamstring muscles and control of the pelvic-femoral muscles. Trunk rotation in this position is also possible. The pelvis rotates over the face-side femur.

Wide abduction of the legs is also possible during long sitting. This posture provides additional positional stability, but it requires marked mobility in the hip adductor muscles. Although this posture provides a wide play area, it does not permit transition mobility.

Most of the time, the 10-month-old baby sits with the legs in a tailor position, which provides stability but also permits transitions. This position reduces the stretch on the hamstrings and permits

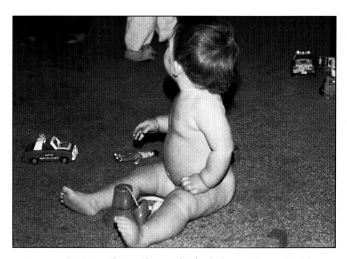

*Figure 10.1. By the tenth month, the baby can long sit with the legs in line with the body. Trunk rotation may still be counterbalanced with active external rotation of the skull-side leg (left).*

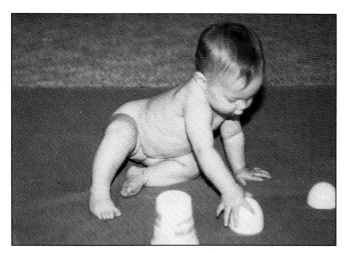

**Figure 10.2.** *The baby extends the trunk forward over the legs to reach for toys. Forward movement of the trunk is also used to transition to quadruped.*

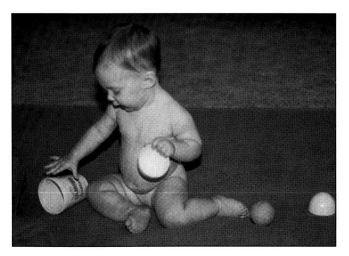

**Figure 10.3.** *Side sitting, assumed by independently internally rotating one hip (left), provides a stable, wide base of support during upper extremity play.*

free movement of the pelvis and extended trunk forward over the legs. This forward movement is used to reach for toys and to transition to quadruped (figure 10.2). These transitions require marked pelvic-femoral mobility.

Side sitting is also frequently used. The baby assumes this position by independently internally rotating one hip (figure 10.3). Side sitting provides a wide base of support during upper extremity play. It is also a position from which the baby can easily transition to quadruped or to tailor or long sitting.

W sitting is still used by some babies. It provides a stable, wide base of support which is used particularly during fine motor manipulative activities (figure 10.4). Most babies do not need to use W sitting for fine motor control, but rather use it as one option. W sitting is not a good position for the hips or the knees. It exaggerates hip internal rotation and stretches the medial ligaments of the knees. This could lead to increased medial femoral torsion, a knock-knee position in standing, and/or knee instability.

The 10-month-old baby can easily transition out of W sitting (figure 10.5). The baby can lift the trunk and shift it laterally over the leg. The leg, accordingly, moves from internal to external rotation. The baby can also rise to kneeling from W sitting by contracting the quadriceps.

Each of these maneuvers occurs with a stable trunk and marked pelvic-femoral mobility and control. These changes in posture occur automatically as the baby reaches for toys, plays with toys, and interacts with the environment.

### Upper Extremities

Increased control of trunk rotation enables the baby to reach across midline (figure 10.2) (Vogtle and Albert 1985). Because of increased trunk control, scapular adduction is no longer needed to reinforce trunk stability during reaching. Subsequently, there is also less posturing with elbow flexion. Increased distal control is seen as slight wrist extension during the reaching phase.

Between the ninth and twelfth months, the infant uses digital activity to manipulate and explore objects. According to Ruff (cited in Corbetta and Mounoud 1990), infants have several exploratory behaviors, depending on the object's properties. Infants visually explore objects with different shapes by rotating the forearm to bring the object into the visual field. Objects with different textures are fingered under visual control. Objects with different weights are banged rather than visually inspected.

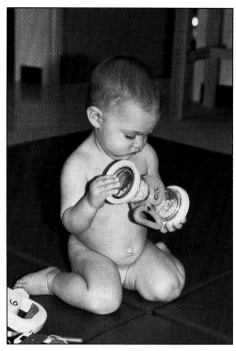

**Figure 10.4.** *Some babies use W sitting for play. It provides a stable base of support, but it is not good for the hips or knees.*

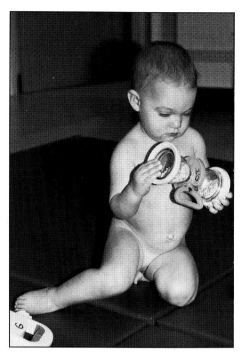

**Figure 10.5.** *The 10-month-old baby can easily transition out of W sitting by lifting the trunk and shifting it laterally over the leg. The weight-bearing leg (left) moves from internal to external rotation.*

The 10-month-old practices a variety of prehension patterns along with release. The baby can use a pincer grasp, in which the distal pads of the thumb and index finger meet (Erhardt 1984; Vogtle and Albert 1985), to pick up a raisin or a piece of cereal.

The baby also uses a "three-jaw chuck" grasp, in which the thumb, index, and third fingers are active and the two ulnar fingers are quiet (Erhardt 1984; Vogtle and Albert 1985; Nash 1991). This grasp is used for self feeding as well as for picking up small toys.

Increased dissociation and quieting of the fingers enables isolation of the index finger (Nash 1990, 1991). During this pattern, the third finger and the two ulnar fingers are quiet. Radial deviation of the wrist is increasingly used to place the index finger during pointing. The isolated finger is used to point to objects and to poke into little holes (Erhardt 1984; Nash 1990, 1991). Pointing is often used to label objects.

Finger control is more refined for grasp than release. Babies are more proficient at taking objects out of a container, but they are beginning to practice release by putting objects into containers. The baby can release a cube into a large container and is beginning to release into a small container (Erhardt 1984; Vogtle and Albert 1985).

The 10-month-old is also practicing release through forearm supination (Nash 1991). As the forearm is supinated, the fingers open and the toy can fall out. The baby needs a surface, often a caretaker's hand, into which to release the toy.

The 10-month-old can use two-handed coordination behaviors for manipulation and exploration (Corbetta and Mounoud 1990). Two-handed coordination is demonstrated when the baby removes a cube from a container while the other hand stabilizes the container. The baby can also bang two objects together and transfer objects from hand to hand.

The 10-month-old can crawl with toys in both hands. This may contribute to the development of the palmar arches (Nash 1991). Usually the toy is held by the radial side of the hand, which shifts the weight to the ulnar side of the hand and facilitates external rotation in the shoulder.

# Crawling and Climbing

Crawling and climbing are major activities for the 10-month-old. These movements demonstrate and develop the baby's coordination between the trunk and the extremities. They also demonstrate and develop the emerging perceptual skills. The baby now has sufficient motor control and body awareness to maneuver the body over, around, or onto obstacles that may obstruct a toy.

Crawling is still the primary means of locomotion. Reciprocal extremity movements and trunk counterrotation enable the baby to move smoothly and quickly across the floor.

If babies encounter obstacles while crawling to a toy, they can continue their forward progression by climbing up onto or over the obstacle (figure 10.6). Through experimentation, they will encounter obstacles of different heights, widths, and stability and will thus be challenged to develop a problem-solving repertoire regarding which obstacles are safe to climb on and which are not (Gibson and Schmuckler 1989). This judgment is developed only through experience and active problem solving. Babies will experience instability and may possibly fall when they climb on unstable objects. Hopefully this information will be filed in the problem-solving repertoire and will alert them the next time they try to climb on a similar object.

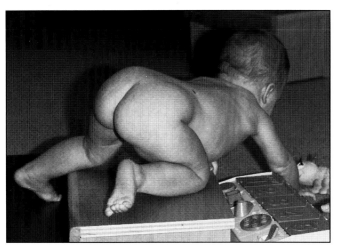

**Figure 10.6.** *If a 10-month-old encounters an obstacle while crawling to a toy, the baby can continue the forward progression by climbing up onto or over the obstacle.*

Objects of different heights and widths challenge the baby in different ways. Motor planning and problem-solving skills are learned as the baby practices reaching up and down with the hands and feet in search of a stable point. Motor planning skills are also learned during climbing as the baby experiments with extremity and trunk placement. The baby must make fine adjustments in posture to remain stable during these maneuvers.

Climbing requires lower trunk stability for upper trunk movements, and upper trunk stability for lower trunk movements. Since one upper and one lower extremity often move simultaneously, dynamic trunk stability is an essential requirement.

Climbing stairs is still an activity that the baby enjoys. Alternate reciprocal extremity movements are used to move up the stairs. The 10-month-old seems to have more perceptual awareness with respect to coming down the stairs. The baby now looks behind (figure 10.7), then lowers over the weight-bearing leg (figure 10.8) so as to tailor sit on the step. From the sitting posture, the baby can bring the arm forward for weight bearing and trunk stability to be able to move the leg. When the baby feels stable, the leg is lowered to the step below (figure 10.9). This is a new activity for the baby, who still needs assistance. However, the baby's attempts to control the lowering process demonstrate an increasing perceptual awareness.

Kneeling without external support is a common occurrence for the 10-month-old (figure 10.10). Contraction of the quadriceps is needed to elevate the body. Hip extensors are needed to stabilize the trunk. If hip flexors, in addition to hip extensors, are still used to stabilize the trunk, there is a slight anterior pelvic tilt and synergistic ankle dorsiflexion.

The 10-month-old can easily transition into and play in half kneeling (figure 10.11). Assumption of this posture demonstrates the baby's increased control of lower extremity dissociation. From this position, the baby transitions back to sitting by lowering the body over the weight-bearing leg. The leg muscles, especially the quadriceps, are active during the lowering. The nonweight-bearing hip remains externally rotated, which provides stability to the pelvis. This was the same maneuver used to come to sit on the stairs (figure 10.8).

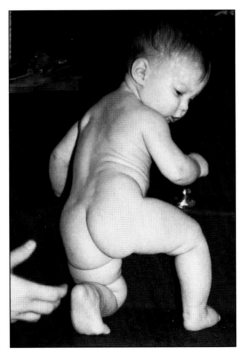

*Figure 10.7.* The 10-month-old seems to have more perceptual awareness in coming down the stairs, now looking to the rear before moving the weight-bearing leg.

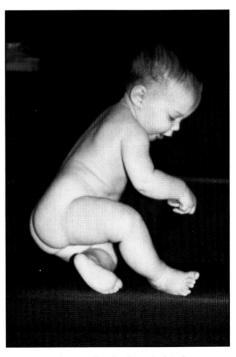

*Figure 10.8.* After looking behind, the baby lowers the body over the weight-bearing leg and comes to a tailor-sitting position.

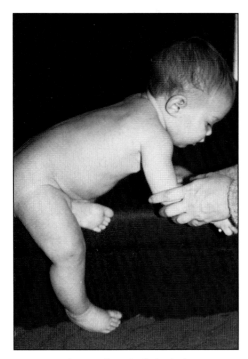

*Figure 10.9*. When the baby feels stable, the baby will lower the leg to the next step below.

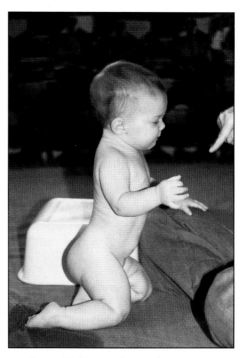

*Figure 10.10*. Kneeling without external support is a common occurrence for the 10-month-old. An anterior pelvic tilt is still seen.

# Rising to Stand

The legs are very active in rising to stand. The upper extremities seem to be used more for balance than for control. From half kneeling, the baby shifts weight forward onto the flexed leg and rises to a single-limb stance (figure 10.12). This demonstrates good concentric control in the quadriceps.

Forward movement of the trunk must be coordinated with extension of the knee. If the forward leg is also slightly abducted, the hip adductors must work to bring the trunk and center of gravity over the weight-bearing foot. When the hip external rotators (such as the gluteus maximus) are active during this process, the weight will shift to the lateral border of the foot. If the hip external rotators are not active, the weight will shift to the medial side of the foot, and the foot will pronate.

# Standing

Once in standing, the baby uses leg muscles and minimal assistance of one hand to control the posture. The arms and hands are free for exploration or manipulation. This eventually enables the baby to stand without upper extremity support. The baby spontaneously relinquishes hand support when presented with an interesting toy that requires two hands. For bilateral hand use to be successful, the baby must preadjust posture for stability.

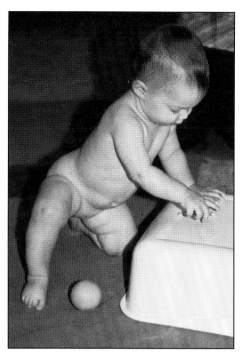 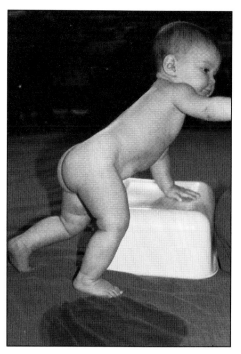

**Figure 10.11.** *The 10-month-old can easily transition into and play in half kneeling. Assumption of this posture demonstrates the baby's increased control of lower extremity dissociation.*

**Figure 10.12.** *In rising to stand, the baby shifts the weight forward from half kneeling onto the flexed leg. The weight-bearing hand is used for balance rather than control.*

Increased ankle movements are noted in standing, especially active plantar flexion. The gastrocnemius muscles are used to plantar flex and invert the calcaneus. Inversion of the calcaneus locks the subtalar joint and subsequently the midtarsal joint of the foot, thus locking the whole foot (Root et al. 1971; Root, Orien, and Weed 1977). From this locked-foot position, the baby's weight is transferred over the metatarsal heads of the foot, enabling the baby to rise on the toes. This elongates the toe flexor muscles. Prior to ten months, the baby's toe flexors were rarely elongated. They were more frequently shortened as the baby flexed or curled the toes during balance activities.

When the baby uses asymmetrical ankle plantar flexion, the posture of the foot, with weight over the metatarsal heads, resembles the lower extremity pattern used in the terminal stance, pushoff phase of mature gait (figures 10.16, 10.17). This ankle-foot pattern seems to reinforce hip and knee extension.

The increased control of the leg muscles, especially graded eccentric control of the quadriceps, enables the baby to lower from a standing posture (figures 10.13, 10.14). The baby can squat on symmetrical legs while stabilizing with the upper extremities (figure 10.13). The weight is shifted posteriorly while the trunk remains extended. Slight forward movement of the tibia over the foot may occur when the baby squats with upper extremity support.

Asymmetrical lowering occurs when the baby tries to reach for a toy (figure 10.14). The baby usually uses one hand for support while the other hand reaches. The weight is transferred to one leg, and eccentric action of the quadriceps is used for the lowering.

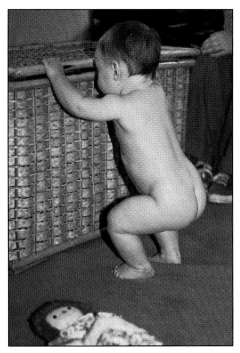

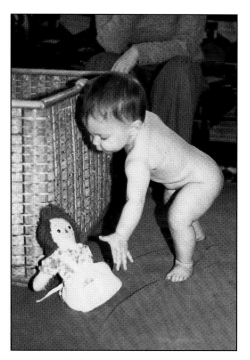

*Figure 10.13.* The 10-month-old can squat on symmetrical legs while stabilizing with the upper extremities. The weight is shifted posteriorly while the trunk remains extended. Slight forward movement of the tibia over the foot may occur.

*Figure 10.14.* Asymmetrical lowering occurs when the baby tries to reach for a toy. One hand is needed for support while the other hand experiments with a new range of reaching.

Reaching for a toy on the floor while standing is a perceptual and motor challenge for the baby (figure 10.14). The baby must experiment with a new range of reaching which presents new challenges to the postural system. To stabilize the posture during this new reaching pattern, the baby must make constant trunk and lower extremity adjustments during the reaching and lowering process. Feedback is used for these adjustments. After practicing this activity, the baby will be able to anticipate the postural requirements and will subsequently establish them prior to the reach (feedforward). However, feedback will still be used to regulate the movement.

# Cruising

The ability of 10-month-olds to control their posture and lower extremities in standing enables them to continue to vary the cruising pattern. They may cruise sideways with lower extremity abduction, as they did in previous months, or they may turn so that they can face the direction in which they are going (figure 10.15). This causes them to walk forward holding on with one hand, rather than sideways holding on with two hands.

In order to face the direction in which they are going, babies must rotate the pelvis over the femur to dissociate the legs (figure 10.15). Dynamic rotation at the

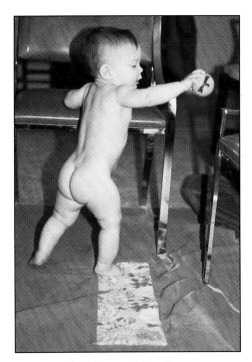

*Figure 10.15.* In cruising, the 10-month-old may turn to face the direction of movement, causing the baby to walk forward holding on with one hand, rather than sideways holding on with two hands.

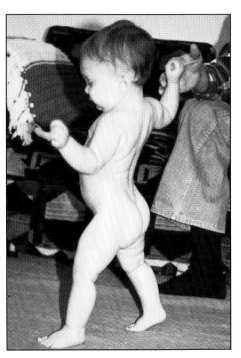

*Figure 10.16.* With one hand held, the 10-month-old often finds stability during early forward walking by using scapular adduction, trunk extension, and an anterior pelvic tilt. Increased pelvic-femoral rotation leads to increased lower extremity dissociation.

pelvic-femoral joint facilitates triplanar movement of the hips during walking. During forward walking, this rotation enables one leg to flex while the other leg extends (sagittal plane), and it enables the legs to come in line with the trunk (frontal plane).

At ten months, cruising around the furniture includes increased perceptual challenges. The baby is starting to move across open spaces and around corners (figure 10.15). Motor planning skills are being developed and practiced in standing as well as other activities.

The 10-month-old's curiosity will lead the baby to attempt cruising around pieces of furniture of different heights and firmness. Each variation causes the baby to actively problem solve how to regulate the body to remain stable and yet move. The more these variations are practiced, the more skillful the baby becomes in meeting new motor challenges.

## Supported Walking

Forward walking along the furniture while holding on with one hand is a natural precursor for forward walking across the floor with one hand held (figure 10.16). The baby often finds stability during early forward walking by using scapular ad-duction, trunk extension, and an anterior pelvic tilt. This pattern may limit the

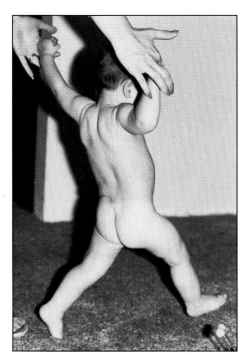

*Figure 10.17. The 10-month-old uses marked trunk extension when walking forward with two hands held. The baby seems to play with trunk extension to increase lower extremity extension and step length.*

degrees of freedom, or fix, the trunk and pelvis, so that the baby can experiment with various hip movements. As pelvic-femoral rotation mobility and control increase, the baby can achieve more lower extremity dissociation during walking.

The 10-month-old also uses marked trunk extension when walking forward with two hands held. Until pelvic-femoral rotation is developed, the baby may play with trunk extension to increase lower extremity extension and step length (figures 10.16, 10.17).

The swing phase of gait is still characterized by marked hip flexion with knee flexion, followed by knee extension and lumbar extension which propels the body forward (figures 10.16, 10.17). The ankle is usually dorsiflexed during swing, suggesting that there is still synchronous action among the hip, knee, and ankle.

Forward movement of the body is also accomplished through extension of the stance leg. The trunk, hip, knee, and ankle extend during terminal stance (figures 10.16, 10.17). The body weight is shifted to and rolls over the metatarsal heads of the foot (figure 10.17). The baby relies on the supporting person while experimenting with the developing leg control.

Standing and walking with one hand held is a new challenge for the baby. To stand with only one hand held, the baby must be able to control the weight shift in the trunk and pelvis with the hip and leg muscles. Balance must be initiated from the base of support, thus the feet. Until now, the baby has relied on the supporter for balance.

It is easier for the baby to shift weight laterally toward the side on which the hand is held (figure 10.16). Flexion of the arm overhead helps to elongate the entire side and thus facilitates a lateral weight shift to that side. Once the weight is shifted, the unweighted leg can move forward.

When shifting the weight away from the hand-held side, the baby must shift the weight in the legs and trunk. Initial attempts often result in a weight shift in the legs but not in the pelvis and trunk. This posture resembles that seen when the gluteus medius is weak (Brunnstrom 1979). This causes dropping of the pelvis and leaning of the trunk toward the unweighted side. The baby is thus very dependent on the external support. With experimentation and decreased reliance on the hand support, the baby will shift the weight in the pelvis and trunk as well as in the legs.

# Indications of Possible Disturbances in Motor Development

By the tenth month, the baby is combining many movement components that developed in previous months. If there is a disturbance in motor development during the tenth month, it will be a continuation of a problem seen in earlier months.

# The Eleventh Month

**B**abies at 11 months continue to practice and perfect the skills started in the tenth month. Gross motor skills enable them to move efficiently on the floor by crawling. They can bring themselves to stand, walk around furniture, or climb on or over furniture. Eleven-month-olds can stand at furniture and manipulate toys with both hands. They usually lean on the furniture to do this, but they are beginning to use both hands while standing freely near the furniture.

Independent standing occurs when the baby is at furniture and when pulling to stand on a person. Independent standing occurs automatically when the baby is absorbed in the task at hand (for example, manipulating a toy or obtaining a bit of cereal). This increased control of the lower extremities enables the baby to walk with one hand held. The control soon leads to attempts at walking with no hands held.

The baby continues to enjoy container play, dropping things in and taking them out. The 11-month-old now has more control of release, and the grasp is changing from the three-jawed chuck to a neat pincer grasp (Erhardt 1984). The baby continues to use a strong index finger approach for poking into small holes and labeling objects. The baby likes to carry objects during crawling and walking.

The 11-month-old uses both hands in games like pat-a-cake, to bang objects together, and to assist with dressing tasks. The baby enjoys toys with small holes, cars that can be pushed, toys with strings, shape sorters, busy boxes, and all sizes of containers (Nash 1991).

## Sitting

The 11-month-old may be observed in quiet sitting when engaged in dressing, eating, or a fine motor task. The baby enjoys mimicking activities that occur in the world and likes to try to assist with dressing and undressing activities (figure 11.1). During these activities, the baby is free to assume many different postures, using long sitting, side sitting, ring sitting, or W sitting.

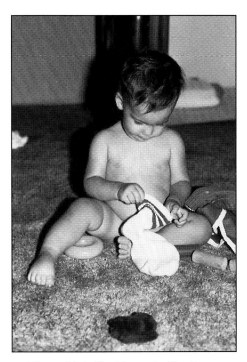

*Figure 11.1. The 11-month-old enjoys mimicking familiar activities. The baby likes to try to assist with dressing and undressing activities. The baby can orient the forearm and hand to align toys and clothing for proper placement while sitting in a variety of postures.*

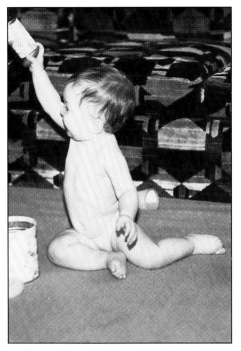

*Figure 11.2. Wide ranges of shoulder abduction and flexion occur freely as increased trunk control provides a stable base from which the baby can move the arms efficiently during play.*

Babies may use wide abduction of the legs to create a wide play area in front of them. But they can tuck the leg under the hips and easily move out of sitting into quadruped (figure 11.7).

Increased trunk control provides a stable base from which the baby can move the arms efficiently while playing. Wide ranges of shoulder abduction and flexion occur freely (figure 11.2). The baby also has more freedom in the elbows and forearms because of the dynamic stability of the shoulder girdles and the increased dexterity of the hands. Therefore the child can easily manipulate a toy with the hands while visually inspecting it. The baby can also orient the forearm and hand to align toys and clothing for proper placement (figures 11.1, 11.3).

If the fine-motor task is difficult, the baby may revert to increased fixing by adducting the arms to the sides and adducting the fingers (figure 11.3). Humeral adduction provides increased upper extremity stability by limiting the degrees of freedom of the shoulder girdle. With increased humeral stability, the baby can experiment with various movements of the elbow and forearm. The baby can now hold a container with one hand while trying to place another container into it (figure 11.3). This is a new task for the baby, one that demonstrates increased control in bimanual cooperation and coordination. It is more difficult than previous tasks because the hands are performing dissociated tasks rather than associated tasks (Corbetta and Mounoud 1990; Fagard 1990). One hand provides stability while the other hand moves.

While sitting, the baby continues to move the extended trunk and pelvis forward as a unit over the femurs. This occurs primarily when reaching forward and when transitioning to quadruped (figure 11.7). The 11-month-old demonstrates increased use of trunk flexion when reaching and when trying to inspect objects visually.

Trunk rotation occurs through a greater range than in previous months and does not interfere with sitting stability (figure 11.4). Trunk rotation enables the baby to reach for objects at the side and behind. Mirroring postures of the upper extremities are seen in these early rotation patterns. This may assure symmetry in the trunk. As the baby practices the movement, less mirroring of the upper extremities occurs.

During the eleventh month, the baby practices more sitting positions which utilize spinal lateral flexion (figure 11.5). The increased range and mobility in lateral flexion of the spine may suggest that the baby is freeing up degrees of freedom in the trunk.

There are various forms of side sitting. When starting with this position, the baby created a very wide base of support with the legs (figure 9.3). Some low-tone babies continue to use this wide base, especially when they are engaged with a fine motor and/or visual-motor task. Side sitting that utilizes a wide base of support actually

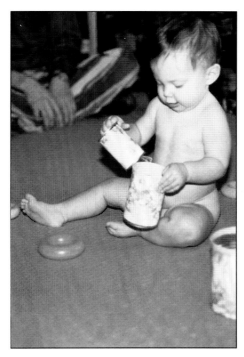 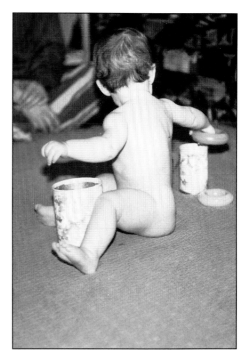

*Figure 11.3.* *If a fine motor task is difficult, the baby may revert to increased fixing by adducting the arms to the sides and adducting the fingers. Humeral adduction provides increased upper extremity stability by limiting the degrees of freedom of the shoulder girdle. With increased humeral stability, the baby can experiment with various movements of the elbow and forearm.*

*Figure 11.4.* *Trunk rotation occurs through a greater range than in previous months and does not interfere with sitting stability. Mirror postures of the upper extremities are often seen in early rotation.*

keeps the trunk and spine symmetrical (figure 11.6). The baby assumes the position by adjusting or rotating the legs under the symmetrical pelvis. The symmetrical pelvis stabilizes the trunk and frees the arms to move in various positions.

When the baby narrows the base of support during side sitting, lateral flexion of the spine increases (figure 11.5). This is accompanied by lateral flexion of the pelvis. The base of support is narrowed when the baby's leg is in line with the trunk (figure 11.5, right leg). Compare this with the baby's right leg in figure 11.6.

# Quadruped

After a brief period of play, most babies will move out of sitting into quadruped (figure 11.7). From quadruped the baby can crawl to other toys or people. This often involves carrying toys. Crawling is still the baby's main means of locomotion.

Container play is not limited to small containers. When presented with a large container, the 11-month-old explores its affordances. The baby in figure 11.8 will try to put herself in and out. Such play increases the baby's motor planning skills, perceptual skills, and awareness of the body scheme. The baby is learning how to maneuver the body to interact with the environment.

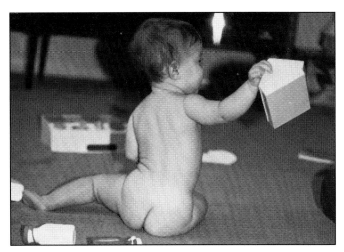

*Figure 11.5. During the eleventh month, the baby practices more sitting positions which utilize spinal lateral flexion. Side sitting is accomplished with a narrow base of support. The right leg is in line with the trunk.*

Once in the container, the 11-month-old continues to experiment with motor skills. The baby will try all of the skills that have been practiced elsewhere. The motor planning and perceptual challenge is increased because of the confined space.

# Kneeling

From quadruped, the baby can easily move into kneeling. Kneeling is accomplished without upper extremity support, through synergistic contraction of the hip extensors and the quadriceps. The hip extensors extend the hips and stabilize the trunk on the femurs. The quadriceps extend the knees and elevate the hips and trunk. When the quadriceps and hip extensors work efficiently in synergy, the ankles relax into plantar flex. Kneeling is frequently used as a part of the reaching pattern (figure 11.9).

# Climbing

Climbing is still one of the favorite activities for 11-month-olds. Most furniture becomes a challenge (figure 11.10). Babies use the same skills to climb up onto the furniture that they used in previous months. This includes a lateral weight shift, elongation on the weight-bearing side, lateral flexion on the unweighted side, and lower extremity dissociation (figure 11.10). Upper extremity strength is also a critical component of climbing.

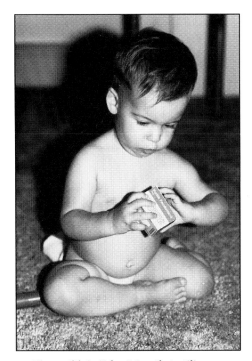

*Figure 11.6. Side sitting that utilizes a wide base of support keeps the trunk and spine symmetrical. This posture is often used by babies with low tone during fine motor tasks.*

Once on the furniture, the 11-month-old has the motor planning and motor skill to maneuver the body from the climbing position to sitting, facing the direction of ascent (figure 11.11, 11.12). This maneuver is similar to the one used on the floor to move from quadruped to sitting.

From quadruped, the baby rotates the pelvis over the weight-bearing leg while simultaneously externally rotating and tucking that leg under the trunk (figure 11.11, left leg). The unweighted leg must actively abduct and externally rotate (figure 11.12, right leg) to reorient the pelvis and trunk. One upper extremity is used for postural stability (figure 11.12, left), while the other upper extremity (right) assists with the trunk rotation.

Fortunately, the baby is beginning to develop perceptual and motor skills that can be used to descend from the furniture (figures 11.13, 11.14). However, these skills usually must be taught to the baby, because moving backward is not a skill that the baby intuitively practices.

To descend from the furniture, the baby turns to quadruped and moves the body backward (figure 11.13). While moving backward, the baby must be aware of where the body is in relation to the furniture. This awareness is especially important in knowing when to let the legs extend and how securely to hold on with the hands (figure 11.14). The baby must also be aware of when the feet have touched the ground, and when to reduce upper trunk stability. These skills and perceptions are learned through practice.

If surfaces of varying heights and firmness are used to practice on, the baby will develop problem-solving skills for an even greater variety of heights and firmness. Babies who do not practice climbing on different surfaces have more difficulty problem solving how to get on and off any surface. In either case, the baby needs supervision during climbing activities.

## Squat: Rising to Stand

By the eleventh month, most babies are attempting to rise to stand without external hand support. The baby usually initiates a rising sequence from quadruped. From quadruped, one leg comes forward into a semihalf-kneeling position (figure 11.15). Then the baby shifts weight onto the hands and one foot and brings the other leg forward to squat. The baby may stay in this squat position and play (figures 11.16, 11.17).

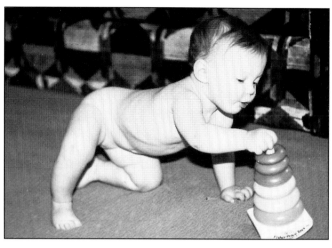

*Figure 11.7. After a brief period of play, most babies will move out of sitting into quadruped. The baby continues to move the extended trunk and pelvis forward as a unit over the femur.*

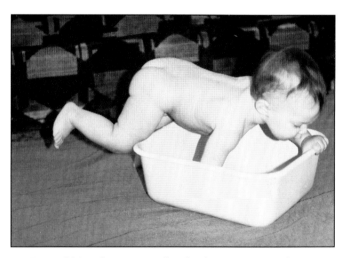

*Figure 11.8. When presented with a large container, the 11-month-old will explore it, crawling over it and trying to fit into it.*

Squatting is a symmetrical position (figures 11.16, 11.17) during which the baby keeps the weight posterior with minimal ankle dorsiflexion. This position, with its marked posterior weight shift, puts a strain on the quadriceps and stretches the gastrocnemius muscles. Subsequently, the hip extensors, abdominals, quadriceps, and ankle dorsiflexors contract in synergy to provide stability. The position also puts demands on the ankles and feet for balance control. Initial attempts to balance are often made with toe curling (figure 11.17).

From the squat position, the baby can rise to stand (figures 11.17, 11.18) by symmetrically extending the knees and hips while stabilizing the body at the ankles and feet (figure 11.18). Rising with symmetry and a wide base reinforces the baby's stability. Strong toe curling may accompany this transition, which may increase lower extremity stability.

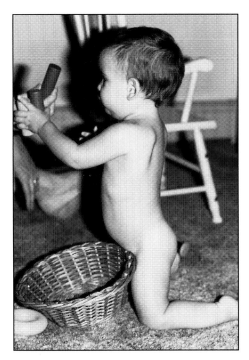

*Figure 11.9*. Kneeling is frequently used as a part of the reaching pattern. Less anterior tilting of the pelvis and more ankle plantar flexion are seen because of increased hip extensor activity.

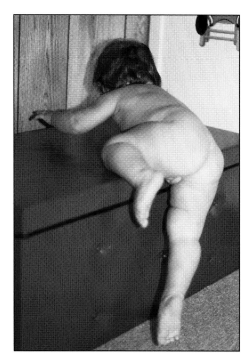

*Figure 11.10*. Climbing is still one of the 11-month-old's favorite activities, and most furniture is seen as a climbing challenge for the baby. A lateral weight shift with elongation of the weight-bearing side (right) is followed by lateral flexion on the unweighted side.

# Furniture: Rising to Stand

With one hand on the furniture, the baby can easily rise to stand through a half-kneeling posture (figures 11.19, 11.20). The baby can shift weight forward onto the flexed leg and lift the body weight with that leg. This requires strength and control in the quadriceps and hip extensors. The ankle and foot are used for balance. The back leg extends synchronously at the hip, knee, and ankle. Once in standing, the baby may assume a wide stance to assure stability.

From standing, the baby can lower to a squat and rise again without difficulty (figure 11.21). This suggests strong control of the quadriceps and hip extensors for both concentric and eccentric contraction. The baby can now use various ranges in squatting. The deeper the squat, the more the quadriceps must work to control the movement and posture. During squatting, the weight is kept posterior and minimal ankle dorsiflexion is used.

The baby may also try asymmetrical lowering (figure 11.22). This maneuver is more difficult because of the dissociated position of the legs. Therefore, hand support is usually needed. Although babies can rise with the strength of the quadriceps of one leg, they have difficulty lowering themselves on one leg. During lowering, the quadriceps must contract eccentrically. The eccentric contraction is more difficult than the concentric contraction.

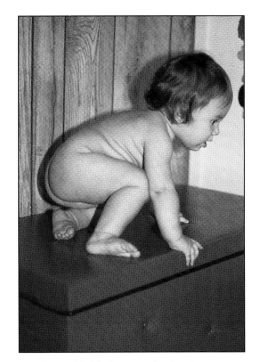

*Figure 11.11.* Once on the furniture, the 11-month-old has the motor planning and motor skill to maneuver the body from the climbing position to sitting. The pelvis and trunk are rotated over the left leg while the leg is simultaneously externally rotated and tucked under the trunk.

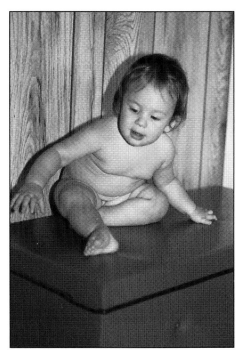

*Figure 11.12.* The unweighted right leg is actively abducted and externally rotated to reorient the pelvis and trunk. The left upper extremity is used for postural stability while the right upper extremity assists with the trunk rotation.

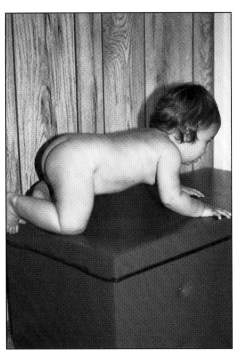

*Figure 11.13.* The baby turns to quadruped and moves the body backward in order to descend from the furniture.

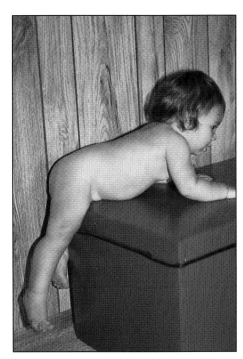

*Figure 11.14.* While moving backward, the baby must be aware of where the body is in relation to the furniture. This awareness is especially important in knowing when to let the legs extend and how securely to hold on with the hands.

The back leg assists during asymmetrical lowering. Weight is shifted to the toes, which become increasingly more dorsiflexed as the baby's weight is lowered to the floor. The back leg sustains some of the weight, which means that the foot must provide stability and mobility during the lowering.

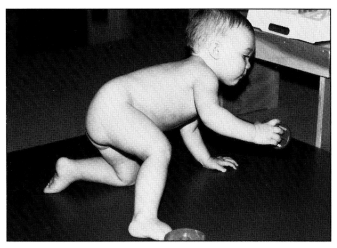

*Figure 11.15. By the eleventh month, most babies are attempting to rise to stand without external hand support. From quadruped, one leg comes forward into a semihalf-kneeling position. Then the baby shifts the weight onto the hands and one foot and brings the other leg forward to squat.*

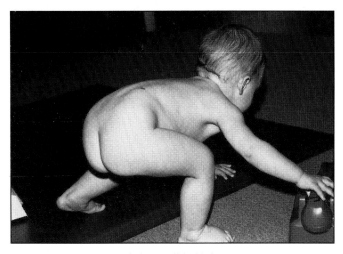

*Figure 11.16. Some babies will hold this squat position and play.*

## Standing

Standing without external support is a new accomplishment for the baby (figure 11.23). It usually occurs automatically when babies become very interested in a toy they want to hold or explore with two hands. Wide abduction of the legs assures a wide, stable base of support. These postural adjustments occur automatically before the baby lets go with the hands.

## Supported Walking

The baby's independence in walking is increasing quickly. Furniture cruising with one hand on the furniture and free walking with one hand held enable the baby to practice lower extremity-pelvic-trunk weight shifting and postural adjustments. In addition, the baby has been using automatic postural adjustments in the lower extremities when engaging both hands on a toy while standing. All of these experiences prepare the baby to step out into space unsupported.

Early attempts by the baby to walk independently often emerge from holding onto an adult's arm (figures 11.24, 11.25). This somewhat unstable support forces the baby to make postural adjustments that are adequate to stay upright and yet move. Scapular adduction is often used to fix and limit the degrees of freedom in the upper trunk. Weight shift is easier toward the hand-support side, enabling elongation on that side while the other leg swings through (figure 11.24). Weight shift of the trunk away from the hand-support side is difficult if the baby is relying on the support. Therefore the weight will be shifted in the legs, but the pelvis and trunk will lean toward the unweighted side (figure 11.25). This may result in a shorter step on that side.

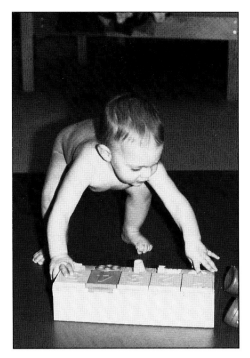

*Figure 11.17.* Squatting is a symmetrical position: the baby keeps the weight posterior, with minimal ankle dorsi-flexion. Toe curling may be used to assist with balance.

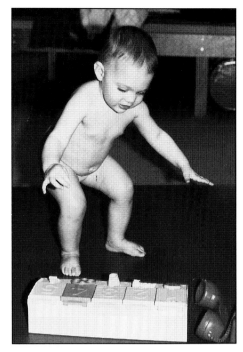

*Figure 11.18.* From the squat position, the baby can rise to stand, symmetrically extending the knees and hips while stabilizing the body at the ankles and feet.

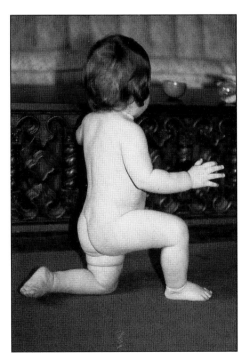

*Figure 11.19.* With one hand on the furniture, the baby can easily assume a half-kneeling posture. The legs are well dissociated with full hip extension on the back leg.

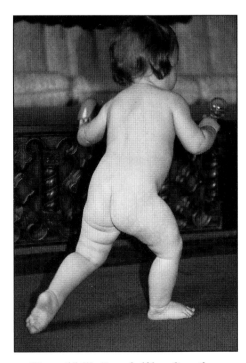

*Figure 11.20.* From half kneeling, the baby can shift the weight forward onto the flexed leg and lift the body weight with that leg. The back leg extends synchronously at the hip, knee, and ankle.

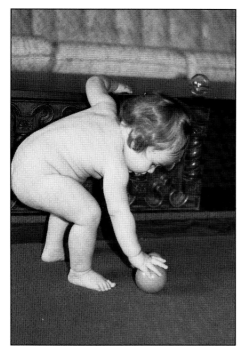

**Figure 11.21.** *From standing, the baby can lower into a squat and rise again without difficulty. The weight is kept posterior and minimal ankle dorsiflexion is used.*

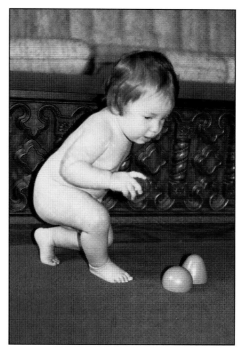

**Figure 11.22.** *The baby may also try asymmetrical lowering, a more difficult maneuver because of the dissociated position of the legs. The back leg sustains some of the weight and some of the control.*

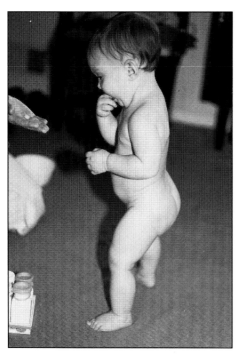

**Figure 11.23.** *Standing without external support is a new accomplishment for the baby. A wide base of support assures postural stability.*

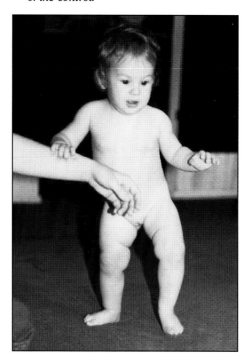

**Figure 11.24.** *Early attempts by the baby to walk independently often emerge from holding onto an adult's arm. Weight shift is easier toward the hand-support side, enabling elongation on that side while the other leg swings through.*

# Unsupported Walking

During initial attempts at independent walking, the baby's movement components tend to regress to those used in early supported walking. The baby assumes a wide base of support with the feet, abducts the arms, and flexes the elbows (Forssberg 1992).

The upper trunk-fixing pattern that the baby uses depends on the goal. The most common pattern of shoulder elevation, scapular adduction, and elbow flexion is used when the baby's goals are more nonspecific. When the baby is walking to a parent, the fixing pattern includes shoulder elevation, humeral flexion, and abduction (figure 11.26).

The lower extremity movements return to the steppage-like gait used in initial hand-held walking. The swing leg is flexed while abducted and externally rotated (figure 11.26). At the end of the swing phase, the baby may begin to extend the knee. The stance leg stays in line with the trunk on the sagittal plane and does not extend (figure 11.26).

Forssberg (1992) reports that, during initial attempts at unsupported walking, there is coactivation of the anterior tibial and lateral gastrocnemius during the stance and swing phases. This coactivation tends to decrease after the first week

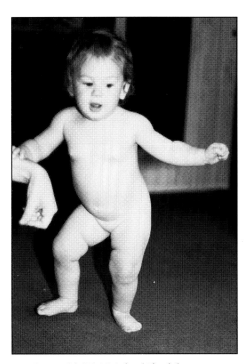

*Figure 11.25.* Weight shift of the trunk away from the hand-support side is difficult if the baby is relying on the support. Therefore the weight will be shifted in the legs, but the pelvis and trunk will lean toward the unweighted side.

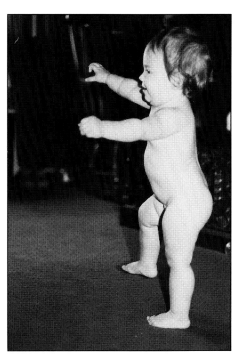

*Figure 11.26.* When the baby is walking toward a specific goal, the upper trunk fixing pattern includes shoulder elevation, humeral flexion, and abduction. Lower extremity movements return to the steppage-like gait used in initial hand-held walking. At the end of the swing phase, the baby may begin to extend the knee.

of independent walking. There is also coactivation of the quadriceps and hamstring muscles in early unsupported walking. This coactivation decreases two or three months after initiation of unsupported walking.

The leg movements are very quick as the baby propels forward. Trunk leaning toward the weight-bearing side is common. This suggests incomplete control of the hip abductors to control the lower extremity-pelvic-trunk weight shift.

Because balance is poor in early walking, the baby moves very quickly and usually falls or is caught in the arms of a parent. This does not discourage the baby or the parents, and walking workouts are practiced until the baby is independent.

# The Twelfth Month

**M**ost 12-month-old babies are very active and very independent. The basic motor skills are all present. Now the babies practice them in old and new ways. New objects in the environment become a challenge for babies as they experiment with the properties of the objects and with their own motor ability. They try old motor schemes on the new objects and develop new schemes when the old ones are insufficient.

## Sitting

During quiet sitting times, the 12-month-old is actively engaged in play activities. The baby enjoys all toys and spends time inspecting them and exploring their properties. Container play is still a favorite endeavor. The baby enjoys challenges such as putting pegs in a hole (figure 12.1), turning objects over (figure 12.2), and turning pages. Positioning and movement of the hand are done primarily from the elbow, utilizing graded flexion, extension, and rotation. The shoulders are quieter and participate more subtly in hand placement (Vogtle and Albert 1985). Smooth rotation of the trunk occurs when the baby reaches across the midline (figure 12.3).

The 12-month-old continues to enjoy mimicking household activities such as dressing and cooking. Household objects, such as pots and pans, are often favorite toys. Play with these objects continues to challenge and develop the baby's perceptual and fine motor skills.

Bimanual activities are performed as mirror movements (Fagard 1990): putting two blocks together, putting two broken pieces of crayon together, tearing tissues. These activities demonstrate the baby's increasing capacity to associate objects (Fagard 1990) and enhance development of bilateral coordination. The 12-month-old continues

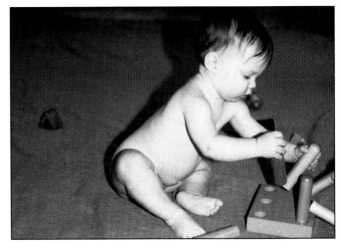

*Figure 12.1.* The 12-month-old enjoys challenges such as putting pegs in a hole. Ring sitting continues to be the most common posture.

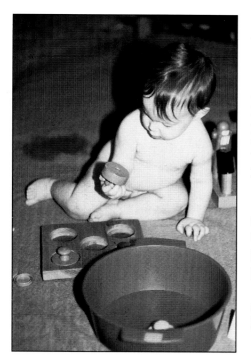

*Figure 12.2. The baby is able to turn objects over and explore them. Positioning and movement of the hand are done primarily from the elbow, utilizing graded flexion, extension, and rotation.*

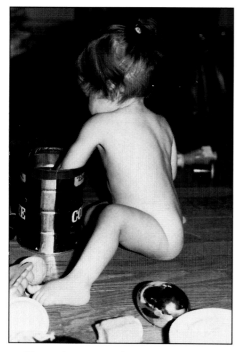

*Figure 12.3. Smooth rotation of the trunk occurs when the baby reaches across the midline. Active external rotation of the leg may still be used to reduce pelvic weight shift.*

to learn about the concept of weight and begins to make appropriate wrist and hand adjustments for different weights (Corbetta and Mounoud 1990).

Fagard (1990) reports that between 12 and 18 months, the hands begin to develop more coordinated asymmetrical roles. One hand is active and the other hand is more passive, providing stability. During these later months, the infant also develops the ability to use the hands in complementary asymmetrical roles (for example, one hand stabilizes a container as the other hand unscrews its lid).

The 12-month-old baby grasps with a superior or fine pincer grasp in which the fingertips and thumb are engaged (Erhardt 1984) (figure 12.4). The palmar arches begin to be visible during this grasp pattern. During reaching, the wrist extends and deviates radially to position the thumb and index finger for grasp (Vogtle and Albert 1985). Release is smooth and graded for large objects but is still clumsy for small objects (Erhardt 1984). Release is accomplished with less wrist flexion (Vogtle and Albert 1985).

# Transitions from Sitting

The 12-month-old moves in and out of sitting. These transitions are easily made to quadruped, kneeling, squatting, and standing.

The baby consistently uses trunk rotation to transition from sitting to quadruped. Utilizing increased trunk control, the baby subtly rotates the trunk and pelvis over the femur and transitions to quadruped. In earlier transitions, the baby initiated the transition from the legs. The baby would flex, abduct, and externally rotate the leg, orienting it in the direction of planned movement. Then the trunk moved symmetrically over the femur (figure 9.13.) Now the trunk initiates the direction of rotation and subsequently moves over the stable leg.

# Quadruped

The baby frequently assumes quadruped with lower extremity dissociation (figure 12.5). From this position the baby can creep, half kneel, or squat. This position requires mobility in the lumbar spine, hip joints, knees, and ankles.

Although crawling is still the baby's primary means of locomotion, it is being replaced by walking. However, the baby will revert to crawling when wishing to move quickly.

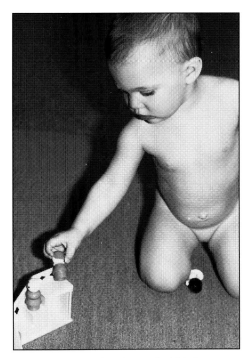

**Figure 12.4.** *The 12-month-old baby grasps with a superior or fine pincer grasp in which the fingertips and thumb are engaged.*

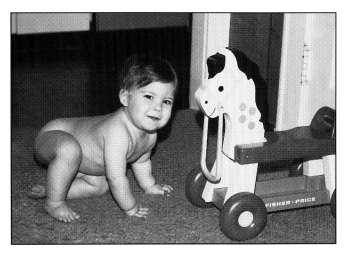

**Figure 12.5.** *The baby frequently assumes quadruped with lower extremity dissociation.*

# Kneeling

Sitting to kneeling and half kneeling are common transitions for the 12-month-old (figure 12.6). Kneeling and half kneeling are often combined with reaching patterns. For the baby to use the hands freely while kneeling and half kneeling, the posture must be dynamically controlled by the hip and lower extremity muscles. The quadriceps control the rise and fall of the body, while the pelvic-femoral muscles stabilize the trunk over the legs. This synergistic postural control occurs automatically because of the baby's prior experience in moving through and stabilizing in these positions.

# Squatting

Some babies transition to a squatting position for play (figure 12.7). Squatting requires marked hip and knee mobility. It stretches the quadriceps and at the same time requires marked quadriceps control to rise out of the position. Activity in the ankles and feet is needed for balance.

The ankle is frequently maintained at 90° during squatting because of the posterior position of the center of gravity (figure 12.7). But as the baby shifts weight (and the center of gravity) forward, ankle dorsiflexion will occur. When the weight is posterior, the ankle dorsiflexor muscles are used for balance. When the weight is shifted forward and the tibia moves forward over the foot, weight is shifted to the metatarsals, and ankle plantar flexor muscles may be used for balance.

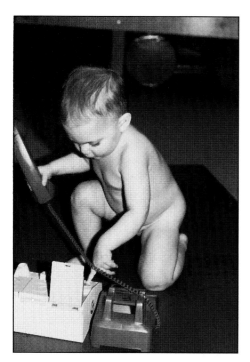

**Figure 12.6.** *Moving from sitting to half kneeling is a common transition for the 12-month-old. The index finger is frequently used for pointing and poking.*

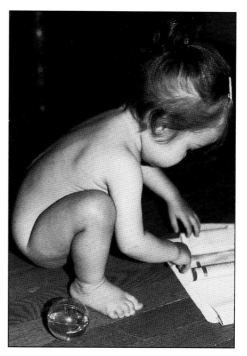

**Figure 12.7.** *Some babies transition to a squatting position for play, which requires marked hip and knee mobility. The ankle is frequently maintained at 90° because of the posterior position of the center of gravity.*

Development of control of the tibia over the foot is important. The ankle and foot muscles are needed for controlled standing and walking. When standing responses are mature, the ankle muscles are the first to respond to postural disturbances and the first to respond in anticipated postural adjustments (Shumway-Cook and Woollacott 1985; Woollacott, Shumway-Cook, and Williams 1989).

# Climbing

Climbing continues to be a favorite activity. The baby will climb onto or into anything perceived as an affordance or explorable. Each object presents a new challenge to the baby. As these enticements are explored, the baby's perceptual and motor systems are challenged and stimulated.

Figures 12.8 through 12.11 illustrate a 12-month-old's increasing skill in planning, organizing, and executing complex motor and perceptual tasks. While standing, the baby has sufficient lower extremity range and control to flex the leg and place a foot onto the step (figure 12.8). The baby can then use the strength in arms and quadriceps to lift the body up onto the step (figure 12.9). Next, the baby must plan how to get into the playpen. Increased lower extremity control and dissociation enable the baby to shift the weight to one leg while abducting and flexing the other leg over the lowered playpen rail while maintaining stability with the hands (figure 12.10). The baby then unweights the upper extremities and lowers into the playpen (figure 12.11).

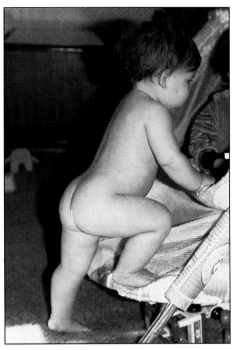

**Figure 12.8.** *While standing, the baby has sufficient lower extremity range and control to flex the leg and place the foot onto a step for climbing.*

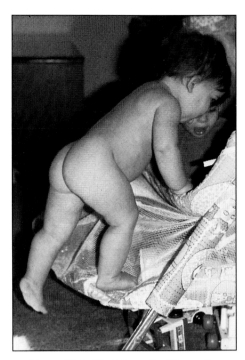

**Figure 12.9.** *The 12-month-old uses the strength in the arms and quadriceps to lift the body up onto the step.*

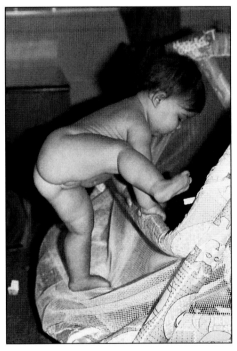

**Figure 12.10.** *Increased lower extremity control and dissociation enable the baby to shift weight to the left leg, abducting and flexing the right leg over the lowered playpen rail while maintaining stability with the hands.*

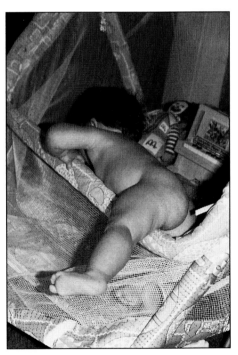

**Figure 12.11.** *The baby then unweights the upper extremities and lowers into the playpen.*

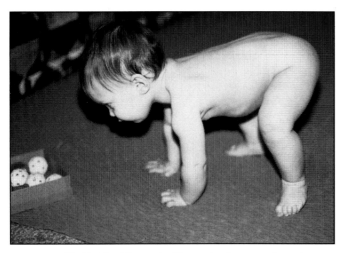

*Figure 12.12. The 12-month-old can rise from quadruped to stand without external support. The baby brings one leg forward so that the foot is placed on the floor. Then, while maintaining the weight on the upper extremities, the baby laterally shifts the weight in the lower trunk onto the foot and brings the back leg forward so that the weight is on the hands and feet.*

# Rising to Stand

The 12-month-old can rise from quadruped to stand without external support. The baby uses the same motor scheme as was used at 11 months of age. From quadruped, the baby brings one leg forward so that the foot is placed on the floor. While maintaining the weight on the upper extremities, the baby laterally shifts the weight in the lower trunk onto the foot and brings the back leg forward, so that the weight is on the hands and feet (figures 11.15, 11.16; 12.12).

To rise to stand, the baby must shift the weight posteriorly to unweight the upper extremities and to stabilize the center of gravity (figure 12.13). The posterior weight shift brings the ankle to neutral (90°) or slight plantar flexion. From this posterior position, the baby raises the trunk toward the upright by extending the hips while the knees remain flexed (figure 12.13). Finally, the baby symmetrically extends both knees and hips to stand upright.

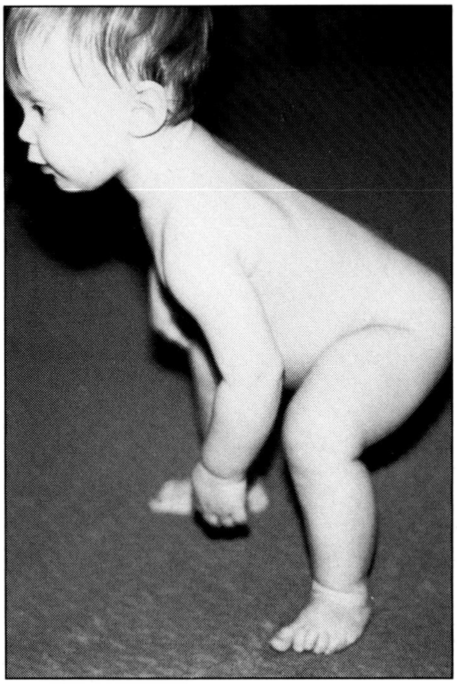

# Standing

By the twelfth month of age, most babies can stand independently without support (figure 12.14). To provide postural stability and limit the degrees of freedom in the legs, the baby may assume a wide base of support with the legs and may co-contract the leg muscles to increase stiffness in the legs.

From standing, the baby can lower the body with or without external support (figure 12.15). To do this, the baby shifts the weight posteriorly, as if sitting down. The baby flexes the hips and knees but not the ankles. The tibia-foot angle stays at 90° or plantar flexes slightly (figure 12.15). During this marked posterior weight shift, the baby must rely on the ankle and foot dorsiflexor muscles for balance. The quadriceps, hip extensors, and abdominals are also active in maintaining control. If the weight is shifted posteriorly without the knees being flexed, the baby will fall to sitting.

While conquering the challenge of rising to stand independently, the baby begins to organize the process of learning how to play with the same toys in standing that are played with while sitting. Standing presents new postural challenges to the baby because the base of support is different. When the baby is sitting, the hips are the base

*Figure 12.13. To rise to stand, the baby must shift the weight posteriorly to unweight the upper extremities and to stabilize the center of gravity. From this posterior position, the baby raises the trunk toward the upright by extending the hips while the knees remain flexed.*

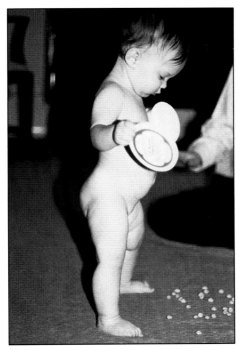

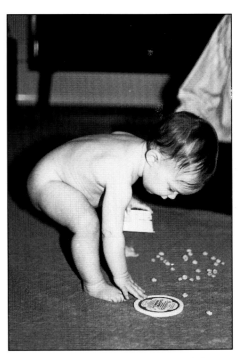

**Figure 12.14.** *By the twelfth month of age, most babies can stand independently without support. A wide base of support is used.*

**Figure 12.15.** *From standing, the baby can lower the body with or without external support. The baby shifts the weight posteriorly, as if sitting down. The hips and knees flex, but the ankle stays at 90° or plantar flexes.*

of support. Therefore, postural control is initiated at the hips. When the baby is standing, the baby's feet are the base of support. Therefore postural control is initiated at the feet. Initial postural stability may be achieved through toe curling.

Changing the postural requirements results in what seems to be regression in upper extremity and fine motor skills (figure 12.16). This regression is transient and is related to the new postural challenges. As the baby experiments with the new postural muscles in the lower extremities, the degrees of freedom in the upper trunk are limited. This produces fixing in the upper extremities and a temporary deterioration in fine motor skills. As the baby practices the new synergistic postural control and develops postural strategies, the baby will increase the degrees of freedom in the upper trunk and upper extremities. Subsequently, the baby will develop control and freedom of movement in the upper extremities while standing. The baby will soon combine this postural control with fine motor manipulation.

One of the favorite play activities at 12 months is container play, and babies will continue this play in standing. As they expand their repertoire with containers, they are just as likely to put themselves—as well as toys—into containers. Standing offers many new opportunities.

In figures 12.17 and 12.18, a 12-month-old demonstrates the ability to weight shift, maintain her balance in single-limb stance, lift her other leg, and perceptually and motorically guide it into the bucket.

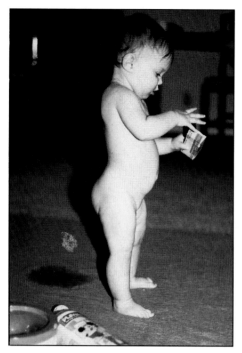

*Figure 12.16. Changing the postural requirements results in what seems to be regression in upper extremity and fine motor skills. The humeri adduct to the side and the wrists flex while the fingers extend during reaching.*

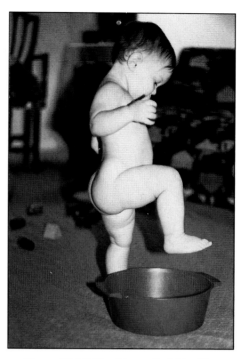

*Figure 12.17. The 12-month-old is able to weight shift and maintain balance in single-limb stance while perceptually and motorically guiding the other leg into the bucket.*

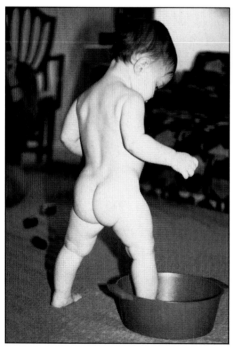

*Figure 12.18. Once the baby has one foot in the bucket, she will try to figure out how to get the other foot in. This presents more motor planning challenges.*

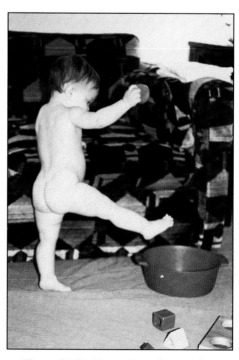

*Figure 12.19. Forward reaching with the leg is a difficult movement for the 12-month-old because it is a triplanar movement and requires dynamic dissociated control of the two legs.*

As she attempts these lower extremity challenges, she once again limits the degrees of freedom in her upper trunk by fixing with trunk extension, scapular adduction, shoulder elevation, humeral abduction, and elbow flexion (figures 12.17, 12.18). Once she has one foot in the bucket, she will try to figure out how to get the other foot in. This presents more motor planning challenges.

As more control in standing is acquired, the baby experiments with reaching with the legs (figure 12.19). Forward reaching with the leg is a difficult movement for the 12-month-old because it is a triplanar movement. The baby must simultaneously control hip flexion, abduction/adduction, and internal/external rotation on the reaching leg, and hip extension, abduction/adduction, and external rotation on the weight-bearing leg.

Through various exploratory games, babies engage in problem-solving activities. They are learning about their bodies, their control of their bodies, and about the environment and what it affords. Each self-initiated challenge seems to reinforce the babies' motor skills and perceptual skills.

Once the container game has started, the baby is often not content until she has tried all possibilities of getting her body into the container (figures 12.20, 12.21). She puts her hands in, and her hands and knees (figure 12.20). Another approach is to try to sit in the bucket (figure 12.21). The baby is analyzing movement strategies, trying to determine which combination of movements will help her reach her goal of getting her body in the bucket. In the process, she is learning about space and her body, and what fits and what doesn't.

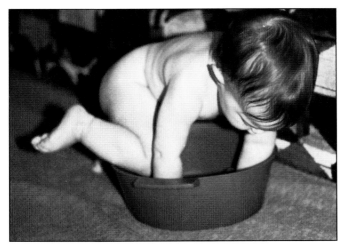

*Figure 12.20. The 12-month-old tries all possibilities of getting the body into the container, starting with the hands, then adding the knees.*

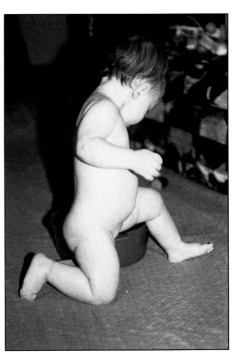

*Figure 12.21. Attempting to sit in the bucket, the baby is analyzing movement strategies, trying to determine which combination of movements will help to reach the goal of getting the body in the bucket.*

# Walking

Most babies walk independently by or during the twelfth month (Sutherland 1984). Early independent walking usually has the following characteristics: a fast speed (Statham and Murray 1971; Sutherland et al. 1980), short stride length (Statham and Murray 1971), short step length (Sutherland 1984), high cadence (Statham and Murray 1971; Sutherland 1984), short swing phase (Statham and Murray 1971; Sutherland et al. 1980; Sutherland 1984; Okamoto 1973), wide base of support (Sutherland 1984; Burnett and Johnson 1971; Forssberg 1992), and no reciprocal arm swing (Sutherland et al. 1980; Okamoto 1973). See Table 12.1 for a summary of the data that have been reported for initial unsupported walking.

## TABLE 12.1.
### Summary of data reported for initial unsupported walking

> The average age of independent walking is 11.2 months (Sutherland et al. 1988).

### Hip Flexion and Extension (Sagittal Plane Movements)

> New walkers show excessive hip flexion throughout the entire gait cycle (Statham and Murray 1971; Sutherland 1984; Forssberg 1992).
>
> Maximum hip flexion is seen during swing.
>
> A few degrees of hip extension (approximately 2°) are seen at terminal stance prior to toe-off (Statham and Murray 1971).
>
> Other investigators report the lack of extension at terminal stance (Okamoto 1973).

### Hip Abduction and External Rotation
### (Frontal and Transverse Plane Movements)

> In new walkers, the hip remains externally rotated throughout the entire gait cycle (Sutherland et al. 1980; Sutherland 1984; Burnett and Johnson 1971).
>
> Increased hip abduction contributes to a wide base of support (Sutherland et al. 1980; Burnett and Johnson 1971; Okamoto 1973).

## Knee Flexion and Extension

In new walkers, knee flexion occurs at the point of foot contact (Sutherland et al. 1980; Burnett and Johnson 1971; Okamoto 1973; Statham and Murray 1971).

In early infant ambulation, the knee remains flexed through midstance; however, the degree of flexion is gradually reduced and extension increases (Sutherland et al. 1980; Okamoto 1973; Statham and Murray 1971).

There is a quick extension of the knee after initial foot contact (Burnett and Johnson 1971). This occurs during the first two weeks of independent ambulation. By the eighth week of independent ambulation, the knee flexes at the point of foot contact.

If the knee remains in extension during midstance, the trunk hyperextends to shift the center of gravity posteriorly and thus maintain balance over the base of support (Burnett and Johnson 1971).

At the end of stance, the knee remains flexed or extends slightly (Statham and Murray 1971; Burnett and Johnson 1971).

## Ankle Flexion and Extension

New walkers have no heel strike. They usually contact the floor with a flat foot or with a plantar-flexed foot (Sutherland 1984; Okamoto 1973; Burnett and Johnson 1971; Forssberg 1992).

Soon the toes extend prior to foot contact. Later, the foot dorsiflexes toward the end of swing, but contact is not made with the heel. The first appearance of a heel strike is observed from the medial border of the foot. Later, it appears when viewed from the lateral border (Burnett and Johnson 1971).

Flat foot or toe contact is followed by ankle dorsiflexion (Statham and Murray 1971).

Ankle dorsiflexion continues through midstance.

Ankle dorsiflexion decreases at the end of stance, but plantar flexion for pushoff does not occur (Statham and Murray 1971; Burnett and Johnson 1971).

The baby's upper extremity patterns vary according to the goal. When the baby is trying to walk to a parent, the shoulders are usually flexed, with the arms outstretched (figure 12.22). If less goal directed, the baby usually reverts to fixing the upper extremities with scapular adduction (figure 12.23).

Hyperflexion of the swing leg and synchronous hip, knee, and ankle joint movements are once again employed in early independent walking (Forssberg 1992) (figure 12.22). Hip, knee, and ankle extension during terminal stance may be amplified by the baby's speed (figure 12.22).

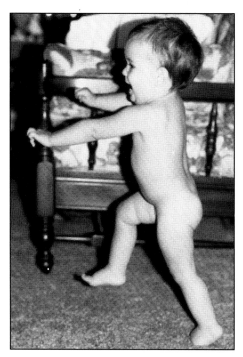

*Figure 12.22*. When the 12-month-old is trying to walk to a parent, the shoulders are usually flexed, with arms outstretched.

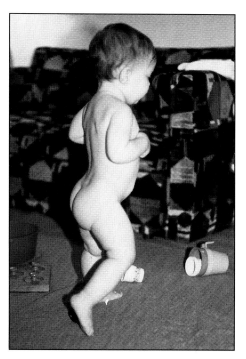

*Figure 12.23*. When less goal directed, the baby usually reverts to fixing the upper extremities with scapular adduction.

Increased postural control in the lower extremities and increased ability to anticipate and make postural adjustments result in decreased fixing with the upper extremities and upper trunk (figure 12.24). Once upper extremity fixing is reduced, the baby can once again carry toys in the hands while walking. However, the baby may still use the pattern of scapular adduction with elbow flexion when less goal directed (figure 12.23).

As the baby practices walking with its continuous weight-shifting and weight-bearing experiences, postural stability improves. This is noted as longer time on the stance leg and thus a slower walking speed. The baby can also stop and start walking as desired.

Very shortly after initiating unsupported walking, the baby becomes quite independent in walking skills. The baby then replaces crawling with walking as the primary means of locomotion.

# Conclusion

This is just the beginning. Babies have learned much about their bodies—what they can and cannot do. They have discovered and explored countless affordances in their environment. This foundation will provide them with a basis to continue the quest to move, learn, and explore.

## *Indications of Possible Disturbances in Motor Development*

Babies who are developing atypically have also learned much about their bodies—what they can and cannot do. This foundation provides them with a basis on which to face the future challenges in their lives. Limited and/or compensatory motor skills often affect the baby's desire to move and explore. Movement may seem to be too difficult and the baby may give up, which often leads to "learned helplessness." Subsequently they make limited discoveries and explore fewer affordances in their environment.

Therapeutic intervention must be geared to enhancing the infant's motor skills—for the purpose of exploration, discovery, and learning. In therapy, it is important to work on kinesiological components, alignment, and synergistic muscle activity. However, it is the interest in interacting with the environment that makes the work and challenges of moving worthwhile. Therefore, therapeutic intervention must address both simultaneously.

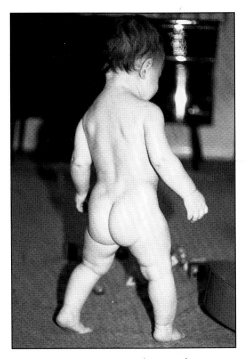

*Figure 12.24. Increased postural control in the lower extremities and increased ability to anticipate and make postural adjustments result in decreased fixing of the upper extremities and upper trunk.*

# References

Adelson, S., and S. Fraiberg. 1974. Gross motor development in infants blind from birth. *Child Development* 45:114-126.

Allen, M. C. 1991. Preterm development. In *Developmental disabilities in infancy and childhood,* edited by A. J. Capute and P. J. Accardo, 69-85. Baltimore: Paul H. Brookes.

Andre-Thomas, and S. Autgaerden. 1966. *Locomotion from pre- to post-natal life. Clinics in Developmental Medicine* no. 24. London: William Heinemann Medical Books, Ltd.

Andre-Thomas, Y. Chesni, and S. Saint-Anne Dargassies. 1960. *The neurological examination of the infant. Clinics in Developmental Medicine* no. 1. Spastics International Medical Publications. London: William Heinemann Medical Books, Ltd.

Aston, A. 1974. *How to play with your baby.* Larchmont, NY: Fountain Publishing Co.

Ayres, J. A. 1972. *Sensory integration and learning disorders.* Los Angeles: Western Psychological Services.

Barnes, M., C. Crutchfield, and C. Heriza. 1978. *The neurophysiological basis of patient treatment.* Vol. 2, *Reflexes in motor development.* Morgantown, WV: Stokes Publishing Co.

Beats, R. K. 1969. Developmental changes in the femur and acetabulum in spastic paraplegia and diplegia. *Developmental Medicine and Child Neurology* 11:303-313.

Bernstein, N. 1967. *The coordination and regulation of movement.* New York: Pergamon Press.

Bleck, E. E. 1987. *Orthopedic management in cerebral palsy. Clinics in Developmental Medicine* no. 99/100. Philadelphia: J. B. Lippincott.

Brazelton, T. B. 1969. *Infants and mothers.* New York: Delta Publishing.

_____. 1973. *Neonatal behavioral assessment scale. Clinics in Developmental Medicine* no. 50. London: National Spastic Society with Heinemann Medical Books, Ltd.; Philadelphia: Lippincott.

Brunnstrom, S. 1979. *Clinical kinesiology.* 3d ed. Philadelphia: F. A. Davis.

Burnett, C., and E. Johnson. 1971. Development of gait in childhood, part II. *Developmental Medicine and Child Neurology* 13:207-215.

Cailliet, R. 1964. *Neck and arm pain.* Philadelphia: F. A. Davis.

_____. 1968. *Low back pain syndrome.* Philadelphia: F. A. Davis.

_____. 1977. *Soft tissue pain and disability.* Philadelphia: F. A. Davis.

Capute, A. J., P. J. Accardo, E. Vining, J. E. Rubenstein, and S. Harryman. 1978. *Primitive reflex profile.* Baltimore: University Park Press.

Corbetta, D., and P. Mounoud. 1990. Early development of grasping and manipulation. In *Development of eye-hand coordination across the life span,* edited by C. Bard, M. Fleury, and L. Hay, 188-216. Columbia, SC: University of South Carolina Press.

Crelin, E. 1973. *Functional anatomy of the newborn.* New Haven, CN: Yale University Press.

Cupps, C., M. G. Plescia, and C. Houser. 1976. The Landau reaction: A clinical and electromyographic analysis. *Developmental Medicine and Child Neurology* 18:41-53.

Daniels, L., M. Williams, and C. Worthingham. 1964. *Muscle testing.* 2d ed. Philadelphia: W. B. Saunders.

Drews, J. E., J. K. Vraciu, and G. Pellino. 1984. Range of motion of the joints of the lower extremities of newborns. *Physical and Occupational Therapy in Pediatrics* 4(2):49-62.

Easton, T. A. 1972. On the normal use of reflexes. *American Science* 60:591-599.

Egan, D., R. S. Illingworth, and R. C. MacKeith. 1969. *Developmental screening 0-5 years. Clinics in Developmental Medicine* no. 30. London: Spastics International Medical Publications in association with William Heinemann Medical Books, Ltd.

Elliott, J. M., and K. J. Connolly. 1984. A classification of manipulative hand movements. *Developmental Medicine and Child Neurology* 26:283-296.

Erhardt, R. P. 1984. *Erhardt developmental prehension assessment.* Laurel, MD: Ramsco Publishing.

Fagard, J. 1990. The development of bimanual coordination. In *Development of eye-hand coordination across the life span,* edited by C. Bard, M. Fleury, and L. Hay, 262-282. Columbia, SC: University of South Carolina Press.

Fantz, R. L., J. F. Faga, and S. B. Miranda. 1975. Early visual selectivity. In *Infant perception: From sensation to cognition.* Vol. 1, *Basic visual processes,* edited by L. B. Cohen and P. Salapatek, 249-345. New York: Academic Press.

Fiorentino, M. 1972a. *Normal and abnormal development: The influence of primitive reflexes on motor development.* Springfield, IL: Charles C. Thomas.

_____. 1972b. *Reflex testing methods for evaluating CNS development.* Springfield, IL: Charles C. Thomas.

_____. 1981. *A basis for sensorimotor development—Normal and abnormal.* Springfield, IL: Charles C. Thomas.

Forssberg, H. 1992. Evolution of plantigrade gait: Is there a neuronal correlate? *Developmental Medicine and Child Neurology* 34(10):920-925.

Forssberg, H., H. Hirschfeld, and V. P. Stokes. 1992. Development of human locomotor mechanisms. In *XXIV Minnesota symposium of child development,* edited by M. Gunner and K. Nelson, 1-12. Hillsdale, NJ: Lawrence Erlbaum Associates.

Fritts, D. 1990. Unpublished lecture notes, NDT Baby Course, Sydney, Australia.

Gentile, A. M. 1987. Skill acquisition: Action, movement, and neuromotor processes. In *Movement science: Foundations for physical therapy in rehabilitation,* edited by J. H. Carr, R. B. Shepherd, J. Gordon, A. M. Gentile, and J. M. Held, 93-154. Rockville, MD: Aspen Publishers.

Gesell, A., and G. S. Amatruda. 1947. *Developmental diagnosis.* 2d ed. New York: Harper and Row.

Gibson, E. J., and M. A. Schmuckler. 1989. Going somewhere: An ecological and experimental approach to development of mobility. *Ecological Psychology* 1:3-25.

Gibson, J. J. 1986. *The ecological approach to visual perception.* Hillsdale, NJ: Lawrence Erlbaum Associates, Inc. (Original work published in 1979.)

Horack, F. B., and L. M. Nashner. 1986. Central programming of postural movements: Adaptation to altered support surface configurations. *Journal of Neurophysiology* 55:1369-1381.

Illingworth, R. S. 1975. *The development of the infant and young child, normal and abnormal.* 6th ed. New York: Churchill Livingston.

Inatsuka, T. T. 1979. Fine motor development. In *Hawaii early learning profile (HELP),* edited by S. Furuno, K. O'Reilly, C. M. Hosaka, T. T. Inatsuka, T. L. Allman, and B. Zeisloft, 109-126. Palo Alto, CA: VORT Corp.

Kapandji, I. A. 1970a. *The physiology of the joints.* Vol. 1, *Upper limb.* 2d ed. New York: Churchill Livingston.

_____. 1970b. *The physiology of the joints.* Vol. 2, *Lower limb.* 2d ed. New York: Churchill Livingston.

_____. 1974. *The physiology of the joints.* Vol. 3, *The trunk and the vertebral column.* 2d ed. New York: Churchill Livingston.

Kelso, J. A. S. 1982. Perspectives and issues in motor behavior. In *Human motor behavior: An introduction,* edited by J. A. S. Kelso, 1-62. Hillsdale, NJ: Lawrence Erlbaum Associates.

Kendall, H., F. Kendall, and G. Wadsworth. 1971. *Muscles: Testing and function.* 2d ed. Baltimore: Williams and Wilkins.

Lehmkuhl, L. D., and L. K. Smith. 1983. *Brunnstrom's clinical kinesiology,* 4th ed. Philadelphia: F. A. Davis Co.

Leonard, C. T., H. Hirschfeld, and H. Forssberg. 1991. The development of independent walking in children with cerebral palsy. *Developmental Medicine and Child Neurology* 33:567-577.

Martin, J. B. 1965. Tilting reactions and disorders of the basal ganglion. *Brain* 88:855-874.

McGraw, M. B. 1945. *The neuromuscular maturation of the human infant.* New York: Hafner Publishing.

Moore, J. 1984. The neuroanatomy and pathology of cerebral palsy. In *Selected proceedings from Barbro Salek Memorial Symposium,* 1-58. Oak Park, IL: NDTA.

_____. 1986. Neonatal neuropathology. In *The high risk neonate: Developmental therapy perspectives,* edited by J. Sweeney. *Physical and Occupational Therapy in Pediatrics* 6(3/4):55-90.

Mueller, H. A. 1972. Facilitating feeding and prespeech. In *Physical therapy services in the developmental disabilities,* edited by P. Pearson and C. Williams, 283-310. Springfield, IL: Charles C. Thomas.

Nash, M. 1990. Unpublished lecture notes, NDT Course, Honolulu, HI.

_____. 1991. Unpublished lecture notes, NDT Baby Course, Villa Park, IL.

Nashner, L. M. 1985. Adaptation of human movement to altered environments. In *The motor system in neurobiology,* edited by E. V. Evarts, S. P. Wise, and D. Bousfield, 106-112. New York: Elsevier Biomedical Press.

Norkin, C., and P. Levangie. 1983. *Joint structure and function: A comprehensive analysis.* Philadelphia: F. A. Davis.

O'Connell, A. L., and E. B. Gardner. 1972. *Understanding the scientific basis of human movement.* Baltimore: Williams and Wilkins.

Okamoto, T. 1973. Electromyographic study of the learning process of walking in one- and two-year-old infants. *Medicine and Sport.* Vol. 8, *Biomechanics* III:328-333.

Prechtl, H. F. R. 1977. *The neurological examination of the full term newborn infant.* 2d ed. Clinics in Developmental Medicine no. 63. Philadelphia: J. B. Lippincott.

Quinton, M. 1976, 1977, 1978. Unpublished lecture notes, NDT courses.

Root, M., W. Orien, and J. Weed. 1977. *Normal and abnormal function of the foot.* Vol. 2. Los Angeles: Clinical Biomechanics Corp.

Root, M., W. Orien, J. Weed, and R. Hughes. 1971. *Biomechanical examination of the foot.* Vol. 1. Los Angeles: Clinical Biomechanics Corp.

Saint-Anne Dargassies. 1972. Neurological symptoms during the first year of life. *Developmental Medicine and Child Neurology* 14:235-263.

_____. 1977. *Neurological development in the full term and premature neonate.* Amsterdam: Elsevier.

Shumway-Cook, A., and M. H. Woollacott. 1985. The growth of stability: Postural control from a developmental perspective. *Journal of Motor Behavior* 17(2):131-147.

Soderberg, G. L. 1986. *Kinesiology.* Baltimore: Williams and Wilkins.

Staheli, L. T. 1980. Medial femoral torsion. Symposium on the child's hip. *Orthopedic Clinics of North America* 11(1):39-49.

Statham, L., and M. Murray. 1971. Early walking patterns of normal children. *Clinical Orthopaedics and Related Research* 79:8-24.

Stockmeyer, S. A. 1967. An interpretation of the approach of Rood to the treatment of neuromuscular dysfunction. In *American Journal of Physical Medicine* vol. 46, no. 1, 900-956. Baltimore: Williams and Wilkins.

Sutherland, D. 1984. *Gait disorders in children and adolescents.* Baltimore: Williams and Wilkins.

Sutherland, D., R. Olshen, E. Biden, and M. Wyatt. 1988. *The development of mature walking.* Clinics in Developmental Medicine no. 104/105. Philadelphia: J. B. Lippincott.

Sutherland, D., R. Olshen, L. Cooper, and S. Woo. 1980. The development of mature gait. *Journal of Bone and Joint Surgery* 62A(3):336-353.

Tachdjian, M. O. 1972. *Pediatric orthopedics.* Vols. 1 and 2. Philadelphia: W. B. Saunders.

Tax, H. R. 1985. *Podopediatrics.* 2d ed. Baltimore: Williams and Wilkins.

Taylor, M. J. 1992. Visual evoked potentials. In *The neurophysiological examination of the newborn infant,* edited by J. A. Eyre, 93-111. Clinics in Developmental Medicine no. 120. New York: MacKeith Press (distributed by Cambridge University Press).

Thelen, E. 1984. Learning to walk: Ecological demands and phylogenetic constraints. In *Advances in infancy research,* vol. 3, edited by V. Collier, 213-250. Norwood, NJ: Ablex.

_____. 1985. Developmental origins of motor coordination: Leg movements in human infants. *Developmental Psychobiology* 18:1-22.

Thelen, E., and D. W. Cooke. 1987. Relationship between newborn stepping and later walking: A new interpretation. *Developmental Medicine and Child Neurology* 29:380-393.

Thelen, E., and D. M. Fisher. 1982. Newborn stepping: An explanation for a "disappearing" reflex. *Developmental Psychology* 18(5):760-775.

_____. 1983. The organization of spontaneous leg movements in newborn infants. *Journal of Motor Behavior* 15(4):353-377.

Thelen, E., D. M. Fisher, and R. Ridley-Johnson. 1984. The relationship between physical growth and a newborn reflex. *Infant Behavior and Development* 7:479-493.

Touwen, B. 1976. *Neurological development in infancy.* Clinics in Developmental Medicine no. 58. Philadelphia: J. B. Lippincott.

Tuller, B., H. L. Fitch, and M. T. Turvey. 1982. The Bernstein perspective: II. The concept of muscle linkage or coordinative structure. In *Human motor behavior: An introduction,* edited by J. A. S Kelso, 253-270. Hillsdale, NJ: Lawrence Erlbaum Associates.

Twitchell, T. E. 1965. Normal motor development. In *The child with central nervous system deficit,* 85-89. Washington, DC: U. S. Department of Health, Education, and Welfare, Children's Bureau.

Vogtle, L., and J. Albert. 1985. Unpublished course handout, NDT.

von Hofsten, C. 1990. A perception-action perspective of the development of manual movement. In *Attention and performance*, vol. 13, edited by M. Jeannerod, 739-762. Hillsdale, NJ: Lawrence Erlbaum Associates.

Walker, J. M. 1991. Musculoskeletal development: A review. *Physical Therapy* 71(12):878-889.

Weisz, S. 1938. Studies in equilibrium reactions. *Journal of Nervous and Mental Disorders* 99:150-162.

Woollacott, M. H., A. Shumway-Cook, and H. G. Williams. 1989. The development of posture and balance control in children. In *Development of posture and gait across the life span*, edited by M. H. Woollacott and A. Shumway-Cook, 77-96. Columbia, SC: University of South Carolina Press.

# Additional Reading

Becker, M. S., and B. S. Banus. 1979. Sensory perceptual dysfunction and its management. In *The developmental therapist*, 2d ed., edited by B. S. Banus, C. A. Kent, Y. S. Norton, D. R. Sukiennicki, and M. L. Becker, 237-275. Thorofare, NJ: Charles B. Slack.

Bly, L. 1983. *The components of normal movement during the first year of life and abnormal motor development.* Monograph. Chicago: NDTA.

Bobath, B. 1967. The very early treatment of cerebral palsy. *Developmental Medicine and Child Neurology* 9:373-390.

_____. 1971. Motor development: Its effect on general development and application to the treatment of cerebral palsy. *Physiotherapy* 57:526-532.

_____. 1985. *Abnormal postural reflex activity caused by brain lesions.* 3d ed. Rockville, MD: Aspen Systems.

Bobath, K. 1980. *A neurophysiological basis for the treatment of cerebral palsy.* Clinics in Neuro-developmental Medicine no. 75. Philadelphia: J. B. Lippincott.

Bobath, K., and B. Bobath. 1984. Neuro-developmental treatment. In *Management of the motor disorders in children with cerebral palsy.* Clinics in Developmental Medicine no. 90. Edited by D. Scrutton, 6-18. Philadelphia: J. B. Lippincott.

Bresson, F., L. Maury, G. Pieraut-Le Bonniec, and S. DeSchonen. 1977. Organization and lateralization of reaching in infants: An instance of asymmetric functions in hand collaboration. *Neuropsychologia* 15:311-320.

Cailliet, R. 1966. *Shoulder pain.* Philadelphia: F. A. Davis.

Caplan, F., ed. 1973. *The first twelve months of life: Your baby's growth month by month.* Princeton, NH: Edcom Systems.

Clark, D. L., J. R. Kreutzberg, and F. K. Chee. 1977. Vestibular stimulation influences of motor development in infants. *Science* 196:1228-1229.

Gesell, A. 1940. *The first five years of life.* New York: Harper and Row.

Parr, C., M. Byrd, D. Routh, and J. McMillian. 1974. A developmental study of the asymmetrical tonic neck reflex. *Developmental Medicine and Child Neurology* 16:329-335.

Saint-Anne Dargassies. 1966. Neurological maturation of the premature infant of 28 to 41 weeks gestational age. In *Human development*, edited by F. Falkner, 306-325. Philadelphia: W. B. Saunders.

Schmidt, R. A. 1982. More of motor programs. In *Human motor behavior: An introduction*, edited by J. A. S. Kelso, 189-217. Hillsdale, NJ: Lawrence Erlbaum Associates.

Schwartz, S., and J. E. Miller. 1988. *The language of toys.* Rockville, MD: Woodbine House.

Thelen, E., and B. D. Ulrich. 1991. Hidden skills. *Monograph of the Society for Research in Child Development* vol. 56, no. 1.

White, B. 1975. *The first three years of life.* Englewood Cliffs, NJ: Prentice Hall.

# Index